MW01037573

Dreams

A Reader on Religious, Cultural, and Psychological Dimensions of Dreaming

Edited by

Kelly Bulkeley

palgrave

DREAMS
Copyright © Kelly Bulkeley, 2001.
All rights reserved. No part of this book may be used or reproduced in any manner whatsoever without written permission except in the case of brief quotations embodied in critical articles or reviews.

First published 2001 by PALGRAVE™
175 Fifth Avenue, New York, N.Y. 10010 and
Houndmills, Basingstoke, Hampshire, England RG21 6XS.
Companies and representatives throughout the world.

PALGRAVE is the new global publishing imprint of St. Martin's Press LLC Scholarly and Reference Division and Palgrave Publishers Ltd. (formerly Macmillan Press Ltd.).

ISBN 0–312–29333-X (cloth)
ISBN 0–312–29334–8 (pbk.)

Library of Congress Cataloging-in-Publication Data
Dreams: a reader on religious, cultural & psychological dimensions of dreaming / Kelly Bulkeley, editor.
p. cm.
Includes bibliographical references.
ISBN 0–312–29333-X—ISBN 0–312–29334–8 (pbk.)
1. Dreams. I. Bulkeley, Kelly, 1962-
BF 1078.D7295 2001
154.6-dc21

2001032755

A catalogue record for this book is available from the British Library.

Design by Letra Libre, Inc.

First edition: December 2001
10 9 8 7 6 5 4 3 2 1

Printed in the United States of America.

Contents

Section II
INDIVIDUALS

Section III
METHODS

Acknowledgments

My thanks go first of all to Gayatri Patnaik, who has expertly and enthusiastically guided this project through its many conceptual incarnations to its final realization as a published book. At a time when scholars are finding it increasingly difficult in the rapidly changing commercial circumstances of academic publishing to find a home for their writings, it is a blessing to have an editor like Gayatri who appreciates a project's potential and is willing to devote her time and energy to the painstaking process of nurturing it to fruition.

I also thank the many overlapping scholarly communities in which I befriended most of the contributors to this book. The University of Chicago is where I first met Wendy Doniger and Bert Cohler, who served as trustworthy guides during my doctoral education and whose influence on my thinking has only grown in the years since then. At Santa Clara University I have had the privilege of teaching with Diane Jonte-Pace and Tracey Kahan and working with them to stimulate interdisciplinary conversations among other faculty members interested in religion and psychology. The Person, Culture, and Religion Group of the American Academy of Religion sponsored a panel at its 1999 meeting on the centennial of the original publication of Freud's The Interpretation of Dreams at which James DiCenso and J. Allan Hobson joined Diane Jonte-Pace in making presentations. Another AAR program unit, the Comparative Studies in Religion Section, sponsored a session at the 2000 meeting entitled "Dreams and Their Interpretation," and I persuaded panelists Lee Irwin, Serinity Young, Jeffrey Kripal, and Marcia Hermansen to contribute chapters for this book. The annual conferences of the Association for the Study of Dreams, which I have faithfully attended since 1988, have been rich and stimulating gatherings of dream researchers from many different fields, among them several authors of coming chapters: Jeremy Taylor, Jane White-Lewis, G. William Domhoff, Barbara Tedlock, Nancy Grace, Waud Kracke, and George Lakoff.

A symposium on the use of Freudian and Jungian theory in religious studies, held at the Graduate Theological Union in the fall of 2000 (organized under the auspices of the GTU's Area 5, Religion and Psychology, chaired by Lewis Rambo), gave me the opportunity to engage Frederick Crews in a "spirited" dialogue about the scientific legitimacy of dream research. Most recently, I have benefited from my association with the Center for Theology and the Natural Sciences here at the GTU, particularly in regard to my thinking about the methodological issues raised in the concluding debate with Crews.

I appreciate the efforts of the editorial staffs at the State University of New York Press and the journals Ethos: Journal of the Society of Psychological Anthropology and Dreaming: Journal of the Association for the Study of Dreams for their permission to reprint the works of Wendy Doniger (SUNY), Waud Kracke, Thomas Gregor, and Roger Lohmann (Ethos) and Barbara Tedlock and George Lakoff (Dreaming).

Any edited anthology is bound to face last-second technical problems, and I could not have brought this book to a timely completion without the assistance of Richard Wilkerson, my web guru at www.dreamgate.com, Kasy Moon, Rick Delaney, and Donna Cherry of the Palgrave editorial staff, my Kensington neighbor Ashley Block, and the helpful employees of Krishna Copy Center on University Avenue in Berkeley.

Finally, this is the place to say how much I appreciate the love and support of my children Dylan, Maya, and Conor and my wife Hilary. It would not be possible for me to continue exploring the nether regions of the dreaming imagination if it were not for their care and affection. Everything I write is ultimately a tribute to their love.

Permissions

Chapter 6 reprinted from "The Role of Dreams in Religious Enculturation Among the Asabano of Papua New Guinea" by Roger Ivar Lohmann in *Ethos* (2000) vol. 28, no. 1, pp. 75–102, by permission of the American Anthropological Association. Not for sale or further reproduction.

Chapter 7 reprinted from "A Content Analysis of Mehinaku Dreams" by Thomas Gregor in *Ethos* (1981) vol. 9, no. 4, pp. 353–390, by permission of the American Anthropological Association.

Chapter 9 reprinted from "Kagwahiv Mourning: Dreams of a Bereaved Father" by Waud Kracke in *Ethos* (1981) vol. 9, no. 4, pp. 258–275, by permission of the American Anthropological Association.

Chapter 14 reprinted from "Western Dreams about Eastern Dreams" by Wendy Doniger in *Among All These Dreamers: Essays on Dreaming and Modern Society,* edited by Kelly Bulkeley, by permission of the State University of New York Press. © 1996 State University of New York. All Rights Reserved.

Chapter 16 reprinted from "The New Anthropology of Dreaming" by Barbara Tedlock in *Dreaming* (1991) vol. 1, no. 2, pp. 161–178, by permission of Kluwer Academic/Plenum Publishers.

Chapter 17 reprinted from "How metaphor Structures Dreams: The Theory of Conceptual Metaphor Applied to Dream Analysis" by George Lakoff in *Dreaming* (1993) vol. 3, no. 2, pp. 77–98, by permission of Kluwer Academic/Plenum Publishers.

For Hilary

Introduction

Contemplating Freud's Navel

There is at least one spot in every dream at which it is unplumbable—a navel, as it were, that is its point of contact with the unknown.

—*Sigmund Freud*[1]

In the one hundred years since the publication of Freud's *The Interpretation of Dreams,* the study of dreams has become a fruitful resource in the investigation of the deepest meaning-making capacities of the human mind. Dreams offer a unique insight into the creative imaginal space where religion, culture, history, and psyche join together in dynamic interplay. The aim of this book is to explore that creative space, to plumb the mysterious depths of the "dream navel," in Freud's haunting words. *Dreams* brings together a collection of provocative writings from scholars in religious studies, anthropology, history, and psychology. The twenty-three chapters highlight the most important theories, the most contentious debates, and the most exciting prospects in this growing field of study. For researchers, teachers, students, and general readers alike, *Dreams* provides a one-volume compendium of the best that contemporary dream study has to offer.

The book is organized into three broad thematic sections: Traditions, Individuals, and Methods. Although nearly every chapter touches on all of these themes, the three major sections distinguish which chapters focus chiefly on (1) the dream beliefs and practices of a particular cultural tradition; (2) the dream experiences of particular individuals; and (3) the methods used to investigate and understand the origins, functions, and meanings of dreaming.

Section I begins with detailed historical studies of dreaming in Buddhism ("Buddhist Dream Experience: The Role of Interpretation, Ritual, and Gender," by Serinity Young), ancient Egypt ("Through the Looking Glass: Dreams in Ancient Egypt," by Kasia Szpakowska), ancient Mesopotamia ("Dreams and Dream Interpreters in

Mesopotamia and in the Hebrew Bible [Old Testament]," by Scott Noegel), and Islam ("Dreams and Dreaming in Islam," by Marcia Hermansen). Following those chapters are investigations of contemporary non-Western dream traditions among the Plains Indians of North America ("Sending a Voice, Seeking a Place: Visionary Dreams Among Native Women of the Plains," by Lee Irwin), the Asabano of Papua New Guinea ("The Role of Dreams in Religious Enculturation Among the Asabao of Papua New Guinea," by Roger Ivar Lohmann), and the Mehinaku of the Amazonian rain forest ("A Content Analysis of Mehinaku Dreams," by Thomas Gregor[2]). The section finishes with a discussion of present-day American musicians who draw on dreams as a source of inspiration in their creative work ("Making Dreams Into Music: Contemporary Songwriters Carry on an Age-Old Dreaming Tradition," by Nancy Grace).

The chapters in Section II focus on the dream lives of particular individuals, with special attention to the hermeneutic process of trying to understand what the dreams of those particular individuals might mean. First is a chapter exploring the dreams of a Kagwahiv man from the Amazonian Rain Forest who is mourning the recent death of his son ("Kagwahiv Mourning: Dreams of a Bereaved Father," by Waud Kracke). Then come two chapters set in contemporary America, one describing the process of dream interpretation as practiced in Jungian analysis ("Reflecting on a Dream in Jungian Analytic Practice," by Jane White-Lewis) and the other describing the interpretive benefits of sharing and discussing dreams in a group context ("Group Work with Dreams: The 'Royal Road' to Meaning," by Jeremy Taylor). Next is a critical reinterpretation of Freud's famous "Botanical Monograph" dream as it relates to the psychoanalytic dream theory he presents in *The Interpretation of Dreams* ("Wish, Conflict, and Awareness: Freud and the Problem of the 'Dream Book,'" by Bertram Cohler). The final chapter of the section offers another critical reinterpretation of a historically significant dream: Queen Penelope's dream, in book 19 of Homer's *The Odyssey,* of her twenty geese being slaughtered by a mountain eagle ("Penelope as Dreamer: The Perils of Interpretation," by Kelly Bulkeley).

The first several chapters of Section III concentrate on the methodological challenges involved in different kinds of dream research. These include the relevance of myth and religious history to modern psychological investigations of dreaming ("Western Dreams About Eastern Dreams," by Wendy Doniger), the role of erotic experience in the study of dreams and mysticism ("The Dream of Scholarship: Some Notes on the Historian of Mysticism as a Dreaming Creative," by Jeffrey Kripal), and the daunting linguistic and cultural impediments to making claims about allegedly universal, transcultural features of dreaming ("The New Anthropology of Dreaming," by Barbara Tedlock). The next several chapters respond to those methodological challenges by proposing a variety of sophisticated research strategies. These include the use of metaphor theory and cognitive linguistics ("How Metaphor Structures Dreams: The Theory of Conceptual Metaphor Applied to Dream Analysis," by George Lakoff), psychoanalysis modified by postmodern philosophy ("Dreams, Inner Resistance, and Self-Reflection," by James J. Dicenso), psychoanalysis modified by feminist theory ("Turning Away at the Navel of the Dream: Religion and the Body of the Mother at the Beginning and End of Interpretation," by Diane Jonte-Pace), quantitative content analysis ("Using Content Analysis to Study Dreams: Applications and Implications for the Humanities," by G. William Domhoff), neuroscientific investigations in the sleep laboratory ("The New Neuropsychology of Sleep: Implications for Psychoanalysis," by J. Allan Hobson), and recent developments in the psychology of consciousness, imagination, and metacognition ("Consciousness in Dreaming: A Metacognitive Approach," by Tracey L. Kahan). The book's final chapter presents a "Dialogue with a Skeptic," in which I and Frederick Crews, a renowned scourge of anything even vaguely psychoanalytic, exchange ideas about the question of whether the study of the religious, cultural, and psychological dimensions of dreaming can be a legitimate scholarly enterprise.

Although I have placed each of the book's chapters into one of these three sections, I do so with the awareness that every chapter has strong affinities with different chapters in other sections. For example, the issue of gender is a prominent concern for Young, Irwin, Jonte-Pace, Taylor, and Tedlock. Religious themes are central in Lohmann, Hermansen, Taylor, Noegel, Irwin, Jonte-Pace, Young, and Doniger. The nature of language, wordplay, and symbolism is a central issue in the chapters by Lakoff, Dicenso, Szpakowska, Noegel, Cohler, Domhoff, and Young. The mystical dimensions of dreaming are of particular interest to Kripal, Doniger, Irwin, Tedlock, and Hermansen. Re-evaluating Freud's dream theory is a primary goal of Hobson, Domhoff, Cohler, Jonte-Pace, DiCenso, Kracke, and Crews. Detailed discussions of the role of self-reflexivity in dream research and interpretation appear in Cohler, Tedlock, Kripal, and Taylor. The spontaneous creativity of dreaming is discussed at length by Grace, Taylor, Kahan, Kripal, and Lakoff.

Along with these multidimensional connections and affinities, certain chapters in the book stand in vivid opposition to each other, and these contrasts mark important debates in the dream studies field. For example, a sharp disagreement about the legitimacy of using content analysis in the cross-cultural study of dreams separates Tedlock's chapter from Domhoff's and Gregor's. Their dispute highlights the difficulty of studying phenomena like dreams, which are both deeply idiosyncratic to the individual dreamer and deeply imprinted by the broader culture in which that dreamer lives. Another example is the issue of lucid dreaming and its religious and psychological significance, which receives dramatically opposing treatment from Doniger, who points to the profound differences between Tibetan Buddhist and contemporary American attitudes toward consciousness in dreaming, and Kahan, whose research highlights the fundamental metacognitive capacities that underlie the phenomenon of lucid dreaming across cultural differences. Yet another intratextual dispute pits Hobson, Crews, and Domhoff, who forcefully reject many of the basic tenets of psychoanalysis, against DiCenso, Jonte-Pace, Cohler, Kracke, White-Lewis, and Taylor, all of whom assert the continuing validity of Freudian and/or Jungian theory. This debate illustrates the need for dream researchers in the twenty-first century to continue struggling with the ambiguous legacy of their forebears from the twentieth century. Still another point of disagreement pits Irwin, Taylor, and Grace, who claim that certain dreams possess a powerfully visionary quality radically transcending the limitations of ordinary consciousness, against Hobson (and perhaps the majority of his neuroscientific colleagues), who argues that current sleep laboratory research shows dreaming to be nothing more than the natural functioning of the brain-mind system. Their dispute on this point shows how the field of dream studies stands squarely in the middle of the broader battle between religion and science in contemporary Western culture.

These crisscrossing lines of agreement and disagreement among the various chapters illustrate as well as anything can the infinite potential for interdisciplinary dialogue in the field of dream studies. Each chapter in *Dreams* has a life of its own with its own distinct questions and concerns, its own special aims and interests. Each chapter points in several different directions, across many different disciplinary boundaries, beckoning readers to follow.

Although I believe the independent dynamism of each chapter makes the book as a whole very stimulating to read, I must confess it has made my life as editor very difficult indeed. As I labored to produce a cohesive and well-shaped collection of chapters, the image kept coming to me that I was playing croquet in the Queen's garden in *Alice's Adventures in Wonderland:*

> Alice thought she had never seen such a curious croquet-ground in her life: it was all ridges and furrows: the croquet balls were live hedgehogs, and the mallets live flamingoes, and the soldiers had to double themselves up and stand on their hands and feet, to make the arches. The chief difficulty Alice found at first was in managing her flamingo: she succeeded in getting its body tucked away, comfortably enough, under her arm, with its legs hanging down, but generally, just as she had got its neck nicely straightened out, and was going to give the hedgehog a blow with its head, it *would* twist itself round and look up in her face, with such a puzzled expression that she could not help bursting out laughing; and, when she had got its head down, and was going to begin again, it was very provoking to find that the hedgehog had unrolled itself, and was in the act of crawling away: besides all this, there was generally a ridge or a furrow in the way wherever she wanted to send the hedgehog to, and, as the double-up soldiers were always getting up and walking off to other parts of the ground, Alice soon came to the conclusion that it was a very difficult game indeed.[3]

The authors gathered in this book are every bit as willful as the hedgehogs, flamingos, and card soldiers populating the Queen's croquet ground. They have their own ideas about how to play "the dream game," and I have done my best to showcase their unique talents and respect their scholarly independence even as I have juxtaposed them with other chapters in order to raise new issues that go beyond what the authors originally intended to address.

The main principle guiding my editorial choices was the "teachability" of each chapter. I have taught courses on dreams for several years to students at the undergraduate and graduate level and I have also given numerous lectures and presentations to general audiences in a variety of nonacademic settings. These experiences have helped me develop what I believe is a good sense for what works and does not work in dream education. *Dreams* presents a collection of writings that "teach well"—each chapter describes in a clear and concise fashion the most interesting findings from an important area of dream research; each chapter offers a forceful argument for certain modes of dream investigation and against others; each chapter makes a significant and thought-provoking claim about the role of dreaming in human life. I do not want to mislead readers into expecting that every chapter will be equally easy to understand, because many are quite demanding in their complexity and sophistication. But I believe the most educationally successful writings are precisely those that reward a reader's patient effort with fresh insights, broadened horizons, and new questions.[4] That is the primary criterion I used in putting *Dreams* together, and I hope teachers, students, and general readers alike find an abundance of those rewards in the following chapters.

A final word should be said about what is not included in this book. *Dreams* is not an encyclopedia; it does not offer a comprehensive summation of every form of dream research. Although I believe the book covers more territory than any other currently available book,[5] I freely acknowledge that I did not have space or opportunity to include articles on many important topics. For example, more could be said about literary treatments of dreaming[6] and the relevance of certain types of literary criticism to dream research.[7] More could be said about dreams in the history of philosophy[8] and the fertile relationship between dreaming and artistic creativity.[9] Full chapters could certainly have been devoted to the dream traditions of ancient Rome,[10] Medieval Christianity,[11] and the indigenous cultures of Australia[12] and sub-Saharan Africa.[13] The dream theories of other twentieth-century psychologists besides Freud and Jung could have been discussed.[14] Fortunately, readers interested in these topics may turn to a number of excellent recent works, which I have cited below.[15]

In the end, *Dreams* does not cover everything in the field because there is no final limit to the scope of dream research. Dreaming is interwoven throughout the entirety of human experience, meaning that the study of dreams is ultimately the study of human life itself.

Notes

1. Sigmund Freud, *The Interpretation of Dreams,* trans. James Strachey (New York: Avon Books, 1965), p. 143, n2.
2. A word should be said about my selection of this particular article by Thomas Gregor, since even he asked me why I preferred it instead of his other excellent articles on the dream life of the Mehinaku ("'Far, Far Away My Shadow Wandered. . . . ': The Dream Symbolism and Dream Theories of the Mehinaku Indians of Brazil," *American Ethnologist* (1981), vol. 8, no. 4, pp. 709–729, and "Dark Dreams about the White Man," *Natural History* (1983), vol. 92, no. 1, pp. 8–14). While I greatly admire those works, his article using the content analysis method to explore Mehinaku dream life is a unique work of interdisciplinary scholarship and one that I hope will stimulate further efforts to combine different dream research methodologies.
3. Lewis Carroll, *Alice's Adventures in Wonderland* (New York: Dilithium, 1988), pp. 154–155.
4. For those interested in more detailed information on resources for dream education and research, contact www.dreamresearch.net, www.asdreams.org, or www.kellybulkely.com.
5. The only other recent book that aims to provide a broad cultural and historical survey of dreaming is *Dream Cultures: Explorations in the Comparative History of Dreaming,* edited by David Shulman and Guy Stroumsa (New York: Oxford University Press, 1999). I would argue that the present book is more accessibly written, treats a wider variety of topics, and stimulates more interdisciplinary dialogue than Shulman and Stroumsa's book—but of course I am hardly an unbiased reviewer. The book against which all dream anthologies must measure themselves is *The Dream and Human Society,* edited by G. E. Von Grunebaum and Roger Callois (Berkeley: University of California Press, 1966). I have tried to emulate von Grunebaum and Callois's success in bringing together the leading exponents of many different fields of dream research. *The Dream and Human Society* gives readers the sense of attending a kind of "summit meeting" of the best dream researchers around, and I have sought to generate that same feeling in the present collection.
6. See Carol Schreier Rupprecht, ed., *The Dream and the Text: Essays on Literature and Language,* (Albany: State University of New York Press, 1999).
7. See Bert States, *Dreaming and Storytelling* (Ithaca: Cornell University Press, 1993).

8. See Christopher Dreisbach, "Dreams in the History of Philosophy," *Dreaming* vol. 10, no. 1 (2000): 31–42.
9. See Naomi Epel, *Writers Dreaming: Twenty-Six Writers Talk About Their Dreams and the Creative Process* (New York: Crown, 1993).
10. See Patricia Cox Miller, *Dreams and Late Antiquity: Studies in the Imagination of a Culture* (Princeton: Princeton University Press, 1994).
11. See Morton Kelsey, *God, Dreams, and Revelation: A Christian Interpretation of Dreams* (Minneapolis: Augsburg, 1981).
12. See G. W. Trompf, *Melanesian Religion* (Cambridge, U.K.: Cambridge University Press, 1990).
13. See M. C. Jedrej and Rosalind Shaw, eds., *Dreams, Religion, and Society in Africa* (Leiden: E. J. Brill, 1992).
14. See Anthony Shafton, *Dream Reader: Contemporary Approaches to the Understanding of Dreams* (Albany: State University of New York Press, 1995).
15. Detailed bibliographic essays on various areas of dream research can be found in my book *Visions of the Night* (Albany: State University of New York Press, 1999), pp. 131–175.

Section I

TRADITIONS

1

Buddhist Dream Experience

The Role of Interpretation, Ritual, and Gender

Serinity Young

Buddhist dream experience is most readily accessed through the rich and varied sacred biographies of India and Tibet. Dreams play a prominent role in these texts: They provide dramatic shifts in the action, underscore the inevitability of subsequent events, and precipitate significant changes in the spiritual and temporal life of the dreamer.[1] Actually, dreaming is an important element for all religions that emphasize biography as a way of defining the spiritual path, such as Confucianism, Islam, Christianity, and so on.[2]

For the most part, the dreams preserved in religious biographies are prophetic dreams: They predict something that will occur in the future. The belief that dreams can be a form of prophecy has existed from very ancient times. But, like all prophecy, they are open to interpretation, the first step of which is to establish that not all dreams are significant, not all dreams are prophetic. This means that dreams in spiritual biographies have already been vetted: Only those deemed to be prophetic are included. Consequently, a survey of dreams in sacred biographies does not offer a random collection of dreams; they have been preselected. They are, so to speak, prepackaged dreams, dreams that have been chosen for preservation because they reveal something that the tradition values. As an example, I would like to start with the most famous dream in Buddhism, the conception dream of Queen Māyā, the Buddha's mother.

Queen Māyā's Dream

The core elements of Māyā's dream are that she sees a magnificent white elephant that, by striking her right side with its trunk, is able to enter her womb. Many versions of this dream are preserved in early Buddhist iconography and texts. In fact, it is one of the earliest images of Buddhist iconography,[3] and representations of this dream kept up an even pace with the spread of Buddhism. It appears in various important sites throughout Buddhist history, such as Sānchī, Bhārut, Sarnath, Amāravati, Nāgārjunakonda, Ajaṇṭā, Gandhara, and sites in Central, Southeast and East Asia.[4]

The importance of this dream, and of dreams in general, is further attested to by its inclusion in most of the biographical texts on the Buddha.[5] The dream and its interpretation are preserved in the *Lalitavistara,*[6] the *Abiniṣkramaṇasūtra,*[7] the *Buddhacarita,*[8] the *Mahāvastu,*[9] and the *Mūlasarvāstivāda Vinaya,*[10] from which it entered the Tibetan canon.[11] It is mentioned in other Tibetan biographies as well; for instance, two editions of Padmasambhava's biography contain references to it.[12]

One of the most elaborate versions of Māyā's dream is contained in the *Nidāna-Kathā* (hereafter *NK*), the standard Theravāda biography of the Buddha. Note the details surrounding the dream, which provide a meaningful context for its interpretation:

> At that time the Midsummer festival (*Asālaha*) was proclaimed in the city of Kapilasvatthu. . . . During the seven days before the full moon Mahāmāyā had taken part in the festivities. . . . On the seventh day she rose early, bathed in scented water, and distributed alms. . . . Wearing splendid clothes and eating pure food, she performed the vows of the holy day. Then she entered her bed chamber, fell asleep and saw the following dream.
>
> The four guardians of the world [gods] lifted her on her couch and carried her to the Himālaya mountains and placed her under a great sāla tree. . . . Then their queens bathed her . . . dressed her in heavenly garments, anointed her with perfumes and put garlands of heavenly flowers on her. . . . They laid her on a heavenly couch, with its head towards the east. The Bodhisattva, wandering as a superb white elephant . . . approached her from the north. Holding a white lotus flower in his trunk, he circumambulated her three times. Then he gently struck her right side, and entered her womb. (*Dakkhinapassaṁ tāḷetva kucchim paviṭṭhasadiso.*)[13]

When Māyā woke up she told the dream to her husband, who sent for learned Brahman priests to interpret it. They predict that Queen Māyā will give birth to a son who will become a universal ruler (*cakkavatti*), unless he abandons his home for the religious life, in which case he will become a buddha.[14]

It is quite remarkable that this dream is so widespread both textually and iconographically, and from such an early period. Here, at the very beginnings of Buddhism, dreaming is central. Indeed, there is the suggestion that without Māyā's dream, there would be no Buddha and hence no Buddhism.

Using this primary Buddhist dream as a springboard, what follows is an exploration of the cultural context of Buddhist dream experience and practice on three levels: dream interpretation in texts, dream rituals, and gender ideologies.

Dream Interpretation

Let me begin by emphasizing that all dreams take place in a cultural context. Despite the sometimes profound feeling of otherness experienced in dreams, they occur within a cultural milieu that shapes their content as well as their interpretation. In other words, people dream within a pattern established by their culture. For instance, Hindus who have not been exposed to Christianity will not dream of the Christian idea of heaven; they will dream within the Hindu cultural pattern. E. R. Dodds, in his study of the ancient Greeks, develops this idea: "[I]n many primitive societies there are types of dream-structure which depend on a socially transmitted pattern of belief, and cease to occur when that belief ceases to be entertained. Not only the choice of this or that symbol, but the nature of the dream itself, seems to conform to a rigid traditional pattern."[15] Significantly, in Tibetan dream rituals dreamers often receive highly detailed instructions on exactly what they should see.

Most important, the original language of the dreamer provides important clues not only to the particular dream itself but to the whole cultural context of dreaming. For instance, South Asians consistently use the verb "seeing" (Sanskrit: √*dṛś,* Tibetan: *mthong*) a dream rather than "having" a dream. Such language expresses the fact that dreams are experienced as given to individuals rather than being created by them and tends to emphasize the external rather than the internal origin of the dream, thereby lending them a divine or demonic authority. To say one has seen rather than had a dream is to suggest that the dreamer is the passive recipient of an objective vision. The literalness of this thinking is expressed in hymn 4.9 of the *Atharva Veda* that appeals to an eye ointment, *añana,* for protection from troubled dreams, and in a Tibetan text from the *Tangyur* (discussed below) that recommends using a certain eye ointment when seeking an auspicious dream. Such ideas are connected to the powerful and pervasive South Asian belief in the redemptive value of *darśana* (Tib.: *lta-ba*)—seeing—particularly in the sense that the deity or holy person *gives darśana* while the worshipper *takes* it; the devotee both sees the deity and is seen by the deity. When this word is also used for dreams, instead of the more usual *svapna* (derived from the verb √*svap,* to sleep), one begins to sense the power of the dream in South Asia in that the dreamer not only sees the dream but can be seen by it.

As I hope will become clear, without the fullest possible understanding of the cultural context of a dream, without understanding how a particular culture values dreams—what it believes is possible within dreams—and without a grasp of its symbol system, an enormous part of its meaning is lost.

As we have seen, the Buddha's biography not only presents the dream, it includes an interpretation. Some of us, however, might have difficulty removing a psychoanalytic lens from our eyes when we think of the sexual implications of a bull elephant,[16] the phallic qualities of its trunk, and the erotic possibilities of the trunk striking her side. Obviously, these elements are present, as are others we can all imagine. My point, though, or rather the Buddhist point, is that we need to take seriously the official interpretation.

In support of the interpretation that it is an actual conception dream, during my research I found that many ancient people believed women could conceive through dreams[17] and some women sought temple incubation dreams as a cure for infertility.[18] The latter is a provocative concept when applied to Queen Māyā, particularly since she may have been forty years old when her first child, the Buddha, was born, and it is while participating in a religious festival that she dreams of being carried to heaven and conceiving.[19] Essentially, Indian culture accepts the possibility that women could conceive through a dream, and there are lists of dream images that define the nature of the child conceived.[20] I will return to conception dreams and the issue of dream interpretation toward the end of this chapter, within the context of gendered dreaming.

Dream Rituals

The text not only tells us what the dream means, it sets it within a religious festival, which leads into my second point, the cultural context of Buddhist dream rituals. You will recall that Queen's Māyā's dream takes place within a ritual context; she has participated in a seven-day religious ceremony and is sleeping apart from her husband. The question I brought to these details surrounding her dream was: Is there any other evidence for ritual dreaming in ancient India at the time of the Buddha?

I found that indeed there were various ritual means to have a dream, such as performing a specific ritual, going to sleep in a sacred place, praying for a dream, or simply concentrating the mind on having a dream before going to sleep. Such dreams are referred to as sought dreams, those that occur when someone consciously seeks a dream, and they have been documented among many ancient people.[21] The progression from spontaneous dream to sought dream is a reasonable development. If one accepts the prophetic value of dreams in general, then, whether the dreams occur spontaneously or as the result of consciously setting out to have a dream, one still has received a prophecy.

An example of evidence for the sought dream, or more specifically of dream incubation in ancient South Asia can be found in an early *Upaniṣad,* the *Chāndogya* (ca. ninth- to seventh-century B.C.E.). This text describes a ritual to gain spiritual and worldly power, and having a dream is a significant part of it. The ritual lasts for a fortnight, and like Māyā's ritual, it invokes the increasing power of the waxing moon by beginning with a sacrificial consecration on the night of the new moon and ending on the night of the full moon. On the last night the officiant drinks a mixture of herbs, honey and curd. Then he or she "cleans the cup and lies down behind the fire either on a skin or the bare ground, remaining silent and unresistant. If he sees a woman [in a dream], he should know that this rite has been successful" (5.2.8–9).

The dream is sought for a prophecy of the ritual's success or failure, and it is a particularly intriguing example when compared to later Buddhist dream practices that seek the approval of dream women, especially *ḍakinīs* (semi-divine women), before proceeding with an initiation. I will return to this role of gender in Buddhist dreaming.

Two other early examples of the practice of sought dreams come from a ritual text of the *Sāma Veda,*[22] and later examples can be found in folklore that dates back to this early period. Part of the cultural context for these practices, part of the valorization of dreams in India, is the well-known myth, so frequently depicted in South Asian art, that we are all participating in God's dream of creation. As the story goes, at the beginning of time nothing existed but a vast ocean and the god Viṣṇu, who slept on the coils of a great snake. As he sleeps he dreams, and a wonderful lotus grows out of his navel from which arises the universe; God's dream is the basis of all that exists, including waking reality. Thus, by entering into the dream state one can possibly enter into direct relationship with God and his creative powers. Indeed, we all do just this whenever we dream in that we create whole worlds out of dream matter.

The great collection of Indian folk stories, Somadeva's *Kathāsaritsāgara,*[23] contains two stories that revolve around sought dreams. In one story a king loses a debate with a Buddhist monk and converts to Buddhism. Later in the story he asks the monk to teach him how to become a Bodhisattva. The monk replies that one must first be free of all sin and there is but one method to be sure of that, doing a *svapna māṇavaka*—seeking a dream. When the king does this and dreams, he is reminded of a minor sin he committed and is told how to expiate it.[24] In this story a *svapna māṇavaka* is a Buddhist technique for producing dreams; yet another story in this collection uses the same term in a Hindu context, when it has a Kṣatriya pandit do a *svapna māṇavaka* in order to have a dream for his king.[25] Examples such as these show how easily ideas about dreams flowed between different South Asian religions as part of the common culture.[26] At the same time, these sketchy remains of dream practices appear to be similar to dream incubation in the Hellenistic world during the same period, of which we know so much more.

This brief compilation of sought dreams from various Indian texts indicates that dreaming was perceived, both by Buddhists and by Hindus, as a way of communicating with deities and a way of knowing the future. Tibetan biographical sources show that these beliefs flourished in Tibet as well.

This tradition of sought dreams continues today as I myself experienced during the weeklong Kālachakra ceremony held at Madison, Wisconsin, in 1981 when His Holiness the Dalai Lama ritually prepared us to have dreams as part of the initiation.[27]

Given the existence of these sought dream practices, I began to look for texts that described dream rituals, texts that contained instructions on having sought dreams, several of which I found in the Tibetan canon. One is entitled *Milam Tagpa (rMilam brTagpa,* The Examination of Dreams), and is dated to sometime before the ninth-century C.E. It is a short text that gives a set of instructions for obtaining two kinds of dreams, those that will generate the thought of enlightenment and those that will bestow empowerments or initiations (*bwang*). It begins with instructions on how to have such dreams, provides five lists of example dreams containing both good and bad predictions, and concludes with instructions for avoiding the ill effects of inauspicious dreams.

The first set of instructions to obtain dreams is as follows: "On a seat of Kuśa grass prepare a pillow of fragrant grasses and put on a garland of [*jatapa*] flowers. Recite mantras [in order to consecrate] milk from a young girl [a nursing mother], and then use it to anoint the eyes."[28] This is an esoteric text, and therefore it does not offer explanations of all its details, those would be given in the oral teachings; however, a few comments may be ventured about this eye ointment. As I mentioned earlier, South Asian and other ancient people use the verb "seeing" (Skt.: √*dṛś,* Tib.: *mthong wa*) a dream rather than "having" a dream. Such language expresses the fact that dreams are experienced as given to individuals rather than created by them. This use of language emphasizes the external rather than the internal origin of the dream, thereby lending them a divine or demonic authority. To say one has seen rather than had a dream is to suggest that the dreamer is the passive recipient of an objective vision. Putting on eye ointment, in other words ritually preparing the eyes, demonstrates how literally they were thinking of dreams in terms of seeing. All around the world applying magical ointments empowers, transforms and protects the body, and that is the case here. Milk is widely used in Indian rituals because of its positive qualities: Unlike any other food milk can be obtained without causing harm to any living creature, animal or vegetable; from churning the Milk Ocean the gods derived *amṛta,* the nectar of immortality; and, of course, a mother's milk is the ultimate symbol of nurturance.

Gender Ideologies

For my third cultural context of Buddhist dreaming, gender ideology, I will return to this milk ritual and to Māyā's dream. Before that, though, a short excursus into the gendered dimension of Indo-Tibetan dreaming may prove helpful.

Since the vast majority of Indo-Tibetan biographies are written by and are about men, there is an abundance of material on men's dreams and very little on women's dreams. Within male dream experience, however, there are frequent and significant appearances by various females, usually divine ones, and occasionally the dreams of certain women were recorded. These two sources of dream data, men's and women's, reveal some important Buddhist perceptions about women's power and powerlessness and male co-optation of that power for their own ends and to render women irrelevant. In short, women are free to be powerful in men's imaginations or psychic experiences, but not in social reality.[29] South Asian men often dream of women who are frightening, awe-inspiring, and powerful, such as the disheveled women who signify death in the epics and the medical texts and the spiritually empowering *ḍākinīs* of Tibetan biographies. When women dream they subtly voice a connection to these powerful and possibly dangerous dream women of the male imagination. In the biographical texts I have studied, women's dreams are often a form of protest against something their husbands want to do, something that the men have not actually articulated but that the women are capable of intuiting through their dreams. Despite the fact that subsequent events prove women's dreams to be accurate prophecies, husbands frequently dismiss and denigrate their wives' dreams. Another powerful literary means of denigrating women's dreams is the presentation of women who lie about their dreams in order to achieve their own, usually evil, ends. Briefly stated, there is a pattern in Buddhist biographies of women's true dreams being ignored and their false dreams being acted upon. At the same time, men have positive and empowering dreams about imaginary, often divine women.

Women and Female Deities in Men's Dreams

A gendered dimension to Indian dreaming has existed from the earliest period. This flows naturally out of Vedic cosmology, where goddesses are connected with natural elements such as the forests and, of relevance here, night; thus goddesses are associated with the mysterious and dangerous (the unfamiliar forests of ancient India), darkness, and sleep. This mythology was given a negative turn in the medical texts of ancient India, where the appearance of women in dreams, particularly disheveled women, or those dressed in red or having dark skin, become portents of illness and even death.[30] Goddesses such as Durgā and Kālī personify these dream women, as do the many female ghouls, ogresses, and wrathful yoginis of South Asian literature; they are all depicted as disheveled, with dark skin and adorned with bloodied body parts; and they have great power, are frightening and unpredictable.[31] Examples of such frightening dream women are found in popular literature as well, such as Valmiki's *Rāmāyaṇa* (composed ca. second century B.C.E.) and the *Mahābhārata* (composed ca. fifth-century B.C.E. to fourth-century C.E.), where dreams of such women predict death.

In contrast to these frightening dream women, as we have seen, the *Chāndogya Upaniṣad* says seeing a woman in a dream after performing a ritual portends the success of the ritual, suggesting that not all dream images of women are negative (5.2.8–9).

The Tibetan tradition also contains both negative and positive female dream images. Negative images abound in their medical texts, where dream women portend illness and death, but by and large the presence of a woman, human or divine, in dreams and the presence of female imagery such as the color red[32] are widespread and have a positive connotation, whether as a singular female image or coupled with reciprocal male imagery. A fertile climate for such dreams was created by Tantric practices that recommend using the things of this world in order to achieve enlightenment, including actual women as well as female imagery, both benign and frightening. However, real women are for the most part passive and silent participants in the male-centered rituals that are conducted in a covert and secretive fashion.[33] In contrast to real women, Tantra emphasizes the iconography and visualization of active and powerful *ḍākinīs* (Tib. *mKha' 'gro ma*)[34] and other female deities, some of whom are distinctly fierce in appearance, dance wildly, and wear necklaces of human skulls.

The term *dākinī* refers to a range of female beings; *ḍākinīs* can be spirit women or historical women who achieved tremendous spiritual power. On rare occasions it is used to describe a highly advanced living woman practitioner. Of significance here, they frequently appear in the dreams of male Buddhist saints. In Tibetan, the term *dākinī* means "sky-goer"—they cross over between realms, that of *samsāra* and *nirvāna* and that of the living and the dead. Consequently, they can confer enlightenment, they can take one beyond death. More broadly, *ḍākinīs* have an important salvational role in that they can bestow *siddhis,* the supernormal powers that lead to enlightenment. Quite often they bestow these through dreams. Appropriately, these divine woman can be actively sought by means of dream rituals.

The *ḍākinīs* point to the well-known theme in world religion and mythology of male dependence on a female guide[35] in order to complete quests, win a goal, or achieve enlightenment. Wisdom and insight (*prajñā*) are feminine terms in South Asian as well as other religious traditions, and they are frequently personified by goddesses or semi-divine women whose aid must be won in order to succeed in gaining spiritual knowledge and/or power.

Women Dreamers

The dreams of women, however, present a totally different pattern. To begin with, the most frequently preserved women's dreams in Buddhist biographies are conception dreams.[36] Given that the conception dream of the Buddha's mother, Queen Māyā, is so well known, it is not surprising that such dreams figure prominently in Buddhist biographical literature; indeed, they are stereotypical. Overall, conception dreams are a mixed metaphor of passivity and power. In most cases the women are passive recipients of fetuses—they are, after all, sound asleep at the time. This passivity is further emphasized by devices such as the "box" that was believed to surround the fetus placed in the womb of Queen Māyā,[37] thus protecting the male fetus from the polluting effects of a women's body. Even so, conception dreams also bespeak primal female powers of generation, suggesting as they do that women do not require men in order to conceive, or at least not human men. I will pick up this theme of maternal power shortly, but before that I want to return to some of the issues surrounding dream interpretation.

In several texts, the authority to interpret dreams was contested ground between Buddhists and Hindus, most obviously in the Pali *Jātaka*s, where Brahmans are portrayed as inadequate and even corruptible interpreters[38]; in the *śārdūlakarnāvadāna,* where a Brahman tests a Buddhist king's knowledge of dream interpretation[39]; and in the *Kathāsaritsāgara,* where authoritative knowledge of dream consciousness shifts between Buddhist and Hindu religious experts. Similarly, in many biographical texts dream interpretation is contested in terms of gender: women dream but men interpret. The ability to interpret dreams correctly is a tremendous source of spiritual and temporal power because, while everyone dreams, few truly understand their dreams. What sets dream interpreters apart is their ability to grasp the whole of reality; they can understand and function within the waking and sleeping worlds, within the real and the illusory. Men acknowledge women's power to access dream realms when they listen to their dreams, but through their interpretations men subvert that power and make sure it does not translate into the waking world.[40]

For the most part, the dreams I am discussing are preserved in literary texts; often they function to shift the action, to set the stage for an inevitable outcome. It is a passive, nonheroic form of acting that is best performed by a woman (or a junior male), and it is a way to harness female power and keep it and women in their place.[41] When Buddhist heroes dream, they reveal their internalization of this female power and also maintain their power as dream interpreters. In all the South Asian texts I have surveyed, the authoritative voice of dream interpretation is a male one.[42]

In Buddhism the pattern of men interpreting the dreams of their wives in order to dismiss them begins with the Buddha's biography. In the *Lalitavistara* (*LV,* Vaidya), his wife Gopā awakens from a frightening dream that predicts the Buddha's imminent desertion of her for the ascetic life. She tells the Buddha her dream and asks what it means. It is a long dream, and the Buddha gives it an equally long and detailed interpretation before telling her a dream he has had and interpreting as well. Several things are going on in this exchange, not the least of which is the Buddha affirming male access to the dream realm both as dreamer and interpreter. The Buddha must reject the obvious meaning of Gopā's dream, loss of her husband and the kingdom's loss of an heir, if he is to go forth into the religious life. Gopā's dream accurately describes the emotional consequences of his desertion; she sees the whole earth shaken and herself naked, with her hair, hands, and feet cut off. The Buddha's dismissal of her fears and his interpretation undermine her prophetic powers and silence the protest implied in her dream: "Be joyful, these dreams are not evil. Beings who have previously practiced good works have such dreams. Miserable people have no such dreams. . . . The omens are auspicious" (*LV,* Vaidya, 141.9–142.28). Yet when compared to the only nightmare in the same text (the demon Māra's), line for line the imagery is the same.[43]

The Buddha's dismissal of his wife's dream is repeated in the *Abhiniṣkramaṇasūtra* (*AS*) and *The Gilgit Manuscript of the Saṅghabhedvastu, Being the 17th and Last Section of the Vinaya of the Mūlasarvāstivādin* (*MSV*), the other main biographical texts in which it appears. In fact, in the *MSV* his wife extracts a promise from him to take her wherever he goes (*MSV,* vol. I, p. 83). Of course, he does not take her with him, and the text glosses this as meaning he promised to take her along to *nirvāṇa* (liberation). This process is even repeated in the very popular *Vessantara Jātaka,* a past life story in which the Buddha and Gopā are called Vessantara and Maddi. In this tale Maddi has a prophetic dream that reveals her husband will give their children away. When she asks him to interpret it, he dismisses it, attributing it to indigestion, and the text goes so far as to say: "with this deceit [*mohetvā*] he consoled her." Of course, the next day he gives the children away.[44]

In these dream narrations the wives fearfully present their dreams—they know they bode ill. In speaking their fears, these women are attempting to dissipate the dream's influence and to protest (at least obliquely) their husbands' power to bring disaster upon them. Even though there were many rituals to offset the harmful effects of dreams, in these scenarios they are not used because the men want the dreams to be fulfilled. In this way the text presents women as powerful dreamers, as capable of receiving prophetic dreams, at the same time it underlines their actual powerlessness: The women cannot avert the fulfillment of their dreams. They do not even resort to widely available ritual means to do so.

The women know what is going on in their lives, they know what is going to happen to them and the ones they love, and they voice their fears and their protest in the only acceptable way they can, through their dreams. Like women in trance, they are not ultimately responsible for their words; dream narrations are a safe way to protest male authority over their lives. Hence the consistent pattern of women who dream, and fully understand the meaning of their dreams, yet ask their husbands to interpret the dreams is shown to be an oblique way of having direct discourse with their husbands. This pattern is also maintained around conception dreams when the wife who dreams asks her husband what it means. This is actually an indirect way of getting their husbands to affirm paternity or to approve the pregnancy. However, when the men dismiss their dreams or interpret them in ways favorable to what they want, women are ultimately silenced and returned to the background of male drama. And the tendency for men to dismiss women's dreams continues in Tibetan biographies, for instance when Padmasambhava dismisses the dreams of his wife Bhāśadharā[45] and in Milarepa's biography where Marpa dismisses the prophetic dreams of his wife Dakmema.[46]

The texts in which women dream show them to be truly prophetic dreamers, which is a kind of power, and one deemed important and acceptable enough to provide major plot shifts. But both the male denial of the dreams and their eventual fulfillment to the frustration of the female dreamer totally co-opts this female power, thus heightening female powerlessness rather than their power as dreamers and interpreters. Despite all this, these incidents tacitly acknowledge women's power to invade men's dreams as well as women's ability to intuit men's intentions through their own dreams and to voice that intuition without fear of repercussions. That dreams are believed to be a special female weapon against men is demonstrated by stories of women lying about their dreams and/or using dreams for deceptive and manipulative ends. Examples of this can be seen in the *Kuṇala Jātaka,* where co-queens bribe Brahman dream interpreters to deny the auspiciousness of the favorite queen's dream, and in the *Chaddanta Jātaka,* where the queen lies about having a dream in order to harm the Buddha. Especially chilling is Queen Tiṣyarakṣita's manipulation of Emperor Aśoka's dreams in his biography, the *Aśokāvadāna.*[47]

Before going further, two related points about the Indo-Tibetan Buddhist biographical tradition need to be restated. First, it is dominated by men as subjects and as authors. Thus all representations of women are filtered through male experience.[48] Second, they do not strive to be factual representations of someone's life; rather they present (and interpret) events that lead to an individual's enlightenment, including visions and dreams. Whether the dreams actually occurred is unknowable. What we can know about these dreams is that they are examples of what male Buddhists thought about dreams and, of relevance here, what they thought about women. These ideas then seeped into the general consciousness of the societies where these stories were read, recited, and retold.

What is at root here is the male dismissal of real women, especially from the lives of monastics, and the internalization of imaginary women, including the co-optation of women's imaginary processes in dreaming. This goes back to Tantra's incorporation of female imagery and female deities and the distancing of actual, living women. Some women were participants in Tantric rites, but this was no union of equals; for the most part they were marginal women who were silent participants and sworn to secrecy.[49] The few exceptions, such as the biography of the female saint Yeshe Tsogyel,[50] a document of questionable historical accuracy, only emphasizes the rarity of biographies about female practitioners when compared to the innumerable biographies of male practitioners.

The male subjects of the biographies I have studied dismiss women's truthful dreams, report the deceptive dreams of women, and themselves dream of women granting them spiritual power. In other words, male Buddhists render real women irrelevant, meaningless and powerless, while they empower women in their imaginations—dream women. In effect, in one motion, male Buddhists both co-opt women's subjectivity for themselves and deny the subjectivity of real women.[51]

Dreams, Death, and Women

Perhaps the most inauspicious imaging of women is in relation to death, a topic also connected to dreaming. Until fairly recent times there was an almost universal belief in the ability of dreams to predict death, a notion that continues to persists among a great variety of people. In South Asia this connection is easily understood because certain dreams were an accepted sign of death in both medical texts and in epic literature, while language itself conspires to conflate dreams, sleep, and death, as in the Sanskrit root √*svap,* which can mean "to sleep" or "to be dead" and is the root for the noun "dream." In Tibet, the practice of Dream Yoga is said to give one entry into the *bardo* state between death and rebirth. Most obviously, people all around the world often dream about the dead, leading to the idea that through dreams we can access the realm of the dead and conversely that death can access us through dreams. Additionally, many people believe that the soul leaves the body during sleep as it does in death, which is why caution must be used in waking a sleeper,[52] and a sleeping body can just as easily be mistaken for a dead body. A famous Buddhist example that plays with this idea is found in the biographies of the Buddha where, on the night of his departure from home, he observes the sleeping women of the harem, leading him to the reflection that he is living in the middle of a cremation ground (*śmaśana*).[53]

Indeed, Hesiod in the *Theogony* (211–213, 756–766) says that Night is the mother of all three: sleep, death, and dreams.[54] Sleep and dreams know death in a way waking consciousness does not because in crossing over the boundaries of waking consciousness they are believed to draw close to that netherworld. This point is brought out in the *Bṛhadāraṇyaka Upaniṣad,* where the discussion on dreams and sleep inevitably leads to the discussion of death (4.3.13–38 and 4.4).

Examples of women's association with death abound in early Buddhist literature,[55] including the just-mentioned sleeping harem women, as well as in the ancient Indian medical texts and popular forms of Indian literature such as epics and folk tales, in which women figure prominently in dreams that predict death, especially dark-skinned women, those wearing red clothes or carrying red flowers, and those having a wild appearance or being strong enough to drag someone away, especially toward the south, the land of the dead. This is actually a description of the goddess of death, Mṛtyu, "a black woman with red garments and red eyes,"[56] as well as of Kālī.

Some of these negative images survive in Tibetan dream narrations,[57] but for the most part they were incorporated into Tantric practices that purposely utilized death imagery, for instance, the frequent recommendation to live and meditate in cremation grounds. In earlier, pre-Buddhist dream interpretation, death imagery was to be feared. In Tantric Buddhism, confronting and overcoming the fear of death is part of the practice leading to enlightenment. Once the Tantric adept has truly realized the impermanence of all existence, the essential emptiness of all phenomena, there is nothing more to fear. In this way the Tantric incorporation of female imaging of death can be seen as a positive valuing of the feminine in that women, through their connection to death, can lead one to enlightenment.[58] Yet this heroic co-optation of frightening female imagery never really leaves the control of men nor ever really advances the lives of actual women. These dream women may terrify male practitioners, but the men are being trained to overcome that fear. In effect, female imagery is used to conquer a fear of female power.[59]

There are many complicated ideas about women, death, and enlightenment in Indo-Tibetan literature. The goal of Tantric Buddhism is to achieve liberation from the endless cycle of being born and dying through ritual techniques and practices that utilize the human body. However, it appears that the female body, at least when utilized by men through actual or symbolic practices, is particularly useful in achieving this end. At the same time, different types of literature gender dreams differently. The ritual texts of the Tibetan Canon emphasize seeing the male body of the buddhas, while the biographies have no such dreams of buddhas—instead they have frequent dreams of female bodies in the form of *ḍākinīs,* and the color red, symbolizing women's fertile powers, figures prominently in their dreams. A third genre of literature, medical texts, say that dreams about women and the color red (blood) predict death.

This association of women and death exists in many cultures through women's biological connection to birth, which inevitably leads to death, through menstruation, in which the shedding of blood does not kill the menstruating woman but can threaten men with its power, usually its polluting power, and by women's dominant roles in death rituals.[60] On the positive side, associating the female with death frequently means associating females with immortality. This is to suggest that female forces have control over life and death to such a degree that they can free one from death. Some symbolical examples of this thinking are reflected in the skull necklaces of *ḍākinīs* and the word *padmabhājana* (lotus vessel) that is used, for example in the *Hevajra Tantra,* to mean both vaginas and skulls.[61] Either actually or symbolically, vaginas and skulls are essential for the Tantric rituals that lead to enlightenment.

Returning to women's ability to give birth, women are also seen as the source of their husband's immortality because they provide the sons so essential to the continuation of ancestor worship.[62] This complex of related ideas reveals the connection between the negative appearances of dream women in medical texts and the positive conception dreams of real women in the biographical literature; women can dream us into existence and when we dream of them they call us back to death. Tantric dream-practices obliquely acknowledge these beliefs when they transform such female dream imagery into *siddhi*-conferring *ḍākinīs,* women who call one to enlightenment. It also brings us back to the *Tangyur* text that used the consecrated milk of a nursing mother as an eye ointment to procure dreams. Mother's milk is the most positive, life-enhancing female image imaginable in a climate that associates women with death.[63] The use of this milk affirms the need for a female guide through the dream realm that hovers between life and death because it is women who successfully traverse this realm *for others* biologically and, by extension, spiritually. Putting a mother's milk on the eyelids enables one to see with the eyes of this primal female power and assures one's return to waking life.

Conclusion

In this chapter I have utilized Queen Māyā's dream in two ways: to open up the cultural context of Buddhist dream experience and practice and to argue that a dream's cultural context is essential to understanding its meaning. I have done this by highlighting three distinct contexts of her dream: its official interpretation, its ritual dimension, and its relation to Buddhist gender ideologies. By looking further afield into additional Indo-Tibetan Buddhist texts and practices I have documented the larger background of these cultural contexts. Yet I have in no way exhausted the dream's meaning or the meaning of dreams in Buddhism. Dreams speak to the individual dreamer, but they also speak to all who hear them. By sharing the dream, we multiply its meaning among all those who hear it. It is my hope that this chapter will encourage further explorations of the complex but rewarding realm of Buddhist dreaming.

Notes

1. For more information on the topic of dreams in Buddhism, see Serinity Young, *Dreaming in the Lotus: Buddhist Dream Narrative, Imagery and Practice* (Boston: Wisdom Publications, 1999).
2. See, for instance, Barbara Tedlock, ed., *Dreaming: Anthropological and Psychological Interpretations* (Cambridge: Cambridge University Press, 1987); G. E. von Grunebaum and Robert Caillois, eds., *The Dream and Human Societies* (Berkeley: University of California Press, 1966); David Shulman and Guy G. Strouman, eds., *Dream Cultures: Explorations in the Comparative History of Dreaming* (Oxford: Oxford University Press, 1999); Kelly Bulkeley, *The Wilderness of Dreams* (Albany: State University of New York Press, 1994).
3. For some of the earliest representations of this dream, which may even occur in the Aśokan Rock Edicts, see Karl Khandalavala, "Heralds in Stone: Early Buddhist Iconography in the Aśokan Pillars and Related Problems," pp. 21–22, and also Biswanarayan Shastri, "The Philosophical Concepts and the Buddhist Pantheon," p. 56, both in *Buddhist Iconography,* no ed. (Delhi: Tibet House, 1989). The dream may also be represented at pre-Aśokan sites in Andra Pradesh, see D. Sridhara Babu, "Reflections on Andra Buddhist Sculptures and Buddha Biography," in *Buddhist Iconography,* pp. 100–101.
4. Early iconographic representations of this dream and its interpretation are briefly discussed in Patricia Eichenbaum Karetzky, *The Life of the Buddha: Ancient Scriptural and Pictorial Traditions* (Lanham, MD: University Press of America, 1992), pp. 11–15. See also her dissertation, Patricia D. Eichenbaum, *The Development of a Narrative Cycle Based on the Life of the Buddha in India, Central Asia, and the Far East: Literary and Pictorial Evidence* (Ann Arbor, MI: University Microfilm International, 1980), and the list in Dieter Schlingloff, *Studies in the Ajanta Painting: Identifications and Interpretations* (Delhi: Ajanta Publications [India]: 1987), pp. 17–18, and 37–38 nn. 30, 32, and 33. See also the important discussion of iconographic representations of the life of the Buddha in John C. Huntington, "Pilgrimage as Image: The Cult of the A·ṭamahāprātihārya, Part I," *Orientations* 18, no. 4 (April 1987): 55–63.
5. See H. Luders, ed., *Bhārhut Inscriptions,* rev. by E. Waldschmidt and M. A. Mehendale (Ootacamund: Govenment Epigraphist for India, 1963), pp. 89–90, for a brief discussion of some of these texts as well as some of the texts that do not include it. For the early Chinese biographies, see Karetzky, *Life of the Buddha,* p. 4.
6. The *Lalitavistara* is available in a Sanskrit edition, edited by P. L. Vaidya (Darbhanga: Mithila Institute, 1985) (hereafter *LV,* Vaidya). An English edition is available through Gwendolyn Bays's translation of Edouard Foucaux's French translation from the Sanskrit, *The Voice of the Buddha: The Beauty of Compassion* (Oakland, CA: Dharma Press, 1983). It was composed anonymously around the beginning of the common era, although it contains much earlier material from the oral tradition.
7. The *Abhiniṣkramaṇasūtra,* trans. by Samuel Beal from the Chinese edition as *The Romantic Legend of Śākya Buddha* (1875. Delhi: Motilal Banarsidass, 1985), pp. 37–39 (here-

after *AS*). This text was probably composed among the Dharmaguptakas, a Hīnayāna school of early Buddhism (Hirakawa, *History of Indian Buddhism,* p. 265), for which a Sanskrit version has been lost.

8. Aśvaghoṣa, *Buddhacarita,* ed. and trans. E. H. Johnston (1936. Delhi: Motilal Banarsidass, 1984), I.4 (hereafter *BC*). It was composed around the beginning of the Common Era. Johnston's edition contains the extant early chapters in Sanskrit, which are translated into English along with an English translation of the later chapters, which are available in Tibetan.
9. Sanskrit edition by É. Senart, *Le Mahāvastu,* 3 vols. (Paris: À L'imprimerie Nationale, 1890) (hereafter *MV,* Senart); the dream is in vol. II, p. 12. English translation by J. J. Jones, is the *Mahāvastu,* 3 vols. (London: Pali Text Society, 1949–56); the dream is in vol. II, p. 11. Jones argues that its long compilation period began in the second century B.C.E. and continued into the third or fourth century C.E. (*MV,* I.xi-xii).
10. *The Gilgit Manuscript of the Saṅghabhedvastu, Being the 17th and Last Section of the Vinaya of the Mūlasarvāstivādin,* ed. Raniero Gnoli (Rome: Istituto Italiano per il Medio ed Estremo Oriente, 1977), vol. I, p. 40 (hereafter *MSV*). This text comes from the Sarvāstivāda school of early Buddhism which spread into Central Asia, Tibet, and China and was completed around the third century C.E., *Māulasarvāstivādavinayavastu,* ed. S. Bagchi, (Darbhanga: The Mithila Institute of Post-Graduate Studies and Research in Sanskrit Learning, 1967), p. xiii.
11. Cited by W. W. Rockhill, *Life of the Buddha* (Varanasi: Orientalia Indica, 1972), p. 15. The Tibetan historian Buston, though, quotes the dream from the *LV.* Buston, *The History of Buddhism in India and Tibet,* trans. E. Obermiller (1932. Delhi: Sri Satguru Publications, 1986), pp. 10–11.
12. Both references occur in the context of the subjects Padmasambhava (traditionally dated to the eighth century) studies, for instance, astrology, during which he learns about the year when "the six-tusked white elephant was incarnated" (*glang-pa thal kar mche drug sprul*), an obvious reference to Māyā's dream, *Padma bka' thang shel brag ma,* no editor listed (Leh: 1968), at f. 65b.1 (hereafter *Padma*). The other says that Padma "was taught all about the year the conception of the Buddha, the year in which the mother of the Buddha dreamt that a white elephant entered her womb, the year of the Buddha's birth, and how these esoterically significant periods have correspondence with the Tibetan calendar," W.Y. Evans-Wentz, *The Tibetan Book of the Great Liberation* (New York: Oxford University Press, 1954, 1968), p. 122.
13. *Nidāna-Kathā,* in *The Jātaka together with its Commentary,* ed. V. Fausböll (London: Trübner and Co., 1877), I.50 (hereafter *NK*). This began as an introduction to the *Jātakas*, but rapidly became the standard Theravāda biography of the Buddha. The dream and its interpretation are translated by T. W. Rhys Davids as *Buddhist Birth Stories* (1880. New York: E. P. Dutton and Co., 1925), pp. 149–151.
14. *NK,* I.51.
15. E. R. Dodds, *The Greeks and the Irrational* (Berkeley: University of California Press, 1951, 1973), pp. 103–104.
16. The elephant has been a rich and enduring motif in Indian art and literature from the time of the Indus valley civilization until the present, in which it usually symbolizes majesty, raw power, and great dignity. (S. K. Gupta suggests some of these associations may be connected to the elephant's usefulness in war, for which there are references dating to the 326 B.C.E. battle against Alexander, *The Elephant in Indian Art and Mythology* [New Delhi: Abhinav Publications, 1983], p. 5.) In Indian myth an elephant, Airāvata, is the mount (*vāhana*) of Indra, king of the gods. Indra is also a rain god, which heightens the elephant's traditional connection with rain, a connection furthered by frequent envisioning of clouds as celestial elephants. (See Heinrich Zimmer, *Myths and Symbols in Indian Art and Civilization,* ed. Joseph Campbell (1946. New York: Harper

and Brothers, 1962), pp. 104–109 and Paul B. Courtright, *Gaṇeśa: Lord of Obstacles, Lord of Reason* (New York: Oxford University Press, 1985), pp. 21–31, for more on the elephant's association with clouds and rain.) That the Buddhists shared this idea is brought out in the *Vessantara Jātaka,* where a white elephant guarantees the prosperity of the kingdom through its magical ability to bring rain.

17. See the discussion of conception dreams in Young, *Dreaming in the Lotus,* pp. 75–85. For more examples of conception dreams from around the world, see the bibliography on conception dreams in Bulkeley, *The Wilderness of Dreams,* p. 234 n. 9, and Otto Rank "The Myth of the Birth of the Hero," reprinted in Robert A. Segal, *In Quest of the Hero* (Princeton, NJ: Princeton University Press, 1990), pp. 3–86.
18. Ernest Jones, *On the Nightmare* (New York: Liveright Publishing Corp., 1951, 1971), pp. 92ff. The seventh-century Indian text, the *Kādambarī* by Bāṇabhaṭṭa, describes various acts performed by Queen Vilāsavatī in order to conceive a son, including sleeping in the temples of the goddess Caṇḍikā and telling her dreams to Brahmans, quoted by David N. Lorzen, *The Kāpālikas and Kālāmukhas: Two Lost Saivite Sects* (1972. 2nd ed., Delhi: Motilal Banarsidass, 1991), pp. 16–17.
19. H. W. Schumann, *The Historical Buddha,* trans. M. O'C. Walshe (1982. London: Penguin Group, 1989), p. 7. *MV,* Senart, I.355–357 and II.3.1 ff., says she was the youngest of the seven sisters Śuddhodana married and that she was in the prime of life when she gave birth twelve years later. In general, see Telwatte Rahula, *A Critical Study of the Mahāvastu* (Delhi: Motilal Banarsidass, 1978), for his lengthy discussion of Māyā, pp. 187–202.
20. See, e.g., the *MV,* II.13 and the *AS,* pp. 38–39. See also the *Kalpa Sūtra,* in Hermann Jacobi, *Jaina Sutras,* 2 vols. (1884, 1895. New York: Dover Publications, 1968), I:247, and Sharma, "Symbolism in the Jinist Dream-World," in Jagdish Sharma and Lee Siegel, *Dream-Symbolism in The Śrāmaṇic Tradition: Two Psychoanalytical Studies in Jinist and Buddhist Dream Legends* (Calcutta: Firma KLM Private Limited, 1980), p. 3.
21. See, for example, the classical study of Native American dreaming: Jackson Steward Lincoln, *The Dream in Primitive Cultures* (1935. New York: Johnson Reprint Corporation, 1970); also see the more recent typology of Native American dreams by Lee Irwin, *The Dream Seekers: Native American Visionary Traditions of the Great Plains* (Norman: University of Oklahoma Press, 1994); the aforementioned Dodds, *The Greeks and the Irrational;* Patricia Cox Miller, *Dreams in Late Antiquity: Studies in the Imagination of a Culture* (Princeton, NJ: Princeton University Press, 1994); Mircea Eliade, *Shamanism: Archaic Techniques of Ecstasy,* trans. Willard R. Trask (1951. Princeton: Princeton University Press, 1972). For some early Jewish practices, see Joshua Trachtenberg, *Jewish Magic and Superstition: A Study in Folk Religion* (1939. New York: Atheneum, n.d.), pp. 241–243.
22. For more information on this text, especially the dating problems, see *Sāmavidhāna Brāhmana,* ed. A. C. Burnell (London: Trübner and Company, 1873), pp. v-x. The rituals are at iii.4.2 and iii.4.3. I have used the commentary, on pp. 82–83, to elucidate some of the text.

    In order to have a prophetic dream, the text recommends:

    1. Place the deity who dwells in the dung (*Saṅkarevāsinīm*) in a basket along with unhusked grains, incense and flowers, and put it on the head. Then lay down in a pure place with the head toward the east and sing the hymn [from the *Sāma Veda*] that begins "*imam uhuvu.*" After this one should remain silent while falling asleep and he or she will see in a dream the fruit (*phala*) of what will come.
    2. Alternatively, place a poison pill (*garagolikaµ*) in a box and sing the hymn that begins "*āyāhi susamā hi ta.*" Then one should remain silent while falling asleep and he or she will see.

    In the first ritual the unhusked grain of seems to stand for the dormant potential of dreaming within us all. As a birth metaphor it stands in sharp contrast to the death imagery of the poison pill in the second ritual. The latter ritual may very well be connected to the widespread South Asian belief that through dreams one can access the realm of the dead in order to learn the secrets of the future.

23. This eleventh-century collection of stories is based on an earlier (ca. first-century C.E.) and now-lost collection, The *Bṛhat-kathā* of Guṇāḍhya, which was Buddhist or at least heavily influenced by Buddhism, and traces of that influence remain in Somadeva's collection. See the discussion in Charles Rockwell Lanman, *A Sanskrit Reader* (Cambridge, MA: Harvard University Press, 1884), pp. 332–333; Arthur A. Macdonell, *A History of Sanskrit Literature* (1899. Delhi: Motilal Banarsidass, 1971); and Maurice Winternitz, *A History of Indian Literature,* 3 vol. (1927. Delhi: Oriental books reprint corporation, 1977), vol. 3, pp. 353–365.
24. Somadeva Bhaṭṭa, *Kathāsaritsāgara,* ed. Pt. Jagadīśa Lāl Śāstrī (Delhi: Motilal Banarsidass, 1960), book 12, chapter 5. Trans. Tawney as *The Ocean of Story,* vol. 6, pp. 76–77.
25. *Kathāsaritsāgara,* Śāstrī, book 1, chapter 6.137. Tawney, *Ocean of Story,* vol. 1, pp. 70–71.
    The term *svapna māṇavaka* also appears in a twelfth-century Indian text on constructing mandalas that was translated into Tibetan and widely used, the *Vajrāvalīnāma-maṇḍalapāyikā* of Abhayākaragupta. This text recommends seeking and examining a dream (Skt.: *svapna māṇavaka;* Tib.: *rMilam brTagpa*) in order to establish that the deities approve the proposed location of the mandala. I am very grateful to (Pema) Losang Chogyen for bringing this to my attention and sharing his notes with me. Before his untimely death in 1996, he was preparing an English translation and a definitive edition of this text through the use of Sanskrit and Tibetan manuscripts.
26. Compare also the similar understandings of dreams in the Indian (Hindu) and Tibetan (Buddhist) medical texts quoted in Young, *Dreaming in the Lotus,* pp. 65–72. This practice of dream ideologies crossing religious lines also occurred in the Hellenistic world among Judaism, Christianity, and Paganism; see Miller, *Dreams in Late Antiquity,* passim.
27. See Young, *Dreaming in the Lotus,* pp. 133–134, for details of these instructions.
28. Tanjur, *Rgyud 'grel: The Corpus of Indian Commentaries on Vajrayana Buddhist Literature Translated into Tibetan* (Delhi: Delhi Karmapae Chodhey, Gyalwae Sungrab Partun Khang, 1982–1985).
29. This truism of gender studies is effectively argued by Rita Gross, "Methodological Remarks on the Study of Women in Religions: Review, Criticism and Redefinition," in J. Plaskow and J. N. Romero, eds., *Women and Religion* (Missoula: Scholars Press, 1974).
30. See the discussion in Young, *Dreaming in the Lotus,* pp. 65–72, and also the copious dream lists from Sangye Gyatso's commentary (the *Vaidūrya sNgon po*) on the Tibetan medical text, *rGyud bŽi,* the *Four Treatises,* translated into English as *Tibetan Medical Paintings: Illustrations to the Blue Beryl Treatise of Sangye Gyamtso (1653–1705),* ed. Anthony Aris, 2 vols. (New York: Harry N. Abrams, Inc., 1992) (hereafter *Tibetan Medical Paintings*).
31. Liz Wilson discusses some female ghouls in early Buddhist literature in *Charming Cadavers: Horrific Figurations of the Feminine in Indian Buddhist Hagiographic Literature* (Chicago: University of Chicago Press, 1996), pp. 58–60; Ann Gold discusses wrathful yoginis in "Gender and Illusion in a Rajasthani Yogic Tradition," in *Gender, Genre and Power in South Asian Expressive Traditions* (Philadelphia: University of Pennsylvania Press, 1991), pp. 102–135. Of course, Tibetan literature is filled with wrathful *dākinīs*, demons and ogresses, see, e.g., Janet Gyatso, "Down with the Demoness," in Janice D. Willis, ed., *Feminine Ground: Essays on Women and Tibet* (Ithaca, NY: Snow Lion, 1989), pp. 35–51.
32. See Young, *Dreaming in the Lotus,* pp. 79–80, for a discussion of the dream symbolism of the color red.
33. See June Campbell's discussion of the secret role of women in Tantra in *Traveller in Space: In Search of Female Identity in Tibetan Buddhism* (New York: George Braziller, 1996), passim.
34. For more information on *ḍākinīs* see Victoria Urubshurow, "Dakinis," *The Encyclopedia of Women and World Religion* (hereafter *EOW*), ed. Serinity Young (New York:

Macmillan, 1998), vol. I, pp. 231–232; Hildegard Diemberger, "Lhakama (*lha-bka'-ma*) and Khandroma (*mkha'-'gro-ma*): The Sacred Ladies of Beyul Khenbalung (*sbas-yul mKan-pa-lung*)," in *Tibetan History and Language: Studies Dedicated to Uray Géza on his Seventieth Birthday,* ed. Ernst Steinkellner (Wien: Arbeitskreis für Tibetische und Buddhistische Studien, Universität Wien, 1991), pp. 137–153; and Nathan Katz, "Anima and mKha'-'gro-ma: A Critical Comparative Study of Jung and Tibetan Buddhism," in *Tibet Journal* 2, no. 3 (1977): 13–43.

35. For a brief discussion and reference to some further examples, see "Wisdom as Feminine" in Serinity Young, *An Anthology of Sacred Texts By and About Women* (New York: Crossroad, 1993), pp. xxi-xxii, and various entries in the index under "Feminine." Katz, "Anima and mKha'-'gro-ma, pp. 13–43, has an interesting discussion of *ḍākinīs* as guides.
36. For more information on women's dreams, see two articles by Carol Schreier Rupprecht: "Women's Dreams: Mind and Body," in *Feminist Archetypal Theory: Interdisciplinary Re-Visions of Jungian Thought,* ed. Estella Lauter and Carol Schreier Rupprecht (Knoxville: University of Tennessee Press, 1985) and "Sex, Gender and Dreams: From Polarity to Plurality" in *Among All These Dreamers: Essays on Dreaming and Modern Society,* ed. Kelly Bulkeley (Albany: State University Press of New York, 1996). See also Miller's discussion of Perpetua's dreams, and Richard L. Kagan, *Lucretia's Dreams: Politics and Prophecy in Sixteenth-Century Spain* (Berkeley: University of California Press, 1990, 1995), a well documented study of a prophetic female dreamer.
37. At least in the popular *LV* version. Tsongkhapa is also protected by a box in his mother's womb; see Robert A. F. Thurman, *The Life and Teachings of Tsong Khapa* (Dharamsala: Library of Tibetan Works and Archives, 1982), p. 5. This dream is also preserved in the *'Jam mgon chos kyi rgyal po tsong kha pa chen po'i rnam thar thub ba stan mdses po'i rgyan gi cag ngo mtshar nor lu'i 'phreng ba shes sbya ba bshugs so* (Sarnath, Varanasi: Mongolian Lama Guru Deva, 1967) (hereafter *'Jam mgon*), pp. 88–89.
38. E.g., the *Kuṇāla, Vessantara,* and *Mahāsupina Jātaka*s.
39. See Young, *Dreaming in the Lotus,* pp. 50–51, for further discussion of this text.
40. Other examples of gendered battles over the power to interpret dreams can be found in Young, "Dreams," *EOW,* pp. 271–273.
41. See Lynn Bennett, *Dangerous Wives and Sacred Sisters: Social and Symbolic Roles of High-Caste Women in Nepal* (New York: Columbia University Press, 1983), pp. 261–308, for an intriguing discussion of Hindu men's control and pacifying worship of the fierce goddess Durgā as a way of confronting and overcoming their anxieties about real women.
42. This despite the fact that the *Kāma Sūtra* lists dream interpretation as one of the sixty-four arts of a courtesan. However, courtesans are a significantly different category of women from wives. The privileging of male dream interpreters in South Asian texts also flies in the face in the prominence of female dream interpreters in many other cultures; see examples in Young, "Dreams," *EOW.*
43. See the discussion of these two dreams in Young, *Dreaming in the Lotus,* pp. 39–41.
44. *The Jataka Together with its Commentary,* Fausböll, vol. VI, pp. 540–541.
45. *Padma,* f.57b.6.
46. Quoted in Young, *Dreaming in the Lotus,* pp. 81–82.
47. John S. Strong, *The Legend of King Aśoka: A Study and Translation of the Aśokāvadāna* (Princeton: Princeton University Press, 1983, 1989), pp. 274–275.
48. Liz Wilson persuasively argues "that the objectification of women for the edification of men is truly a pan-Buddhist theme." See *Charming Cadavers,* p. 4.
49. Serinity Young, "Tantra," *EOW,* vol. 2, pp. 957–958, and Campbell, *Traveller in Space,* passim.
50. Keith Dowman, *Sky Dancer: The Secret Life of the Lady Yeshe Tsogyel* (London: Routledge and Kegan Paul, 1984).

51. Luce Irigaray is one of the most elegant articulators of the male co-optation of women's speech and subjectivity. See, for example, "The Three Genres," in *The Irigaray Reader,* ed. Margaret Whitford (Cambridge, MA: Blackwell Publishers, 1991), pp. 140–153, and *Sexes and Genealogies* (New York: Columbia University Press, 1993), passim. In a Buddhist context, this point is made repeatedly by Wilson, *Charming Cadavers,* passim, and by Campbell, *Traveller in Space,* passim, especially pp. 189–191. See also Campbell's discussion of Irigaray in relation to female identity in Tibetan Buddhism, ibid., passim.
52. On this belief in India, see William Crooke, *The Popular Religion and Folklore of Northern India,* 2nd ed. (1896. Delhi: Munshiram Manoharlal, 1968), vol. I, p. 231.
53. See, for example, *LV,* Vaidya, 148.25–149.2. This imagery is duplicated in the story of Yasa, one of the earliest Buddhist monks. This and similar stories are recounted in Wilson, *Charming Cadavers,* pp. 77–82.
54. Cited by Jonathan Z. Smith, in "Sleep," *The Encyclopedia of Religion,* ed. Mircea Eliade (New York: Macmillan, 1987), pp. 361–364. This article contains many useful comments on the connections among dreams, sleep, and death.
55. See Wilson, *Charming Cadavers,* passim, which is devoted to this topic.
56. *MBh.* 12.248.13–21, etc., cited and translated by Wendy Doniger O'Flaherty, *The Origins of Evil in Hindu Mythology* (Berkeley: University of California, Press, 1976, 1980), p. 228. For more Indian goddesses associated with death, see Mary Storm, "Death," in Young, *Encyclopedia of Women and World Religion,* vol. I, pp. 243–244.
57. For example, René de Nebesky-Wojkowitz includes a black woman in his list of dreams foretelling death that he collected in Sikkim in the 1950: *Oracles and Demons of Tibet: The Cult and Iconography of the Tibetan Protective Deities* (1956. Graz, Austria: Akademische Druckü. Verlagsanstalt, 1975), p. 466.
58. See Wilson, *Charming Cadavers,* passim, for the negative configuring of this imagery in early Buddhism.
59. Bennett, *Dangerous Wives,* pp. 261–308, makes this point in relation to male worship and propitiation of fierce female deities in Nepal.
60. See, for example, Françoise Pommaret's discussion of the Tibetan *'dos log,* mostly female mediums who travel to hell, talk to the deceased, and return with messages, "Returning from Hell," in Donald S. Lopez, Jr., ed., *Religions of Tibet in Practice* (Princeton, NJ: Princeton University Press, 1997), pp. 499–510. For more general comments on women and death in world religion, see Storm, "Death," and Gail Holst-Warhoff, "Mourning and Death Rituals," both in Young, *EOW,* respectively vol. I, pp. 243–244, and vol. II, pp. 682–685.
61. Cited by James H. Sanford, "The Abominable Tachikawa Skull Ritual," *Monumenta Nipponica,* vol. 46, no. 1 (spring 1991): 14. See passim for the conflation of women and death in this ritual.
62. There is a brief discussion of these ideas within the context of world religions in Young, *An Anthology of Sacred Texts,* pp. xx-xxi.
63. See Wendy Doniger O'Flaherty, *Women, Androgynes and Other Mythical Beasts* (Chicago: University of Chicago Press, 1980), for her discussion of the connections between women and death, passim, and the ambiguities of women's milk, pp. 53–55.

References

Primary Sources

Abhiniṣramaṇasūtra. Trans. by Samuel Beal from the Chinese version as *The Romantic Legend of śākya Buddha* (1875. Delhi: Motilal Banarsidass, 1985).

Aris, Anthony, ed. *Tibetan Medical Paintings: Illustrations to the Blue Beryl Treatise of Sangye Gyamtso (1653–1705),* 2 vols. (New York: Harry N. Abrams, 1992).

Aśvaghoṣa. *Buddhacarita,* ed. and trans. E. H. Johnston (1936. Delhi: Motilal Banarsidass, 1984).
Buston. *The History of Buddhism in India and Tibet,* trans. E. Obermiller (1932. Delhi: Sri Satguru Publications, 1986).
Chāndogya Upaniṣad, in *One Hundred and Twelve Upaniṣads and Their Philosophy,* ed. A. N. Bhattacharya. Parimal Sanskrit Series, no. 26 (Delhi: Parmial Publications, 1987).
Dowman, Keith. *Sky Dancer: The Secret Life of the Lady Yeshe Tsogyel* (London: Routledge and Kegan Paul, 1984).
Evans-Wentz, W. Y., ed. *The Tibetan Book of the Great Liberation* (New York: Oxford University Press, 1954, 1968).
The Gilgit Manuscript of the Saṅghabhedvastu, Being the 17th and Last Section of the Vinaya of the Mūlasarvāstivādin, ed. Raniero Gnoli (Rome: Istituto Italiano per il Medio, ed Estremo Oriente, 1977).
rGyud bŹi. A reproduction of a set of prints from the eighteenth-century Zun-cu ze blocks, from the collections of Dr. Raghu Vira, by O-rgyan Namgyal (Leh: S. W. Tashigangpa, 1975).
Jacobi, Hermann, trans. *Jaina Sutras,* 2 vols. (1884, 1895. New York: Dover Publications, 1968).
'Jam mgon chos kyi rgyal po tsong kha pa chen po'i rnam thar thub ba stan mdses po'i rgyan gi cag ngo mtshar nor lu'i 'phreng ba shes sbya ba bshugs so (Sarnath, Varanasi: Mongolian Lama Guru Deva, 1967).
Lalitavistara, ed. P. L. Vaidya (Darbhanga: Mithila Institute, 1958).
Lalitavistara, translated as *The Voice of the Buddha: The Beauty of Compassion* by Gwendolyn Bays (Oakland: Dharma Press, 1983).
Le Mahāvastu, ed. É. Senart (Paris: A L'imprimerie Nationale, 1890).
Le Mahāvastu, translated as *Mahāvastu* by J. J. Jones, 3 vols. (London: Pali Text Society, 1949–1956).
Mūlasarvāstivādavinayavastu, ed. S. Bagchi (Darbhanga: Mithila Institute of Post-Graduate Studies and Research in Sanskrit Learning, 1967).
Nidāna-Kathā, in *The Jātaka Together with its Commentary,* ed. V. Fausböll (London: Trübner and Co., 1877).
Nidāna-Kathā, translated as *Buddhist Birth Stories* by T. W. Rhys Davids (1880. New York: E. P. Dutton and Co., 1925).
Padma bka' thang shel brag ma (Leh, India: 1968).
Sāmavidhāna Brāhmana, ed. A. C. Burnell (London: Trübner and Co., 1873).
Sangye Gyatso. *Bai ḍūr Sṅon po,* ed. T. Y. Tashigangpa (Leh, India: 1973).
Somadeva Bhaṭṭa. *Kathāsaritsāgara,* ed. Pt. Jagadīśa Lāl Śāstrī (Delhi: Motilal Banarsidass, 1960), book 12, chapter 5. Trans. C. H. Tawney as *The Ocean of Story* (London: Chas. J. Sawyer, Ltd., 1924).
Strong, John S. *The Legend of King Aśoka: A Study and Translation of the Aśokāvadāna* (Princeton: Princeton University Press, 1983, 1989).
Tanjur. *Rgyud 'grel: The Corpus of Indian Commentaries on Vajrayana Buddhist Literature Translated into Tibetan* (Delhi: Delhi Karmapae Chodhey, Gyalwae Sungrab Partun Khang, 1982–1985).
Thurman, Robert A. F. *The Life and Teachings of Tsong Khapa* (Dharamsala: Library of Tibetan Works and Archives, 1982).

Secondary Sources

Babu, D. Sridhara. "Reflections on Andra Buddhist Sculptures and Buddha Biography," in *Buddhist Iconography* (Delhi: Tibet House, 1989), pp. 97–101.
Bennett, Lynn. *Dangerous Wives and Sacred Sisters: Social and Symbolic Roles of High-Caste Women in Nepal* (New York: Columbia University Press, 1983).
Bulkeley, Kelly. *The Wilderness of Dreams* (Albany: State University of New York Press, 1994).
Campbell, June. *Traveller in Space: In Search of Female Identity in Tibetan Buddhism* (New York: George Braziller, 1996).

Courtright, Paul B. *Gaṇeśa: Lord of Obstacles, Lord of Reason* (New York: Oxford University Press, 1985).

Crooke, William. *The Popular Religion and Folklore of Northern India,* second. ed. (1896. Delhi: Munshiram Manoharlal, 1968).

Diemberger, Hildegard. "Lhakama (*lha-bka'-ma*) and Khandroma (*mkha'-'gro-ma*): The Sacred Ladies of Beyul Khenbalung (*sbas-yul mKan-pa-lung*)," in Ernst Steinkellner, ed. *Tibetan History and Language: Studies Dedicated to Uray Géza on his Seventieth Birthday* (Wien: Arbeitskreis für Tibetische und Buddhistische Studien, Universität Wien, 1991).

Dodds, E. R., *The Greeks and the Irrational* (Berkeley: University of California Press, 1951, 1973).

Eichenbaum, Patricia D. *The Development of a Narrative Cycle Based on the Life of the Buddha in India, Central Asia, and the Far East: Literary and Pictorial Evidence* (Ann Arbor: University Microfilm International, 1980).

Eliade, Mircea. *Shamanism: Archaic Techniques of Ecstasy,* trans. Willard R. Trask (1951. Princeton: Princeton University Press, 1972).

Gold, Ann. "Gender and Illusion in a Rajasthani Yogic Tradition," in *Gender, Genre and Power in South Asian Expressive Traditions* (Philadelphia: University of Pennsylvania Press, 1991), pp. 102–135.

Gross, Rita. "Methodological Remarks on the Study of Women in Religions: Review, Criticism and Redefinition," in J. Plaskow and J. N. Romero, eds., *Women and Religion* (Missoula: Scholars Press, 1974).

von Grunebaum, G. E., and Caillois, Robert, eds. *The Dream and Human Societies* (Berkeley: University of California Press, 1966).

Gupta, S. K. *The Elephant in Indian Art and Mythology* (New Delhi: Abhinav Publications, 1983).

Gyatso, Janet "Down with the Demoness," in Janice D. Willis, *Feminine Ground: Essays on Women and Tibet* (Ithacan NY: Snow Lion, 1989), pp. 35–51.

Holst-Warhoff, Gail. "Mourning and Death Rituals," in Young, *EOW,* vol. II, pp. 682–685.

Huntington, John C., "Pilgrimage as Image: The Cult of the Aṣṭamahāprātihārya, Part I," in *Orientations* vol. 18, no. 4 (April 1987): 55–63.

Irigaray, Luce. *Sexes and Genealogies,* (New York: Columbia University Press, 1993).

———. "The Three Genres," in *The Irigaray Reader,* ed. Margaret Whitford (Cambridge, MA: Blackwell Publishers, 1991), pp. 140–153.

Irwin, Lee. *The Dream Seekers: Native American Visionary Traditions of the Great Plains* (Norman: University of Oklahoma Press, 1994).

Jones, Ernest. *On the Nightmare* (New York: Liveright Publishing Corp., 1951, 1971).

Kagan, Richard L. *Lucrecia's Dreams: Politics and Prophecy in Sixteenth-Century Spain* (Berkeley: University of California Press, 1990, 1995).

Karetzky, Patricia Eichenbaum. *The Life of the Buddha: Ancient Scriptural and Pictorial Traditions* (Lanham, MD: University Press of America, 1992).

Katz, Nathan. "Anima and mKha'-'gro-ma: A Critical Comparative Study of Jung and Tibetan Buddhism," *Tibet Journal* vol. 2, no. 3 (1977): 13–43.

Khandalavala, Karl. "Heralds in Stone: Early Buddhist Iconography in the Aśokan Pillars and Related Problems," in *Buddhist Iconography* (Delhi: Tibet House, 1989), pp. 19–41.

Lanman, Charles Rockwell. *A Sanskrit Reader* (Cambridge, MA: Harvard University Press, 1884).

Lincoln, Jackson Steward. *The Dream in Primitive Cultures* (1935. New York: Johnson reprint corporation, 1970).

Lorzen, David N., *The Kāpālikas and Kālāmukhas: Two Lost Saivite Sects,* second ed. (1972. Delhi: Motilal Banarsidass, 1991).

Lüders, H., ed. *Bhārhut Inscriptions,* rev. by E. Waldschmidt and M. A. Mehendale (Ootacamund: Govenment Epigraphist for India, 1963).

Macdonell, Arthur A. *A History of Sanskrit Literature* (1899. Delhi: Motilal Banarsidass, 1971).

Miller, Patricia Cox. *Dreams in Late Antiquity: Studies in the Imagination of a Culture* (Princeton: Princeton University Press, 1994).

Nebesky-Wojkowitz, René de. *Oracles and Demons of Tibet: The Cult and Iconography of the Tibetan Protective Deities* (1956. Graz, Austria: Akademische Druckü Verlagsanstalt, 1975).

O'Flaherty, Wendy Doniger, *The Origins of Evil in Hindu Mythology* (Berkeley: University of California Press, 1976, 1980).

———. *Women, Androgynes and Other Mythical Beasts* (Chicago: University of Chicago Press, 1980).

Pommaret, Françoise. "Returning from Hell," in Donald S. Lopez, Jr., ed., *Religions of Tibet in Practice* (Princeton: Princeton University Press, 1997), pp. 499–510.

Rahula, Telwatte. *A Critical Study of the Mahāvastu* (Delhi: Motilal Banarsidass, 1978).

Rank, Otto. "The Myth of the Birth of the Hero," reprinted in Robert A. Segal, *In Quest of the Hero* (Princeton: Princeton University Press, 1990), pp. 3–86.

Rockhill, W. W. *The Life of the Buddha* (Varanasi: Orientalia Indica, 1972).

Rupprecht, Carol Schreier. "Sex, Gender and Dreams: From Polarity to Plurality" in Kelly Bulkeley, ed., *Among All These Dreamers: Essays on Dreaming and Modern Society* (Albany: State University Press of New York, 1996).

———. "Women's Dreams: Mind and Body," in Estella Lauter and Carol Schreier Rupprecht, eds., *Feminist Archetypal Theory: Interdisciplinary Re-Visions of Jungian Thought* (Knoxville: University of Tennessee Press, 1985).

Sanford, James H. "The Abominable Tachikawa Skull Ritual," *Monumenta Nipponica* vol. 46, no. 1 (spring, 1991): 1–20.

Schumann, H. W. *The Historical Buddha,* trans. M. O'C. Walshe (1982. London: Penguin Group, 1989).

Schlingloff, Dieter. *Studies in the Ajanta Painting: Identifications and Interpretations* (Delhi: Ajanta Publications [India]: 1987).

Sharma, Jagdish. "Symbolism in the Jinist Dream-World," in Sharma, Jagdish and Siegel, Lee, *Dream-Symbolism in The Śrāmaṇṇic Tradition: Two Psychoanalytical Studies in Jinist and Buddhist Dream Legends* (Calcutta: Firma KLM Private Limited, 1980).

Shastri, Biswanarayan. "The Philosophical Concepts and the Buddhist Pantheon," in *Buddhist Iconography,* pp. 52–59.

Shulman, David, and Strouman, Guy G., eds. *Dream Cultures: Explorations in the Comparative History of Dreaming* (Oxford: Oxford University Press, 1999).

Smith, Jonathan Z., "Sleep," in *The Encyclopedia of Religion,* vol. 13. Mircea Eliade, ed. (New York: Macmillan Publishing Company, 1987), pp. 361–364.

Storm, Mary. "Death," in Young, *EOW,* vol. I, pp. 243–244.

Tedlock, Barbara, ed. *Dreaming: Anthropological and Psychological Interpretations* (Cambridge: Cambridge University Press, 1987).

Trachtenberg, Joshua. *Jewish Magic and Superstition: A Study in Folk Religion* (1939. New York: Atheneum, n.d.).

Urubshurow, Victoria. "Dakinis," in Young, *EOW,* vol. I, pp. 231–232.

Wilson, Liz. *Charming Cadavers: Horrific Figurations of the Feminine in Indian Buddhist Hagiographic Literature* (Chicago: University of Chicago Press, 1996).

Winternitz, Maurice. *A History of Indian Literature,* 3 vols. (1927. Delhi: Oriental books reprint corporation, 1977).

Young, Serinity. *An Anthology of Sacred Texts By and About Women* (New York: Crossroad, 1993).

———. *Dreaming in the Lotus: Buddhist Dream Narrative, Imagery and Practice* (Boston: Wisdom Publications, 1999).

———. "Dreams," in *The Encyclopedia of Women and World Religion,* Serinity Young, ed. (New York: Macmillan, 1998), vol. I, pp. 271–273.

———. "Tantra," *EOW,* vol. II, pp. 956–959.

Zimmer, Heinrich. *Myths and Symbols in Indian Art and Civilization,* ed. Joseph Campbell (1946. New York: Harper and Brothers, 1962).

2

Through the Looking Glass
Dreams in Ancient Egypt

Kasia Szpakowska

The image of Egyptian magicians, dream interpreters, incubation temples, and the dreams of pharaohs have become so much a part of popular Western culture that it may come as a surprise to learn that, until quite recently, there has been no comprehensive treatment of ancient Egyptian dreams.[1] This chapter presents a summary of that research and offers a historically based model for studying the dreams of a long-lasting culture with no living witnesses.

The first scholar to explore the topic of dreams in ancient Egypt was Aksel Volten,[2] who focused his attentions on publishing a demotic dream book dating to the Greco-Roman period. Although Volten mentions a few other earlier texts, his primary concern was to explore the issue of dream interpretation. In 1956 A. Leo Oppenheim[3] widened the scope of research on dreams and their interpretation to include the entire ancient Near East. As an Assyriologist, his source materials were largely Akkadian and Sumerian texts, and indeed the work was originally planned as a publication of the "Assyrian Dream Book." He expanded his coverage, however, to encompass a wider variety of dream reports, including a selection of Egyptian texts. His subsequent analysis has become a crucial study of dreams in the ancient Near East, and his division of dreams into a typology of message dreams, symbolic dreams, and mantic dreams suggests one useful method of approaching this topic.

Nevertheless, while Oppenheim's treatment of dreams in ancient Egypt is valuable, it remains limited in two ways. First, he failed to sufficiently distinguish the native Egyptian texts from non-Egyptian documentation or to take into account the time period and cultural context of texts. For example, he included a discussion of "The Famine Stela," a text purportedly describing the dream of King Djoser (ca. 2630–2611 B.C.) but which was actually written during the Greek period, possibly under the reign of Ptolemy V (205–180 B.C.). Although this stela is written in the Egyptian language, the content reflects the Hellenistic understanding and the format of dreams differs dramatically from that of Egypt twenty-five centuries earlier. Second, his examples from Egypt included only those that were well known at the time, namely the dream books and royal message dreams in which a deity revealed himself to pharaoh.

A few years later Serge Sauneron[4] published his seminal summary that until now has remained the main resource for information on dreams in ancient Egypt. He added a new dimension to the study of dreams from the ancient world by exploring the emotional response of the dreamer and by differentiating between dreams that arose spontaneously and those that were invoked. His analyses, however, were quite brief, and since the publication of his study in 1959, a number of important new texts have been discovered, necessitating a re-examination of all the material. More recently, John Ray[5] added to our knowledge of Hellenistic dream interpretation and incubation techniques by publishing the archive of Hor of Sebennytos.

The work of these scholars provides a firm foundation on which to ground new inquiries and inspired me to undertake the first comprehensive investigation into the function and role of dreams in pharaonic Egypt. This investigation looked at issues not previously considered by scholars, such as nightmares and the nondivinatory role of dreams, in addition to the more familiar mantic and royal dreams. My approach was to try to capture the Egyptians' own perceptions of dreams, as revealed not only through texts that were composed specifically to be read by the public but also by private scraps of letters, songs, musings, and even medical documents. While previous research had focused on the role of dreams in Greco-Roman Egypt or in terms of non-Egyptian documentation, I focused strictly on the ancient Egyptian sources against the backdrop of Egyptian history, from the earliest extant references to dreams (ca. 2150 B.C.) up to Egypt's Late Period (approximately 664 B.C.). At this point in time, the references to dreams changed dramatically in tone, function, and form of expression, and likely reflect beliefs and attitudes originating from external sources. From this historical perspective, I was able to perceive the underlying patterns affecting the attitude toward and reception of dreams over time. A timeline is included at the end of the chapter to help illustrate where these trends occurred within the context of Egyptian history and religion.

Still today, when many people discuss dreams in ancient Egypt they refer to Joseph's dream interpretation mentioned in Genesis 41:1–36 or of dream incubation[6] as practiced in the temples during the Greco-Roman period. Indeed, in its later years ancient Egypt acquired quite a reputation for its interest in dreams, suggesting a long tradition in the study of dreams. But if we look at the internal Egyptian evidence prior to the Hellenistic period a rather different picture emerges. The ancient Egyptian civilization lasted for approximately 3,500 years—a singularly long span of time. It is probable that a culture would undergo serious and quantifiable changes over the centuries, and these changes could manifest themselves in a variety of ways. Although the Egyptian culture was remarkably static through the many centuries, it was not stagnant. Change was inevitable, and whether shaped by internal or by external circumstances, these fluxes are imprinted in the shifting conceptions of and attitudes toward dreams in ancient Egypt. Because the evidence for these dreams is based on written reports, they were strictly bound by the literary decorum of the time and only document the dreams of those individuals who either knew how to write themselves or had the means to hire a scribe to record their dreams for them.

From the time of Egypt's unification under one ruler (ca. 3100 B.C.) through the Pyramid Age, which saw the birth of autobiographical inscriptions and religious texts, right up until Egypt's first real political upheaval—the "First Intermediate Period"

(2150–2055 B.C.)—not a single mention of dreams has survived. When a dream finally does make its way into the textual corpus it is of immediate interest, for the terms used to indicate dreams can offer a clue as to how the Egyptians perceived them. The earliest word, and one that is retained even in the Coptic language of present-day Egypt,[7] is *resut,* which means literally "awakening." Egyptian words are usually written as a combination of phonetic signs, plus a sign or "determinative" at the end, indicating the semantic category of the word. Interestingly, *resut* is most often determined by an open eye, which is also used for words related to visual perception (such as "see," "be vigilant"). The other term meaning dream was *qed,* which derived from the word "sleep." When this word meant "sleep," it was followed by the sign of a bed, but when it meant "dream," it used the same open eye sign as *resut.*[8] An Egyptian could also refer to a dream indirectly by saying that someone came and spoke while the person was sleeping, or that he saw or heard something and then woke up.

Also worth noting is the fact that the ancient Egyptians did not have a verb for dreaming, only a noun. In their terminology, one could see something "in a dream" or see "a dream." In other words, a dream was the object of a verb of visual perception—it was something seen, not done. In a sense, it was not an event arising from within the dreamer or an activity performed by an individual; rather, it had an objective existence outside the will of the passive dreamer. In particular, the use of the phrase "seeing in a dream" also indicates that the dream was considered as an alternate state or dimension in which the waking barriers to perception were temporarily withdrawn.

The earliest currently known references to dreams can be found in texts known as "Letters to the Dead."[9] These letters (most dating from the First Intermediate Period) were written to a deceased relative or acquaintance, usually requesting some sort of favor on behalf of the living individual, and then left in the tomb of the addressee. The dream in these texts functioned as a sort of liminal zone, a transparent area between the walls of two worlds that allowed beings in separate spheres to see each other. In one letter, for example, an ailing man begs his late wife to end his pain and asks that he be allowed to watch her doing so, in a dream.[10] Unfortunately, we have no way of knowing if the suffering husband ever did succeed in seeing his wife in a dream. In another letter, the writer refers to unwanted dream visitations from a dead acquaintance.[11] To stop them, he writes a letter to his deceased father urging him to intervene and to forever prevent the other man from watching him in these unwanted dreams. The letter does not provide any details of the content of these dreams other than the appearance of the dead acquaintance, and this is typical of dream references from the Pharaonic period. Rather than describing a dream as a narrative, the Egyptian references mention only a brief image, like a snapshot into another world. These particular examples treat the dream as a transparent liminal zone, with two-way windows allowing the living to see the dead and the dead to watch the living. More specifically, the dreams allow people on earth to communicate with the inhabitants of the Netherworld.

The Egyptian Netherworld was inhabited by the dead and by the gods, but the gods would not appear in dreams until centuries later. The letters above refer to nonroyal individuals having visual communication with the dead. Approximately 500 years after the writing of these letters, in the time span known as the Second Intermediate Period (1780–1570 B.C.) Egypt was once again torn apart by political upheaval, this time instigated by the rulership of foreigners on Egyptian soil. Due to a lack of physical remains, little is known from this time, but the subsequent reunification of Egypt ushered in a period of unparalleled wealth and power, countered by complex international relations with the other growing superpowers of the ancient Near East. In this period known as the New Kingdom (1570–1069 B.C.) Egyptians experienced fundamental changes in their worldview, and these are reflected in their perception of dreams. The written record indicates that dreams acquired both an increased importance and a variety of new functions.

The New Kingdom pharaohs introduced dreams into their royal biographies as a means of access not to the dead but to the gods. This use coincided with the increased use of oracles both on the royal level, where they were used to legitimate the pharaoh's divine destiny, and among lower levels of society, where the belief in predestination played an increasingly important role in an individual's daily life. The use of dreams was still limited, for only three royal dreams were reported, which progressively increased in intimacy and complexity over time. In one dream, the god Amun came before the pharaoh Amunhotep II (Dynasty 18) during a battle and gave him confidence.[12] Later, the nineteenth-dynasty pharaoh Merneptah saw the god Ptah, who told the king to take a sword and promised to banish his fear in the upcoming battle.[13] Interestingly, although both of these dreams involved divine manifestations during battle, they did not play a role in either king's victory—according to the texts, neither king was in danger of losing the battle prior to the dream, and both triumphed as expected.

The third example is the well-known dream of Thutmosis IV, who fell asleep at the foot of the sphinx and discovered the sun god Ra-Harakhty speaking to him in a dream.[14] The god complains that his monument (the sphinx) has been neglected and promises Thutmosis that if he cleans it, he will be crowned king. Note that this dream was recorded well after the crowning of Thutmosis as king. The Egyptians did not use dreams to choose a king, nor did kings seek dreams to help them make decisions. Rather, the function of these dreams seemed to affirm and stress the exclusive relationship between the king and the gods. At this time, the pharaohs wanted to make it clear that the gods communicated directly only with them, within the private milieu of dreams. These dream reports occurred not in the context of religious works or myths but were included in texts that were meant to represent a reality situated in the concrete world.[15]

While the Egyptian royal dreams have been characterized as typical of message dreams in the ancient Near East,[16] such a description obscures the fact that these dreams were not typical of the Egyptian literary tradition until the New Kingdom, when they make their first, rare appearance.[17] With the exception of the dream of Tanutamani (see below), the other dreams usually cited as examples of Egyptian royal dreams are Late Period and Hellenistic pseudepigraphic descriptions attributed to earlier pharaohs, which bear little resemblance to the dream anecdotes recorded centuries earlier.[18]

By the end of the New Kingdom, the importance of dreams as a venue for divine communication had increased not only for the pharaoh but for nonroyal individuals as well. This becomes apparent in two hymns that describe direct contact between upper-class men and a deity in a dream. In the *Biography of Ipwy,* the dreamer described his dream as follows:[19]

> It was on the day that I saw her beauty,
> my mind was spending the day in festival thereof,
> that I beheld the Lady of the Two Lands in a dream
> and she placed joy in my heart.
> Then I was revitalized with her food . . .

The deity referred to in this text was Hathor, a popular goddess of love, beauty, dance, and joy. Another text describes how the same goddess actually spoke directly to another Egyptian, Djehutiemhab.[20] He recorded this momentous occurrence for posterity within his tomb, as a verse in a hymn to Hathor:

> You are the one who has spoken to me yourself, with your own mouth:
> "I am the beautiful Hely,[21]
> my shape being that of Mut.
> I have come in order to instruct you:
> See your place—fill yourself with it,
> without travelling north,
> without travelling south."
> while I was in a dream,
> while the earth was in silence,
> in the deep of the night.

Whereas a few centuries earlier the recording of divine dreams was restricted to the pharaoh, these spontaneous dreams could now be included in texts as an apparently sanctioned venue for communication between the divine world and the world of the nonroyal elite. In pharaonic Egypt, at least until the Late Period, it is no coincidence that the only dreams having enough impact to merit being written down were those involving inhabitants of the Netherworld—the dead and the gods.[22] The divine dreams in particular were deemed important enough to record in detail, for they established the dreamer as a member of an exclusive club—as one who had been in direct contact with the gods. The reality of these dreams was taken for granted and the genuineness of the experience in the eyes of the dreamers was substantiated by the fact that they did not require interpretation to be understood.

The only evidence of dream interpretation at this time comes in the form of a single dream book, discovered in a cache of documents in Der el-Medineh.[23] Reconstructed and published by Gardiner in 1935,[24] this compilation is contained on *P. Chester Beatty* III, recto 1–11 and, like the preceding Hathor hymns, probably dates to the reign of Ramesses II.[25] As it is currently the only oneiromantic manual that has been found in pre-Hellenic Egypt, it is worth examining in detail. This papyrus outlines a total of 227 dreams and their interpretations and is divided into three sections. The first is comprised of the visual images of dreams and their interpretation; the second is a spell to counter a bad dream; and the third begins with a detailed description of the physical and behavioral characteristics of men who are called "followers of Seth,"[26] followed again by their dreams and interpretations. This division of dreams into at least two distinct psychological types of men who apparently saw different dreams and required separate interpretations is intriguing. Unfortunately, the latter portion of the text is broken and only four of the dreams of the followers of Seth remain. The beginning of the text is also missing, leaving us without any description of the counterpart of the "Sethian" man, and we remain uninformed as to what his temperament would have been or whether more categories are missing.

Each dream and interpretation is composed of the initial premise "If a man sees himself in a dream," written in a vertical column, followed by horizontal lists of dream images, an evaluation of the dream as "good" or "bad," and finally an interpretation. Both the image seen and the interpretation of each of the dream passages refer to events or images that were within the realm of possibility in the Egyptian worldview.

The relationship between a visual image and its interpretation in this dream book was largely based on linguistic and cultural associations, reminiscent of the patterns and categorizations that Bert O. States suggests dreams follow.[27] The use of wordplay, including puns, assonance, paranomasia, metonymy, and metaphors, abounds in the dream book.[28] One example would be "If a man sees himself in a dream consuming the flesh of a donkey (*'at*); good, it means that he will become great (*s'at*)."[29] The wordplay in this example consists of assonance between the words *'at* and *s'at*. One of the most intricate is "If a man sees himself in a dream sailing (*faj-tchaw*) downstream (*khed*); bad, it means a life of running backward."[30] The pun stems from the combination of *faj-tchaw* "carrying the wind" (in other words "sailing"), which is the normal way of travelling upstream on the Nile (the winds flow north to south in Egypt) and *khed,* which means traveling downstream (south to north) with the flow of the Nile. The mental image of a boat using sails to go downstream would have been disturbing and thus would have provoked an interpretation of a life going the wrong way as well.

The dream book contains other common divinatory schemes, such as symbolism (i.e., the use of symbols familiar to an Egyptian of that time) and the pairing of similars or of opposites, as in "If a man sees himself in a dream seeing himself dead; good, it means a long life is before him."[31] Other relationships seem to be based on myths, satires, or proverbs. For example: "If a man sees himself in a dream consuming the flesh of a crocodile; good, it means consuming the possessions of an official."[32] There is a play here on the greediness of officials and the greediness of crocodiles to which officials are often compared. Some of the dreams might seem familiar to a modern reader: "If a man sees himself in a dream and his teeth are falling out under him; bad, it means that one of his underlings will die."[33] Others remain obscure: "If a man sees himself in a dream guarding monkeys; bad, it means that change is ahead of him."[34]

Although these dream images may not offer any insights into the psychology of an individual Egyptian, they certainly reveal the cares, wishes, and concerns of the specific segment of the population for which they were intended. (The inhabitants of this village were rather well off and literate—not necessarily representative of the majority of Egyptians.) It appears that nourishment, wealth, prestige, and the impact of the divine world were of greatest concern to the villagers, while emotions and recreational activities were much less important.

This dream book has received much attention, but it should be noted that it is currently the only evidence for dream interpretation until the end of the Nubian dynasty (650 years later) and that there is no evidence that specialists in dream interpretation existed in the New Kingdom. Even this dream book is suspect, for it is not clear that it was ever actually used. It is possible that it was kept as a curiosity or as a literary exercise and did not necessarily require a specialist to be used. For nearly the first 2,000 years of Egypt's history, there is no extant evidence for the mantic use of dreams nor for rituals designed to solicit dreams.[35]

While the divine dreams were invariably described as positive, dreams in general were far more often described in a negative light. Dreams appear in the earliest teaching texts, written ca. 2100 B.C. Their authors recognized that dreams could be used as metaphors to accentuate that which is insubstantial, ephemeral, or uncontrollable. In one set of teachings, the author warned the reader against abusing friendship by approaching the women of the friend's household. The negative repercussions of even a brief moment of such improper behavior were considered serious, and the author warned that "a split second, the likeness of a dream, and death is reached on account of knowing her."[36] Here the more negative aspects of a dream as an unsettling, insubstantial, and untrustworthy phenomenon inspires its use as an analogy for improper behavior. The distinct temporal distortion of a dream made it an ideal metaphor for the ephemeral nature of earthly life and led to the earliest-known attestation of the now-popular phrase: "Life is but a dream."[37]

The dream made an important appearance in the fictional "Tale of Sinuhe," a popular tale of the adventures of a man who fled Egypt upon hearing of the untimely death of the pharaoh.[38] Sinuhe attempted to explain his unjustified flight by claiming that "I don't know what separated me from my place. It was like the unfolding of a dream—like a man from the Delta seeing himself in Elephantine, a man of the marshlands in Nubia." The dream was used to emphasize and excuse the irrationality of the hero's behavior and the dreamer was portrayed as a passive viewer of a scenario that unfolds before him and over which he had no control.

As these examples show, dreams were not necessarily viewed as positive experiences. Medical texts include several prophylactic spells designed to resist bad dreams. Similarly dreams appeared as undesirable, even hostile forces to be guarded against and repelled in the so-called execration texts.[39] These lists of menacing people and forces were written on bowls or figures that would be smashed or buried, thus rendering them harmless. In these texts, the dreams were classified with hostile speech, plots, and other militant acts and were treated somewhat as potential weapons of war.

The textual evidence consistently reveals certain characteristics of the ancient Egyptian perception of nightmares. The descriptions, even though they are inexplicit and vague, seem to match the symptoms of what are currently called common anxiety dreams or nightmares rather than the more troubling and rare phenomenon "night terrors" or *pavor nocturnus.*[40] The typical elements of ancient nightmares consisted of "bad things," "red/buried things," and a desperate feeling of terror. The cause of nightmares was not ascribed to any particular demon, but rather to the hosts of hostile dead and other denizens of the Netherworld. These entities were blamed for a variety of ailments and conditions, and spells could be used both prophylactically and as a remedy to combat them. In one of these spells, the dreamer is urged not to reveal the content of the nightmare but to let the physician drive out the "bad things" that caused the nightmare and then to rub his face with a poultice of bread and herbs which have been marinated in beer and myrrh. These prescriptions are generally difficult to distinguish from other medical spells, and the Egyptians themselves did not feel the need for a distinction. The need to protect the vulnerable sleeper from nightmares is reflected in the fashioning of bedposts, headboards, and headrests decorated with apotropaic spells and/or protective genies. The spells often referred to fire-spitting cobras who, along with other types of genies, could be depicted exhaling flames. Fire was a particularly effective weapon, for it not only brightened the night but it destroyed the chaotic enemies of order.

Egypt, unlike its Mesopotamian neighbors, never incorporated dreams into myths nor a god of dreams into its pantheon, neither as a deity personally responsible for the nocturnal antics of his minions nor as a specific protective deity responsible for protecting the sleeper from nightmares. By the Greek period, a god known as Bes had acquired a reputation for facilitating good dreams,[41] but, during the time in question, the representation of that deity was used purely as a weapon-wielding genie to ward off bad dreams.

At the end of the New Kingdom, Egypt was once again divided with several rulers simultaneously claiming sovereignty. Sometime in the early years of the Third Intermediate Period, a series of texts now called "Oracular Amuletic Decrees" came into vogue.[42] Mass-produced and designed to be worn as amulets, these hollow cylinders contained a decree by a deity or deities promising to keep the bearer safe from a list of specified dangers, including dreams. One typical example reads: "We will make all dreams which she has seen, good ones. We will make all dreams which she will see good ones. We will make all dreams which any man, any woman, any people of any kind in the entire land saw for her, good ones." Another amuletic text reveals that the deities "cause his dreams to be good. We will drive away their bad intent which is in them."

This corpus unveils a series of properties of dreams as they were comprehended in the Third Intermediate Period: they could be seen by both men and women; they were qualified as having been seen in the past and the future; deities had the ability to change the nature of dreams already seen and as yet unseen; others could see or be caused to see dreams for an individual; and dreams could have an intent. These texts also reflect the marked change that occurred in the worldview of the ancient Egyptian culture during the transitional Third Intermediate Period. From this time on, deities played an expanding role in the daily life of Egyptians, apparently even to the point of determining the quality of their dreams.

The twenty-fifth dynasty of Nubian kings ushered in the Late Period, a span of time when Egypt struggled and failed to maintain its independence against a rising Assyrian empire. The last pharaoh of the twenty-fifth dynasty, Tanutamani, introduced yet another element of dreams into the royal discourse—the symbolic dream.[43] In this dream, the pharaoh saw two snakes, one on either side of him. The dream was interpreted for him as representing Upper and Lower Egypt, over which the pharaoh had total dominion. But while this dream has been often discussed, sometimes even in comparison with the symbolic dream of the pharaoh in Genesis, the dream of Tanutamani remains the only instance of a royal symbolic dream found in the Egyptian sources.

It is clear that a dramatic change occurred in the Late Period treatment of dreams in Egypt. From this time on, solicited oracles and spontaneous wondrous signs (including dreams) were woven into the fabric of Egyptian society.[44] In the Late Period, a series of foreign powers, including Assyria and Persia, were able to conquer and rule Egypt. New ideas and divinatory practices entered the mainstream of Egyptian society through the process of diffusion. A general feeling of insecurity among Egyptians led to a demand for increased divine guidance in many forms, including oracular dreams. As these once-autonomous mechanisms for divine discourse gradually became institutionalized, the power structure shifted in favor of those who controlled the mechanisms. By the time of the Libyan dynasty, the oracle was required to legitimize the rule of the pharaoh, thus guaranteeing that the real power rested with those who physically manipulated the oracle—the priesthood of Amun.[45] In a similar fashion, the divine message dream of pharaoh, the meaning of which was immediately comprehensible to the dreamer, was replaced by the first occurrence of a symbolic dream—a dream whose meaning was enigmatic and required a third party for interpretation. Although the interpreter was not specified in this instance, it is likely to have been a priest of Amun, at whose instigation the pharaoh[46] attributed the source of the dream as Amun-Ra. During the Late Period, dreams as phenomena requiring interpretation by an outside agency became standard and dream solicitation and interpretation became officially sanctioned and institutionalized in specific sanctuaries.[47] With the loss of Egypt's independence to the Persians, the textual references to dreams in the Late Period increased, and from the Ptolemaic period Egypt was renowned for its dream interpreters and incubation temples.

In contrast to some of Egypt's contemporary Near Eastern neighbors in the third to second millennia, there is an obvious lack of attested dream narratives, journeys, or epics and a distinct indifference toward the ritual use of dreams for divination or incubation. In contrast, dreams were seen as ideal metaphors and literary devices from the dawning of the art of *belle-lettres* and were recognized as a unique plane of reality between the world of the living and the Netherworld. The dark sides of dreams were also acknowledged and feared, with apotropaic spells, rituals, and talismans designed to repulse nightmare-causing demons and other terrors in the night.

It is unlikely that psychology can offer any sort of unified theory applicable to the study of dreams in the ancient world without taking into account the cultural and temporal matrix in which these dreams were formed. Psychoanalysis fails in light of the lack of individual background. There are no narrative descriptions of dreams, only short snapshots (i.e., Amenhotep II, "His Majesty rested, and the majesty of the god Amun, Lord of the Thrones of the Two lands, came before His Majesty in a dream, in order to give valor to his son, Aa-Kheperu-Ra, his father Amun being the protection of his body, guarding the ruler").[48] These passages tantalize but fail to reveal the individual personality of the dreamer.

Having a combined literary/psychological approach, such as that used by Bulkeley in analyzing the dreams in the Mesopotamian epic of Gilgamesh, could possibly prove to be more fruitful.[49] It could easily be applied to the Ptolemaic Egyptian dream texts, which provide narratives of dream content in stories and long descriptions that were then interpreted. Unfortunately, these are completely lacking in the earlier Pharaonic Egyptian texts, which for the most part do not describe the dreams in any detail. Used cautiously, however, a literary/psychological approach could also enhance the reading of earlier texts that lack extended dream narratives. For example, in one letter to the dead, a son (Heni) wrote to his dead father, concerning his father's dead servant Seni.[50] Heni writes:

> Pay close attention! It is useful to pay attention to the one who provides for you, on account of these things which your servant Seni does: for causing me, your servant to see him in a dream in the one Sole City with you.
>
> Indeed, it is his own character that drives him away. Indeed, that which happened against him, did not happen by the hand of me, your servant. [Nor] was it an end of all that would happen. Indeed, it is not I who first caused wounds against him. Others acted before I, your servant, [did]. Please, may his lord be protective, and do not allow him to do harm. May he be guarded in order that he may be done with watching me, your servant, forever.

Clearly, this was a troublesome dream for Heni, who expressed guilt and anxiety concerning his relationship with Seni. This type of emotional dream is precisely the type of dream that is often recalled by the dreamer,[51] and it must have been compelling for Heni to go to the expense of putting it in writing. That the dream may have caused Heni some sort of mental anguish is linguistically indicated as well. In the phrase "do not allow him to do harm," the word "harm" is written with a particular determinative,[52] one usually associated with abstract "bad things."[53] This determinative may have been chosen to indicate that the harm being done was not physical but abstract, the kind of emotional stress that could be caused by an unpleasant dream. By combining a psychological analysis with a traditional literary approach, without losing sight of its historical context, it may be possible to gain a deeper insight into an individual text.

Bulkeley has noted that "When people face a crisis that either challenges their spiritual beliefs or reveals those beliefs to be inadequate, powerful dreams often emerge: dreams that respond to the crisis, integrate the painfully conflicting elements in the dreamer's life, and give the dreamer a new energetic sense of spiritual purpose that he or she carries back into the waking world."[54] By examining the recorded dreams within their cultural context it appears that this statement can be applied to Ancient Egyptian individuals as well.[55] It seems that dreams find their way in the textual record at critical junctures in Egyptian history. The unfortunate paucity of material offers little more than a glimpse into the perception of ancient Egyptian dreams, but it is sufficient to show that uses of dreams by individuals can be a looking glass onto the social and historical tensions affecting the society as a whole, even if the dreamers themselves did not believe their dreams to be of great importance.

Modern research focusing on the biological nature of sleep and dreams has questioned the boundaries between waking and dreaming,[56] suggesting a more fluid relationship that might have sounded familiar to an ancient Egyptian. Throughout Egypt's history, a dream was often a frightening phenomenon, arising not from within the individual but from a liminal zone between the living and the dead—a spontaneously generated phenomenon that could be seen but not manipulated or invoked. Its function varied through time, both reflecting societal mores and being influenced and shaped by external contacts. In ancient Egypt, dreams were sometimes terrifying, sometimes awe-inspiring, but always disturbing.

Notes

I would like to thank Kelly Bulkeley for helpful discussions, Angel Gulermovich for her careful reading and editing of drafts, and Shawn Higgins for his help in designing the time charts.

1. K. Szpakowska, *The Perception of Dreams and Nightmares in Ancient Egypt: Old Kingdom to Third Intermediate Period,* Ph.D. diss., University of California, Los Angeles, 2000, *UMI* Microform 9973224. This work is currently being revised for publication and includes an appendix with the author's transcription and translation of all the known texts mentioning dreams, including those cited in this chapter.
2. A. Volten, *Demotische Traumdeutung (Pap. Carlsberg XIII and XIV verso),* (Analecta Aegyptiaca III; Kopenhagen: Einar Munksgaard, 1942).
3. A. L. Oppenheim, *The Interpretation of Dreams in the Ancient Near East* (Transactions of the American Philosophical Society, New Series 46/3; Philadelphia, PA: American Philosophical Society, 1956): 179–355. A new work has recently been published which complements and expands the work on Mesopotamian dreams begun by Oppenheim: S. A. L. Butler, *Mesopotamian Conceptions of Dreams and Dream Rituals* (Alter Orient und Altes Testament 258; Münster: Ugarit-Verlag, 1998).
4. S. Sauneron, "Les songes et leur interpretation dans l'Egypte ancienne," *Sources Orientales* II (Paris, 1959), 18–61.
5. J. D. Ray, *The Archive of Hor* (Texts from Excavations 2; London: The Egypt Exploration Society, 1976).

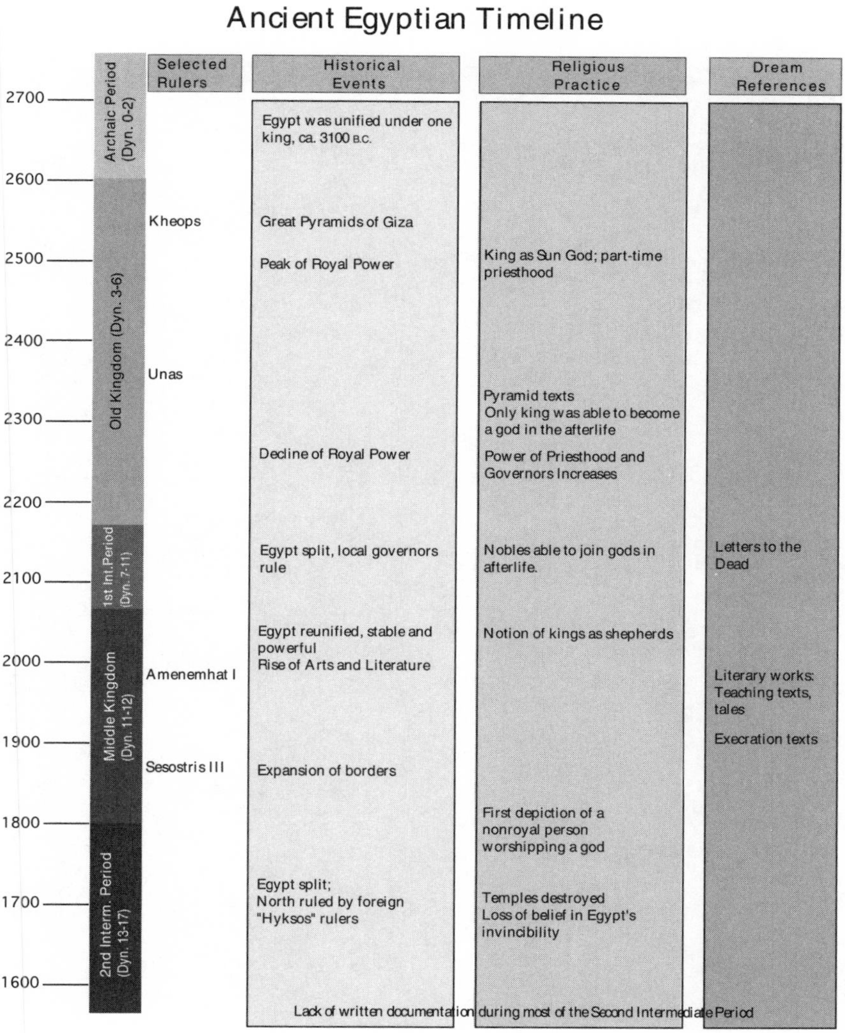

Source: Kasia Szpakowska and Shawn Higgins

6. The practice of sleeping in a temple or another sacred spot in order to solicit a dream is called incubation.
7. Coptic was the language and script used by the Copts (Egyptian Christians) from ca. 300 A.D. The Coptic language uses the ancient Egyptian grammar but is written with Greek letters plus five additional letters from Demotic, an ancient Egyptian script. It continues to be used today as a liturgical language.
8. The word *qed* appeared with the meaning of dream only during a specific time period and in a specific genre of texts.
9. The major publications of these texts are: A. H. Gardiner and K. Sethe, *Egyptian Letters to the Dead: Mainly from the Old and Middle Kingdoms* (London: The Egypt Exploration Society, 1928); A. H. Gardiner, "A New Letter to the Dead," *Journal of Egyptian*

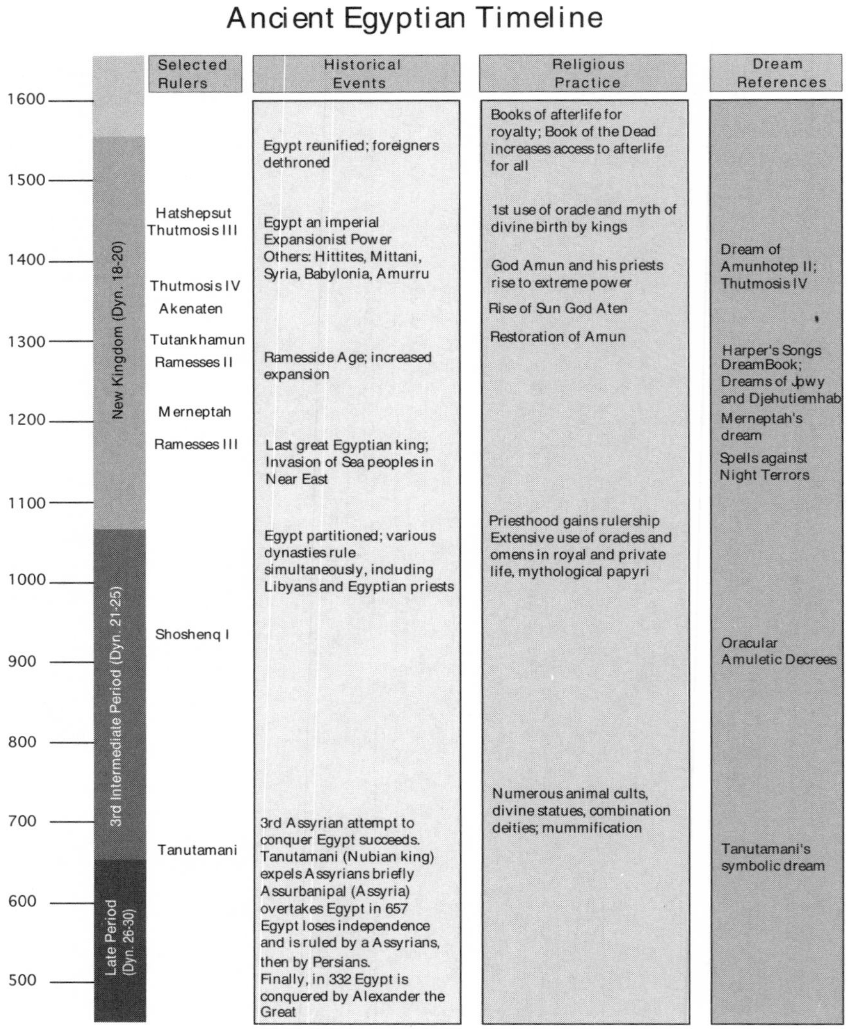

Ancient Egyptian Timeline
Selected Rulers
Historical Events
Religious Practice
Dream References
1600
1500
1400
1300
1200
1100
1000
900
800
700
600
500
New Kingdom (Dyn. 18-20)
3rd Intermediate Period (Dyn. 21-25)
Late Period (Dyn. 26-30)
Hatshepsut
Thutmosis III
Thutmosis IV
Akenaten
Tutankhamun
Ramesses II
Merneptah
Ramesses III
Shoshenq I
Tanutamani
Egypt reunified; foreigners dethroned
Egypt an imperial Expansionist Power Others: Hittites, Mittani, Syria, Babylonia, Amurru
Ramesside Age; increased expansion
Last great Egyptian king; Invasion of Sea peoples in Near East
Egypt partitioned; various dynasties rule simultaneously, including Libyans and Egyptian priests
3rd Assyrian attempt to conquer Egypt succeeds. Tanutamani (Nubian king) expels Assyrians briefly Assurbanipal (Assyria) overtakes Egypt in 657 Egypt loses independence and is ruled by a Assyrians, then by Persians. Finally, in 332 Egypt is conquered by Alexander the Great
Books of afterlife for royalty; Book of the Dead increases access to afterlife for all
1st use of oracle and myth of divine birth by kings
God Amun and his priests rise to extreme power
Rise of Sun God Aten
Restoration of Amun
Priesthood gains rulership Extensive use of oracles and omens in royal and private life, mythological papyri
Numerous animal cults, divine statues, combination deities; mummification
Dream of Amunhotep II; Thutmosis IV
Harper's Songs DreamBook; Dreams of Jpwy and Djehutiemhab
Merneptah's dream
Spells against Night Terrors
Oracular Amuletic Decrees
Tanutamani's symbolic dream

Source: Kasia Szpakowska and Shawn Higgins

Archaeology 16 (1930): 19–22; W. K. Simpson, "The Letter to the Dead from the Tomb of Meru (N 3737) at Nag' ed-Deir," *Journal of Egyptian Archaeology* 52 (1966): 39–50; W. K. Simpson, "A Late Old Kingdom Letter to the Dead from Nag' Ed-Deir n 3500," *Journal of Egyptian Archaeology* 56 (1970): 58–62; M. Guilmot, "Lettre à une épouse défuncte (Pap. Leiden I, 371)," *Zeitschrift für Ägyptische Sprache und Altertumskunde* (Leipzig, Berlin) 99 (1973): 94–103; E. F. Wente, "A Misplaced Letter to the Dead," *Orientalia Lovaniensia Periodica, Löwen* 6/7 (1975/1976): 595–600. Translations can conveniently be found in E. Wente, *Letters from Ancient Egypt* (*Society of Biblical Literature: Writings from the Ancient World,* vol. 1; Atlanta: Scholars Press, 1990).

10. The "Letter on a Stela," Wente, "A Misplaced Letter to the Dead," (1975/1976), pp. 595–600. A detailed analysis in transliteration and translation of this text, the other texts

mentioned in this chapter, and all other textual references to dreams from Egypt prior to the Late Period can be found in the appendix of my dissertation *The Perception of Dreams and Nightmares in Ancient Egypt*.

11. The "Letter to the Dead Nag'ed Deir 3737," Simpson, "The Letter to the Dead from the Tomb of Meru (N 3737) at Nag' ed-Deir," pp. 39–50.
12. The dream portion can be found on lines 20–22 of Amenhotep II's Memphis Stela. The hieroglyphic text can be found in W. Helck, *Urkunden der 18. Dynastie* (Urkunden des ägyptischen Altertums IV, Heft 19; Berlin: 1957), IV, 1306, 11–1307, 2. An English translation of the campaign can be found in P. Der Manuelian, *Studies in the Reign of Amenophis II* (Hildesheimer ägyptologische Beiträge 26 Gerstenberg: Hildesheim, 1987), 225–226.
13. This passage is found in lines 28–30 of the Karnak description of Merneptah's Libyan War campaign. The text publication can be found in K. A. Kitchen, *Ramesside Inscriptions* (Oxford: B. H. Blackwell Ltd., 1968–1991), IV, 5; l. 10–15. An English translation can be found in B. G. Davies, *Egyptian Historical Inscriptions of the Nineteenth Dynasty* (Documenta Mundi: Aegyptiaca 2 Jonsered: Paul Aströms, 1997), 156–157.
14. The entire stela was published in C. M. Zivie, "Giza au deuxième Millénaire," *Bibliothèque d'Étude* 70 (1976). Translations of this text can be found in many works, including B. M. Bryan, *The Reign of Thutmose IV* (Baltimore and London: The Johns Hopkins University Press, 1991).
15. G. Posener, *De la divinité du Pharaon* (Paris: Imprimerie Nationale, 1960), 88.
16. Oppenheim, *The Interpretation of Dreams in the Ancient Near East,* 187–192.
17. In certain other cultures, the oneiric call to office seems to have been much more prevalent and to have served a clearly political purpose. Modern examples seem to express a much stronger political sentiment than that expressed in the New Kingdom royal dream accounts, which did not play such a prominent role in the pharaoh's kingship. See, for example, K. Ray, "Dreams of Grandeur: The Call to Office in North-Central Igbo Religious Leadership," in *Dreaming, Religion and Society in Africa,* ed. M. C. Jedrej and R. Shaw (Studies on Religion in Africa; Leiden: E. J. Brill, 1992), 61, and J. S. Mbiti, "God, Dreams and African Militancy," in *Religion in a Pluralistic Society,* ed. J. S. Poke (Leiden: E. J. Brill, 1976), 38–47.
18. The most famous of these later accounts include the "Dream of Sethos," the "Dreams of the Ethiopian Kings," the "Dream of Ptolemy Soter," the "Hunger Stela," and the "Dream of King Nectanebo." To this list can be added the "Prince of Bakhtan" which does not describe pharaoh but a royal prince. Translations of these texts can be found in Oppenheim, *The Interpretation of Dreams in the Ancient Near East,* pp. 251–253, and in Sauneron, "Les songes et leur interprétation," pp. 21–31.
19. This dream is part of the *Biography of Ipwy* (l.5–7), originally published in H. Satzinger, "Zwei Wiener Objekte mit bemerkenswerten Inschriften," in *Mélanges Gamal Eddin Mokhtar* (ed. P. Posener-Kriéger; Cairo: Institut français d'archéologie orientale du Caire, 1985), 249–254.
20. For the publication of the tomb see K.-J. Seyfried, *Das Grab des Djehutiemhab (TT 194),* (Theben 7; Mainz am Rhein: Philipp von Zabern, 1995). The text publication can be found in J. Assmann, "Eine Traumoffenbarung der Göttin Hathor," *Revue d'Égyptologie* 30 (1978), 22–50, and K. A. Kitchen, *Ramesside Inscriptions* (Oxford: B. H. Blackwell Ltd., 1968–1991), VII,153.
21. A nickname of the goddess.
22. I refer here only to those texts that actually describe dreams that had been seen, in contrast to texts that simply refer to dreams in the abstract.
23. This is the modern name given to the ancient village located on the west bank of Thebes, near the Valley of the Kings. It was inhabited by the highly literate and elite scribes, builders, and craftsmen who worked on the royal tombs during Egypt's New Kingdom.

24. A. H. Gardiner, *Hieratic Papyri in the British Museum, Third Series: Chester Beatty Gift,* 2 vols. (London: British Museum, 1935).
25. The paleography and terminology suggests it was written in the early years of the reign of Ramesses II, perhaps ca. 1279–1257 B.C.
26. Seth was the god of disorder, associated with the desert. The Sethian type of man was described as a rather sensual, temperamental, uncouth man, possibly with red hair.
27. States suggests that rather than being linked by symbolism, "all images in dreams become contaminated by their 'similars,' which is to say by other members of the same category (metonymy) or by their resemblance to things in categories outside them (metaphor)" (States, *Seeing in the Dark: Reflections on Dreams and Dreaming* [New Haven: Yale University Press, 1997], 157).
28. Due to the idiosyncrasies of ancient Egyptian, an Egyptian pun could consist of a play based on sounds, meaning, and signs (A. Loprieno, "Puns and Word Play in Ancient Egyptian," in *Puns and Pundits: Wordplay in the Hebrew Bible and Ancient Near Eastern Literature,* ed. S. B. Noegel [Bethesda: CDL Press, 2000], 3–20). See also S. B. Noegel, chapter 3 of this volume, and K. Szpakowska, *The Perception of Dreams and Nightmares in Ancient Egypt.*
29. *P. Chester Beatty III,* r. 2.21. This reference and the following are based on translations in K. Szpakowska, *The Perception of Dreams and Nightmares in Ancient Egypt.*
30. Ibid., r. 8.3.
31. Ibid., r. 4.13.
32. Ibid., r. 2.22. Crocodiles and officials are again associated in r. 5.11 and r. 5.17.
33. Ibid., r. 8.12. In Egyptian there is a wordplay between the words for "falling under" and "underling," which I have attempted to retain.
34. Ibid., r. 9.27. There is no obvious wordplay here, and I cannot fathom the relationship between image and meaning.
35. Oracles in general are latecomers to the Egyptian world (J. D. Ray, "Ancient Egypt," in *Divination and Oracles,* ed. M. Loewe and C. Blacker [London: George Allen & Unwin, 1981], pp. 174–190).
36. Maxim 18 of the Teaching of Ptahhotep. English translations of this popular text can easily be found in compilations of Egyptian literature, such as R. B. Parkinson, *The Tale of Sinuhe and other Ancient Egyptian Poems 1940–1640 BC* (Oxford: Clarendon Press, 1997).
37. The phrase is found in New Kingdom Harper's Songs and was literally "As for a lifetime done on earth, it is the time of a dream." Two versions of this song have been found—one in the tomb of Neferhotep published in R. Hari, *La tombe thébaine du père divin Neferhotep (TT50),* (Collection Epigraphica Geneva: Editions de Belles-Lettres, 1985), and one in the tomb of Djehutimes published in L. Kákosy and Z. I. Fábián, "Harper's Song in the Tomb of Djehutimes (TT 32)," *Studien zur altägyptische Kultur* 22 (1995), pp. 211–227.
38. The complete text has been found on seven papyri dating to the Middle Kingdom, and more than twenty dating to the New Kingdom (S. G. Quirke, "Archive," in *Ancient Egyptian Literature: History and Forms* [ed. A. Loprieno; Leiden, New York, Köln: E. J. Brill, 1996], 379–401; R. B. Parkinson, "Teachings, Discourses and Tales from the Middle Kingdom," in *Middle Kingdom Studies* [ed. S. Quirke; New Malden: Sia Publishing, 1991], pp. 91–122).

    Some of the most accessible translations of this text can be found in M. Lichtheim, *Ancient Egyptian Literature,* (I: The Old and Middle Kingdoms; Berkeley: University of California Press, 1973), 222–235 and in R. B. Parkinson, *The Tale of Sinuhe and Other Ancient Egyptian Poems 1940–1640 BC* (Oxford: Clarendon Press, 1997).
39. Many of these texts are published in K. Sethe, *Die Ächtung feindlicher Fürsten, Völker und Dinge auf altägyptischen Tongefässscherben des Mittleren Reiches* (Abhandlung der Preussischen Akademie der Wissenschaften 1926; Berlin: Akademie der Wissenschaften, 1926).

Their possible use in rituals has been discussed in R. K. Ritner, *The Mechanics of Ancient Egyptian Magical Practice* (Studies in Ancient Oriental Civilization 54; Chicago: The Oriental Institute of the University of Chicago, 1993), 140–155.

40. C. Fisher et al., "A Psychophysiological Study of Nightmares," *The Journal of the American Psychoanalytic Association* 18 (1970): 747–782; E. Kahn, C. Fisher, and A. Edwards, "Night Terrors and Anxiety Dreams," in *The Mind in Sleep: Psychology and Psychophysiology,* pp. 437–447; A. Spielman and C. Herrera, "Sleep Disorders," in *The Mind in Sleep,* ed. James and Antrobus, 25–80; R. L. Van de Castle, *Our Dreaming Mind* (New York: Ballantine Books, 1994), 347.
41. G. Michaeilidis, "Bès au divers aspects," *Bulletin de l'Institut d'Égypte* 45 (1963–1964): 70–73.
42. Originally published in I. E. S. Edwards, *Oracular Amuletic Decrees,* (Hieratic Papyri in the British Museum 4th Series, II volumes; London: 1960).
43. Found on the Dream Stela of Tanutamani in N. C. Grimal, *Quatre Stèles Napatéennes au Musée du Caire: JE 48863–4866, Textes et Indices* (Mémoires publiés par les membres de l'Institut Français d'Archéologie Orientale du Caire 106; Cairo: Institut Français d'Archéologie Orientale du Caire, 1981).
44. P. Vernus, "La Grande Mutation Idéologique du Nouvel Empire: Une nouvelle théorie du pouvoir politique du démiurge face à sa création," *Bulletin de la Société d'égyptologie de Genève* 19 (1995): 69–95.
45. Ibid., p. 94. See also A. Loprieno, "Le Pharaon reconstruit. La figure du roi dans la littérature égyptienne au 1er millénaire avant J.C.," *Bulletin de l'institut français d'archéologie orientale* 142 (June 1998): 20–21, for the differences between the Libyan and the Ethiopian responses to the problem of legitimation in the Third Intermediate Period.
46. Tanutamani Dream Stele 29–31.
47. It was at this time, for example, that the Oracle at the Siwa Oasis was established—where the Macedonian conqueror Alexander the Great would later be declared a legitimate Egyptian pharaoh.
48. Lines 20–22 of the Memphis Stela of Amenhotep II.
49. K. Bulkeley, *Visions of the Night: Dreams, Religion, and Psychology* (Albany: State University of New York, 1999), pp. 77–91.
50. This is an excerpt from the "Letter to the Dead Nag'ed Deir 3737," Simpson, "The Letter to the Dead from the Tomb of Meru (N 3737) at Nag' ed-Deir," pp. 39–50.
51. E. Hartmann, *The Nightmare: The Psychology and Biology of Terrifying Dreams* (New York: Basic Books, 1984), 41–44. Emotion, including guilt, can be a motivating force behind a dream (States, *Seeing in the Dark,* 235–250). For dreams as a venue for working out troubles, see H. Fiss, "Experimental Strategies for the Study of the Function of Dreaming," in *The Mind in Sleep,* ed. Ellman and Antrobus, 311.
52. Egyptian words were usually followed by a sign indicating their semantic frame of reference. Words having to do with motion, for example, have the determinative of walking legs.
53. This determinative is the little sparrow (Gardiner G37). A detailed analysis of this passage can be found in Szpakowska, *The Perception of Dreams and Nightmares in Ancient Egypt,* 314–316 and K. Szpakowska, "A Sign of the Times," *Lingua Aegyptia* 6(1999), 163–166.
54. Bulkeley, *Visions of the Night,* 22.
55. For a historical approach to dreams see P. Burke, *Varieties of Cultural History* (Cambridge: Polity Press, 1997), 23–42.
56. L. N. Weinstein, D. G. Schwartz, and A. M. Arkin, "Qualitative Aspects of Sleep Mentation," in *The Mind in Sleep,* ed. Ellman and Antrobus, pp. 172–213.

3

Dreams and Dream Interpreters in Mesopotamia and in the Hebrew Bible [Old Testament]

Scott Noegel

The dream comes with much implication.

—*Qohelet 5:2*

Although the subject of ancient Near Eastern dreams has received scholarly attention for some time,[1] recent years have seen a resurgence of interest in the topic. In part this is due to the appearance of several previously unpublished texts,[2] a scholarly desire to update the available resources on the subject,[3] and the currently prevailing academic preference for comparative interdisciplinary inquiry, which has moved the study of the ancient Near Eastern dreams beyond its hitherto nearly entirely descriptive mode.[4] What has emerged from this renewed interest is a new appreciation for the subtleties of dreams, the divinatory, ontological, and ideological contexts of their interpretations, and the variety of methodological frameworks that can be used to understand them. While not every framework has proven useful for elucidating the topic beyond what we already know,[5] the cumulative impact provides new directions for research.

I divide the topic of dreams and their interpretations into two sections: the Mesopotamian evidence and that found in the Hebrew Bible.[6] Throughout I shall adopt A. Leo Oppenheim's typology[7] and distinguish "message" dreams, in which a god or important figure appears in a dream and delivers an auditory missive to the dreamer (often to legitimate, support, or ease the political, national, or military concerns of the dreamer), from "symbolic" dreams, in which the dreamer witnesses enigmatic visual images that require an interpreter upon awakening. Oppenheim also classified separately those dreams that involve prognostication as "mantic" or "prophetic."

Although Oppenheim's work offers a useful starting point, it is important to stress the limits of his typology and of others based on it. Not only does his work make no distinction between literary and historical texts, but, as we shall see, not every dream account fits neatly into one of the two (or three) categories, and there is considerable overlap between them. For example, there are symbolic dreams that require no interpreter, and message dreams that do. There are prophetic message dreams and also prophetic symbolic dreams. Oppenheim's typology also presupposes that the peoples of the ancient Near East, like we do today, conceptually distinguished symbolic modes of discourse from nonsymbolic modes, but the religio-mantic conception of the written word throughout the ancient Near East argues against this.[8] Mesopotamians use the same word, for example, for "visual portent or sign" and "cuneiform sign,"[9] and for diviners, both animal viscera and the stars constituted the "writing of the gods."

I begin by surveying the Mesopotamian evidence, since it is attested much earlier and is much greater than the biblical evidence, in terms of the number and type of relevant textual materials available to us. Unlike the Bible, which preserves only literary accounts of dreams and their interpretations, Mesopotamian dream accounts appear in a variety of textual genres including ritual, oracular, epistolary, historical, dedicatory, and literary texts. We cannot use our abundant evidence, however, to gauge the popularity of oneiromancy in Mesopotamia, for in the scholarly academies dream interpretation never achieved the status of other forms of divination such as extispicy (divining from animal viscera) and later astrology, which were viewed more reliable and less subjective and, therefore, were used to authenticate a dream's interpretation. This is especially evident in the neo-Assyrian period (744–539 B.C.E.) in which kings preferred other divinatory experts in their courts.[10]

Our earliest evidence for dreams in Mesopotamia is a Sumerian[11] relief known as the Stele of Vultures.[12] This now-fragmentary monument was erected by King Eanatum I (ca. 2454–2425 B.C.E.) of Lagash (or possibly his nephew Enmetena)[13] to laud his military success over neighboring Umma. The text recounts how, after appearing beside Eannatum's head (a widespread literary topos in message dream accounts),[14] the god Ningirsu[15] guaranteed the king's victory. Since the stele was carved after the campaign and describes the king as over nine feet tall and created by the god himself, we must see it as tendentious fiction. However, we would be mistaken if we thought of it only as royal propaganda. The stele was discovered in the temple precinct and not on the border of Lagash,[16] suggesting that the cult of Ningirsu had considerable interest in preserving the dream account. The Ningirsu priesthood probably stood to benefit as much from sanctioning the king with Ningirsu's promise as from the campaign itself.

Another Sumerian dream account appears in the mythological text known as "Lugalbanda in the Mountain Cave."[17] In this story, the hero Lugalbanda falls ill while on a military campaign and is left behind in a cave. After surviving the sickness by fervent prayer, Lugalbanda undergoes a series of tribulations that mark his transformation into a savior-holy man. At one point, Lugalbanda lies down to induce dreaming, and the dream god Anzaqar[18] promptly appears issuing a rather vague command.

> The reddish brown bull—who [*will bind*] it for me?
> Who will pour me the sheep's fat?
> He must possess my own axe, whose fine metal is metal of the skies;
> He must possess my side-arm, made of iron![19]

Anzaqar then commands Lugalbanda to wrestle and kill the bull and present its innards "before the rising sun." In all respects, the dream is puzzling. Lying somewhere between a message dream and a symbolic dream, the text legitimizes the hero by representing, in H. Vanstiphout's words, "a first test of Lugalbanda's suitability for holiness, and at the same time his calling to the same."[20]

The verses leading to the dream offer insight into Sumerian conceptions of dreams.

> Dream—a door cannot hold it back, nor can a doorpost;
> To the liar it speaks lies; to the truthful the truth.
> It can make one happy or make one lament;
> It is a closed archive basket of the gods . . .

Of particular note is the comparison to a sealed basket of cuneiform tablets, a well-known practice in juridical contexts, which classifies dreams as secret legal texts[21]—a point to which we will return.

The Sumerian Legend of Sargon, king of Akkad (ca. 2334–2279 B.C.E.), reports how the young Sargon, while serving as a cupbearer for King Urzababa in Kish, had a disturbing message dream, which he promptly reported to the king upon awakening.

> There was a single young woman, she was high as the heaven,
> she was broad as the earth
> She was firmly set as the [bas]e of a wall.
> For me she drowned you in a great [river], a river of blood.[22]

As soon as the king heard this, he realized that Sargon would replace him as king, which, of course, he eventually did.[23] According to J. Sweek, "The text strongly identifies Sargon as the chosen one, becoming king without design or impious rebellion of his own."[24]

In the following centuries, one finds a number of individualized message dream narratives in Mesopotamian royal inscriptions of varying types (e.g., votive steles, clay nails, prisms, and dedicatory bricks). Most date to the reigns of the neo-Assyrian king Assurbanipal (668–627 B.C.E.)[25] and the neo-Babylonian king Nabonidus (555–539 B.C.E.). Since some of these inscriptions were deposited out of human view for the gods, they must have had more of a religious function than a political one. On the other hand, even genuine acts of piety can constitute propaganda, since witnesses were present during the rituals that accompanied the deposition of such texts.

A dream report relating to the neo-Assyrian king Assurbanipal reads as follows. One night, before a battle, the king prayed to the goddess Ishtar for guidance. That same night, a priest dreamed he saw the goddess Ishtar holding a bow and sword and promising victory, which he then related to the king. Although not stated explicitly, the inscription appears to record an incubation practice, that is, a provoked dream omen.[26] The text's political aspects are apparent, but again, we must be careful not to sever it entirely from its religious context.

It is easier to identify the propagandistic function of another dream dating to this king's reign. This unique account tells us that the night before crossing the torrential Idid'e River, Assurbanipal's troops all experienced the same dream in which Ishtar offered comforting words: "I shall go in front of Assurbanipal, the king whom I myself have created!" The next morning, we are told, they crossed bravely and safely.[27]

Propagandistic concerns also are clear in dream narratives dating to Nabonidus. In addition to one report in which the king is encouraged to build the sanctuary of the moon god Sîn at Harran, one stele reports how the deceased king Nebuchadnezzar II appeared to Nabonidus in a dream and deciphered another (presumably) symbolic dream.[28] (The dream itself is lost.) The account aims to set Nabonidus up as Nebuchadnezzar II's legitimate successor. The dream is fascinating not only because it preserves one of two cases in which someone deceased appears in a dream but because the dream depicts an astronomical omen involving the moon, Jupiter, and "the Great Star." It is thus an omen within an omen. It also is a rare example of a dream being interpreted within a dream, an occurrence that signaled prophetic significance throughout the Near East.[29]

Several Mesopotamian literary texts contain what have been described as message dreams, but upon closer look they defy easy classification. *Ludlul bel nemeqi* (lit. "Let Me Praise the Lord of Wisdom") is a case in point.[30] This Babylonian poem describes the experience of a righteous sufferer who has three dreams, each of which suggests that his health will be restored.[31] Although the dreams require no interpreter, they depict mysterious images, including a young man of remarkable stature, an incantation priest sent to cleanse the dreamer, a young woman of shining visage, and an exorcist carrying a tablet—the very tablet upon which the poem is written.[32]

The 750-line Epic of Erra[33] similarly underscores our inability to classify literary message dreams according to the accepted typology. After extolling the attributes of the god Erra, the poet concludes by stating that Erra revealed the entire text to him in a dream, which he recorded faithfully—a statement that constitutes a claim of divinatory privilege. The reference, like the tablet in *Ludlul bel nemeqi,* also helps to contextualize Mesopotamian literary dreams by reminding us that mantic professionals were responsible also for the production of literary texts. As I shall show below, this information is especially useful for contextualizing literary symbolic dreams and for conceptualizing Mesopotamian literature generally.

The site of Mari, on the mid-Euphrates, has produced a number of message dreams dating to the eighteenth century B.C.E. Sometimes labeled "prophetic" dreams, these texts are in actuality missives sent by officials that report the message dreams of seers that have import for the royal house. Since the dream accounts appear in epistolary contexts, a propagandistic function can be ruled out. Nevertheless, the political import of the texts remains. One dream, in which a deceased priest appears, will demonstrate.

> He [the seer] saw the following: "You will not rebuild this deserted house. If the house is rebuilt, I will make it collapse into the river." The day he saw the dream, he said nothing to anyone. The next day he again saw the following dream: "It was a god. You will not rebuild this house. If you rebuild it, I will make it collapse into the river." I now hereby dispatch to my lord the fringe of his garment and a lock from his head . . . from that day, this man has been ill. (Sasson (1983), pp. 283–293)[34]

This dream illustrates three patterns found frequently in message dream accounts. The first is the twice-experienced dream, which signaled divine communication throughout the Near East. The second is that of the seer's commitment to a social, if not legal, contract that forces him to report all potentially significant divinatory observations to the king. The letter implies, in fact, that the seer's illness was due to his not reporting the first dream.[35] The third pattern is the reference to the seer's fringe and hair lock, known especially at Mari, which is meant as proof that the said seer, in fact, did experience the dream. This illustrates the potential political power invested in mantics of good reputation and suggests that such "proof" would not be necessary if attempts to falsify dreams were unknown.

The political import of message dreams for the royal house is also obvious in Assurbanipal's annals, which record the king's experiences during a political revolt provoked by his brother, then king of Babylon. In the dream the god Sîn warns: "Upon all those who plot evil against Assurbanipal, king of Assyria, and resort to [actual] hostilitites, I shall bestow a miserable death, I shall put an end to their lives through the quick dagger of [war], conflagration, hunger, pestilence."[36]

Two other literary accounts of message dreams appear in the famous Epic of Gilgamesh, but they are problematic.[37] The first is the dream of Gilgamesh's friend Enkidu, presumed present (on the basis of the Hittite version)[38] in the broken sections of the Assyrian version. It describes Enkidu's appearance before the divine council where he learns of his imminent death. The second is the god Ea's disclaimer that he did not explicitly "leak" news of the impending deluge: "It was not I who disclosed the secret of the great gods. I caused Atra-hasis to examine a dream, and he perceived the secret of the gods" (XI:186–187). The former dream's appearance in the Assyrian version is too fragmentary to be useful, and the latter dream poses difficulties because the description of dreams as divine secrets and the so-called message of the dream itself classify it more as a symbolic dream.[39]

Symbolic dreams are more widely attested in Mesopotamia than message dreams and appear more often in epic literature than in historical texts. The earliest, a Sumerian cylinder inscription known as Gudea A,[40] reports how Gudea, ruler of the city of Lagash (ca. 2130 B.C.E.), experienced two enigmatic dreams, the first in which a colossal man spoke words of indistinct meaning. Puzzled by the experience, he boarded a boat to Nin, the dwelling of the goddess Nanshe. It is she, or perhaps a priestess through whom the goddess speaks, who interprets his dream as meaning that he will build the god Ningirsu's temple. Afterward, Gudea gets a "second opinion" by having an extispicy (inspection of the entrails of sacrificial victims for divinatory meaning) performed.

In the Sumerian poem "Dumuzi's Dream," the god Dumuzi experiences a bewildering dream influenced by the South wind.[41]

> An owl had caught
>   a lamb in the sheepcote,
> A falcon had caught
>   a sparrow in the reed of the fence . . .
> The churns lay on their sides,
>   poured out no milk,
> The cups lay on their sides,
>   Dumuzi lived there no more,
> The winds only swept the fold.[42]

Upon awakening, his sister Geshtininna affirms his (worst) nightmare by interpreting the dream as portending his death. After several attempts to escape this fate, including a transformation into a gazelle, Dumuzi is eventually captured and killed.

The epistolary texts of Mari preserve at least one symbolic dream, although again the current typology is not helpful.[43] The letter in question reports a dream of the female seer Addu-duri as reported to King Zimri-Lim (ca. 1775 B.C.E.). No interpretation follows, but the symbolic nature of the dream and its ambiguity suggest that we include it here.

> Tell my lord: Addu-duri, your maidservant, says: Since the *shulmum* of your father's house, I have never had a dream [such as] this. Previous portents of mine [were as] this pair. In my dream, I entered Belet-ekallim's chapel; but Belet-ekallim was not in residence. Moreover, the statues before her were not there. Upon seeing this, I broke into uncontrollable weeping. This dream of mine occurred during the night's first phase [lit. during the evening watch]. I resumed [dreaming], and Dada, the priest of Ishtar-pishra, was standing at the door of Belet-ekallim['s chapel], but a hostile voice kept on uttering: "*tura dagan, tura dagan.*" This is what it kept on uttering . . . [44]

Of interest is the word *shulmum,* a pun that means both "restoration" and "destruction" of a royal line. The dream's concluding words, *tura dagan, tura dagan,* also are ambiguous and suggest both "O Dagan return (here)/come back/reconsider" and a proper name connected with a Mari king who ruled over a century before Zimri-Lim.[45] Thus, the entire letter[46] teems with ambiguity, which, J. Sasson notes, "may have drained him [Zimri-Lim] of any will to act purposefully."[47] Since the omen was of considerable political import, ambiguity probably served to safeguard the diviner. Ambiguous omens from the practice of extispicy offer analogies. U. Jeyes notes: "By couching his words in a subtle, not to say ambiguous manner, he could avoid committing himself and his profession in a disastrous way."[48]

In the Epic of Gilgamesh,[49] the hero experiences two symbolic dreams in close succession, which his mother, the goddess Ninsu, interprets.

> The stars of heaven gathered [?] to me, and a meteorite [*kitsru*] from [the god] Anum fell on top [*tseri*] of me I tried to lift it, but it was too heavy for me. I tried to budge it, but I could not budge it. The land of Uruk gathered around it, the young men kissed its feet, I took responsibility [?] for it, they loaded it on to me, I lifted it and brought it to you. . . .
>
> Of spacious Uruk an axe [*hatssinn*] was thrown down, and they gathered around it. The axe looked somehow strange. I saw it and I was glad. I loved it as a wife, and I doted on it. I took it and placed it at my side [*ahiya*].[50]

The Mari letter above illustrated how the ambiguity inherent in symbolic dreams can safeguard diviners when not interpreted or when rendered equivocally. The interpretation of Gilgamesh's dreams shows us yet another side to the interpreter's use of ambiguity. It reveals how words that possess multiple meanings can provide clues to a dream's interpretation. The interpretation of Gilgamesh's mother, for example, hinges on the polysemy inherent in the words used to convey the dream. Gilgamesh stated that the *kitsru* landed "on top" (*tseri*) of me, which his mother interprets as representing a man "born of the steppeland (*tseri*)," a figure whom we learn to be Enkidu. In effect, she has heard in the preposition *tseri* on top the homophonous noun *tseri* "steppeland."[51] Additional puns connect the objects in his second dream and its interpretation,[52] and they are more than literary whimsy or sophisticated intertextuality. They are accurate depictions of a divinatory hermeneutic at work.

Two more examples will demonstrate, taken from later in the epic when Ea warns Utnapishtim in a dream: "spurn property (*makkura zerma*), keep living beings alive"

(XI:26). Two puns occur here: "spurn" (*zerma*), which also can be read as "construct" (*sêrma*); and "property" (*makkura*), which suggests "boat" (i.e., *makura*).[53] In essence, Ea issued two polysemous secrets with one breath: "forsake property and build an ark!"

Later, when Ea tells Utnapishtim that the chief god Enlil promises to "provide" (*zananu*) the people with an "abundance" (*nuhshu*) of "wheat cakes" (*kukki*) and "wheat" (*kibāti*), Utnapishtim divines other meanings in these words: an "excessive" (*nuhshu*) "storm" (*zananu*) of "darkness" (*kukkû*) and "heaviness" (*kibittu*) XI:45–47.[54] Thus, the flood survivor's great wisdom, which earns him the epithet Atrahasis "exceedingly wise" (XI:188), springs from his ability to "hear" between the lines.

We obtain further insight into the socio-religious context of divinatory ambiguity from Babylonian and Assyrian scholarly commentaries,[55] wherein one finds esoteric meanings hermeneutically extracted from texts via wordplay. Many of the text's colophons label the hermeneutics, and the texts to which they are applied, as "secret words" (*amat nitsirti*) and "secrets (*pirishtu*) of the gods," the same expressions that appear in Utnapishtim's statement to Gilgamesh and Ea's words to Utnapishtim.[56] In a technical sense then, the dream secrets of Ea, which Utnapishtim relates to Gilgamesh, accurately portray the privileged divinatory ambiguity of diviners.

Such a realistic rendering of the punning techniques of dream interpreters in literary texts underscores the close connection between divinatory experts and the production of literary texts[57] and raises serious questions concerning what constitutes "literature" (and "literary patterns") in these cultures. Not only does the epic realistically characterize Utnapishtim as a dream interpreter,[58] performing his rituals at night,[59] but the redactor of the epic, Sîn-leqqi-uninni, was an exorcist. We should not be surprised, therefore, that this "literature" accurately reflects mantic hemeneutics.

In addition to literary, epistolary, and historical texts, we possess a collection of dream oracles known as the Babylonian *Dream Book,*[60] of which roughly one hundred oracles have survived out of an estimated five hundred. The series opens by invoking the god of dreams Zaqīqu (also called MA.MÚ)[61] and, much like the Egyptian *Dream Book,*[62] organizes dreams into thematic categories along with their interpretations. Just a few of the themes include: urinating, having sex, flying, visiting certain temples and towns, seeing the dead and the divine, ascending to the heavens, descending to the underworld, carrying objects, standing or sitting in a particular place, turning into various animals, eating and drinking particular items, making objects, performing a particular occupation, seeing animals, being given objects, seeing astronomical bodies, and felling trees and plants.

The *Dream Book,* however, is more than a collection of dreams, for they represent an attempt on behalf of the divinatory establishment to standardize and control dreams. Indeed, the very format and organization of the compendium, like that of lexical lists, demonstrate a desire "to present a systematic and ordered picture of the world."[63] The *Dream Book* also tells as us much about the interpreter's hermeneutical options, as it does about the loves, fantasies, and fears of the average Mesopotamian (unlike message dreams, which are associated typically with kings).[64] Some of the compendium's interpretive strategies include the use of contemporary associations; the pairings of similars or of opposites; learned readings of cuneiform signs; a consideration of the dreamer's occupation, state of mind, status, and personal situation; and a polarity between dreams and their meanings, that is, if one dreams a bad thing, it means a good thing (hence, "If the god utters a curse against the man; his prayers will be accepted").[65] In some cases, the basis for interpretation remains bewildering.

Much like the literary portrayals of symbolic dreams, the compendium often displays punning relationships between the protasis (what is dreamed) and the apodosis (what the dream means).[66] So, "If a man dreams that he is eating a raven [*arbu*]; he will have income [*irbu*]," and "If [someone] has given him *mihru*-wood; he shall have no rival [*māhiru*]." Often the interpretation is based on an erudite reading of cuneiform signs used to record the dream.[67] Although punning certainly was not the only hermeneutic in existence, it served as one of the most pervasive tools of all Mesopotamian mantics in all periods. Thus, we find it in many other divinatory arts, including abnormal birth omens, extispicy, astronomical omens, augury, and magic stones.[68] Such a divinatory preoccupation with ambiguity recalls the words of Sigmund Freud:

> The whole range of wordplay is thus put at the service of the dream activity. The part played by words in the formation of dreams ought not to surprise us. A word being a point of junction for a number of conceptions, it possesses, so to speak, a predestined ambiguity.[69]

Since Freud studied biblical, Talmudic,[70] and Greek dream interpretation,[71] we cannot take his comment as a statement of interpretive universals.[72] Nevertheless, it stands as a telling witness to the legacy of Mesopotamian divinatory practices.

The religious cosmology that undergirds Mesopotamian divinatory disciplines allows us to appreciate more fully the act of dream interpretation by contextualizing it within a belief system in which words index power.[73] G. Contenau explains:

> Since to know and pronounce the name of an object instantly endowed it with reality, and created power over it, and since the degree of knowledge and consequently of power was strengthened by the tone of voice in which the name was uttered, writing, which was a permanent record of the name, naturally contributed to this power, as did both drawing and sculpture, since both were a means of asserting knowledge of the object and consequently of exercising over it the power which knowledge gave.[74]

When viewed in this context, one cannot see the ubiquitous use of divinatory punning and other so-called literary devices as stylistic features. For if words constitute loci of power, then words with multiple associations have greater potential for such power. Hence the need in Mesopotamia for highly literate professionals trained in handling the power inherent in the divine word.

Moreover, to understand how words of power function within dream contexts, we must recognize that acts of divination constitute acts of divine judgment. Not only do diviners use the word *purussû,* meaning "legal decision" or "verdict," to refer to an omen's prediction,[75] divinatory texts in general share in common with legal codes the formula *if x, then y.*[76] From a juridical perspective, wordplays and erudite readings that connect protases to apodoses constitute vehicles for demonstrating and justifying divine judgment.[77] Insofar as they underscore the tie between the sign and its prediction, they illustrate the principle and process of *lex talionis,* "the law of retribution." J. Bottéro describes: "In Mesopotamia . . . each phonetic similarity was to be considered serious and very significant: two realities whose names coincided were bound as closely together as their designations."[78]

Thus, the dream oracles and literary accounts of symbolic dreams not only affirm Mesopotamian theological and legal principles, they embody them; and their punning interpretations are more performative than literary, since words index power and since flourishment is only the result of a pun's *talion* function. Moreover, insofar as correlations between protases and apodoses reflect mantic efforts to demonstrate that theological principles continue to function (i.e., there is no such thing as coincidence), they register and dispel mantic insecurities. In this sense, dream interpretation in Mesopotamia represents less a preoccupation with ambiguity than an attempt at rendering ambiguity into a projected and authoritative reality.

Complementing the compendium of symbolic dreams are a variety of ritual texts dating mostly from the neo-Assyrian period and onward, called *namburbû*.[79] The ritual techniques mentioned in the *namburbû* vary according to the specific goals of the practitioner. Typically they invoke the gods of fire, light, or magic.[80] Techniques include the use of amulets, figurines, substitution, deity invocation, purification of the dreamer, and incantations. Some rituals purify the sleeper and his environment in preparation for the dream state or instill the dreamer with a good dream. Others aim to provoke dreams that disclose and manipulate the future. Still others exorcise demons and the potentially harmful consequences of bad dreams. The belief in the efficacy of such mechanical measures, one must admit, negates any role for individual moral or religious responsibility. It also directly contradicts the Mesopotamian religious worldview in which fate governs all things.[81] Such incongruencies, however, were either not apparent or unimportant to the Mesopotamians themselves.

We can tell these rituals were as important to the interpreter as to the dreamer, because the first and last two tablets of the *Dream Book* contain *namburbû* incantations. One such *namburbû* transforms a bad dream into a good one by pleading the dreamer's case before the sun god: "Shamash, you are the judge—judge my case! You are the one who makes the decisions—decide my case! Change the dream I had into a good one!"[82] Note the legal language in the incantation, which again illustrates Mesopotamian conceptual links among dream interpretation, divinatory rituals, performative utterances, and divine jurisprudence. In fact, the performance of legal practices sometimes appears in the ritual ceremonies themselves, which often include oath formulae.

Dream rituals also served a medical function.[83] Mesopotamian divinatory professionals promoted the belief that cultic purity ensured good health, and so consequently, bad dreams were blamed on a dreamer's impiety, which in turn caused "the abscence of the protective canopy of his personal deities."[84] The loss of this protection opened the door for demons and deceased spirits, the agents of evil, false, and sexual dreams.[85] The ambiguous nature of symbolic dreams, therefore, was cause for concern, and forgetting one's dream spelled disaster, because one needed to know the dream in order to perform the proper ritual. Thus, important *namburbû*s involved washing one's hands in bed, or recounting the dream and transferring it to a substitute figurine, which was then destroyed. Sometimes figurines were buried in a room's corner or placed at the dreamer's head. In the case of dream apparitions, substitute figurines were encircled by flour,[86] an act that parallels the rituals performed when one is visited by demons or ghosts. Such rituals aimed to transfer contamination and outwit demons.

Namburbû rituals would begin on an empty stomach "in the early morning, on the day [after] the dream was seen . . . , before the dream's evil took ahold of its victim."[87] Dream-provoking rituals took place on auspicious days. Typically the expert performed the *namburbû* on or over the dreamer's bed, sometimes near the bed's head, with one of the dreamer's feet placed on the ground while he or she lies in bed. The very act of interpreting dreams, like the *namburbû* rituals, was therapeutic.[88]

By "solving" the puzzling dream, the interpreter "dissolved" its harmful consequences and thus "resolved" the dreamer's health.

We can explain the close connection among divinatory, legal, hermeneutical, medical, and religious aspects of dream interpretation by considering the interdisciplinary skills required of mantic experts. S. Parpola explains:

> In my opinion it is essential to consider these disciplines not in isolation but as integral parts of this larger whole, and to realize that as parts of an integrated system of thought, the different subdisciplines of the 'wisdom' were in constant contact and interaction with each other.[89]

Indeed, there is so much overlap between various disciplines[90] that today it is difficult to distinguish the various mantic professionals and the textual genres they have left us.[91] Take, for example, the terms used for dream interpreters. Mesopotamian texts specify three, or possibly four, different individuals. The first is the *barû,* a term most often associated with extispicy, but also with oil, incense, and bird divination.[92] *Barû* were organized into highly learned guilds with masters and apprentices.[93] A second figure is the *sha'ilu,* who, though apparently highly literate, was perhaps of a lower social status—which might explain, or be explained by, his or her frequent connection to necromancy.[94] Although more men are attested than women for both groups, women dream interpreters do appear, as we have seen already.[95] Despite attempts to distinguish the *barû* from the *sha'ilu,*[96] the textual evidence conflates their roles. Both groups practiced a variety of divinatory arts. By the neo-Assyrian period, dream interpretation also fell partially under the domain of the LÚ.MASH.MASH, a Sumerian term rendered into Akkadian by either *ashipu* "medical practitioner, conjuror" or *mashmashshu* "exorcist."[97]

This brings us to ancient Israelite views on dreams, a topic that we must consider within the greater ancient Near East. Unlike Mesopotamia, the Hebrew Bible (Old Testament) preserves no omen or ritual texts; all of its dream accounts occur in literature, making it difficult to reconstruct any ritual or mantic contexts. Moreover, far from representing a monolithic attitude toward dreams and their interpretation, the Bible's dream accounts constitute a pastiche of sometimes varying traditions, often folkloristic in origin, woven together over a long period of time. Biblical dream accounts, therefore, cannot be seen as wholly historical and cannot be divorced entirely from their redactional,[98] polemical, and literary contexts. When seen from a literary perspective, dreams, however categorized, often appear to govern the narrative's compositional structure[99] and to serve theological agendas.

In Mesopotamia, dreams had associations with the underworld and derived from the god of dreams or demons. The Israelites' monolatristic[100] belief system left little room for any agent (mechanical or divine) other than Yahweh, the God of Israel, in the dreaming and interpretive process. Still, the Israelites saw dreams as divine in origin.[101] The Israelites also shared in common with Mesopotamians three elements fundamental to the conceptual framework of divinatory and prophetic discourse: a socio-religious conception of deity as judge; a belief in the performative power of words[102]; and the presence of *lex talionis* as a productive legal, theological, and literary principle.[103] The shared conceptual framework allows us to see in the Bible a similar divinatory conception of words as indices of power and vehicles of divine judgment, even though the elements of divinatory ritual praxis as we know them in Mesopotamia are absent.

Where the Bible differs radically from the conceptual views of Mesopotamia[104] is in its literary and theological, if not polemical, characterization of the interpreter. Not only is effort taken to distance interpreters from all acts of magical praxis, and thus keep them in accord with legislation that forbids "foreign" religio-mantic acts (Deut. 13:2–6, 18:9–15), but the Bible consistently portrays foreigners as not having the divine wisdom, like Israelites, to decipher enigmatic dreams. Despite the presence of a host of mantic professionals, it takes the Israelite Joseph to interpret the dreams of Pharaoh and his prisoners (Gen. 40–41), and Daniel must interpret the dreams of the Babylonian king (Dan. 2 and 4). Even Joseph's family is able to understand his enigmatic dreams (Gen. 37). The only exception to this pattern is the dream of the Midianite soldier (Judg. 7:13–15), which a fellow soldier interprets. Even here, however, the dream positions the import of its interpretation at an Israelite advantage.

Israelite ideological concerns notwithstanding, the Bible's accounts of message dreams resemble their Mesopotamian counterparts in terms of content and purpose. The account of Solomon's dream in 1 Kings 3:1–15 (= 2 Chron. 1:7–13) informs us that the king offered a sacrifice at a high place at Gibeon, and, while spending the night in the shrine (possibly as an incubation rite),[105] experienced a theophoric dream in which Yahweh granted him a "wise and discerning mind" as well as riches and glory. The story's structure and message reminds us of the many of the Mesopotamian historical texts discussed above. Like the Mesopotamian kings, this dream aims to remove doubt concerning Solomon's fitness to rule.

Similar motives appear in the Bible's other message dream accounts, most of which occur in Genesis. The story of the dream of Abimelech king of Gerar (Gen. 20:3–7) explains how the foreign king took Abraham's wife, believing her to be his sister. During the night, God appeared to Abimelech and told him not to touch her, for she was Abraham's wife, and that if he restored her, Abraham would intercede for him and save his life, since he was a prophet. On a literary level, the dream reinforces Abraham's role as a prophet. On an ideological level, it illustrates how Yahweh assumes an active role in saving the founding father of the Israelite religion.

The account of Jacob's dream at Bethel (Gen. 28) is at once a symbolic dream (Jacob sees what appears to be the steps of a ziggurat with angels ascending and descending it) and a message dream. As such, it again attests to the difficulties of the current typology. The message of the dream reads as follows:

> I am Yahweh, the God of your father Abraham and the God of Isaac: the ground on which you are lying I will assign to you and your offspring. Your descendants shall be as the dust of the earth; you shall spread out to the west and the east, to the north and the south. All of the families of the earth shall be blessed by you and your descendants.

Upon awakening, Jacob erects a stone and anoints it with oil, naming the place Bethel (lit. "House of God"). Despite the dream's images, which have concerned exegetes for centuries,[106] the dream's divine legitimation of both Jacob and Bethel is more obvious.

Jacob's dream in Gen. 31:10–13[107] similarly illustrates how Yahweh aids his patriarchs. One night, while Jacob was frustrated with the treatment he received from his uncle Laban, God instructed Jacob in a dream how to procure better yields from his flocks. "Note well that all the he-goats that are mating with the flocks are streaked, speckled and mottled; for I have noted all that Laban is doing to you." Exactly how Jacob followed God's advice is unclear, since the pericope describing the flock manipulation is confusing and involves a subtle shuffling of live stock.[108] Still, the story's ideological message is clear—Yahweh ensures the patriarch's success and has a proactive hand in the history of Israel.

1 Samuel 3 tells the story of the prophet Samuel, who while serving in the Shiloh temple as a boy experienced a dream in which Yahweh promised the complete annihilation of the House of Eli, the rather scandalous family then functioning as overseers of the Ark of the Covenant. The story introduces the reader to Samuel for the first time and functions to characterize him as a true prophet: "Samuel grew up," we are told, "and Yahweh was with him: He did not leave any of Samuel's predictions unfulfilled. All Israel, from Dan to Beersheba, knew that Samuel was a trustworthy prophet of Yahweh" (3:19–20).

I could survey other message dream accounts (e.g., Gen. 15:1–16, 26:24, 31:24, 46:1–4; Num. 22:8–13, 19–21),[109] but their common ideological gist, I think, is by now clear. Like message dreams in Mesopotamian historical and literary works, biblical message dreams serve to legitimate the political, national, or military concerns of the dreamer, who is invariably someone of great importance.

Ideological concerns are present also in the Bible's accounts of symbolic dreams, most of which appear in the Joseph story and the book of Daniel's Aramaic portions. In nearly every case the text uses a dream to demonstrate God's creative hand in Israelite history or to bolster and contrast a biblical figure's character and abilities, which are invariably centered within the theological discourse of Yahweh and his covenant, with the inabilities of foreign kings and mantic professionals.

It is of note that scholars see the formulaic style and consistent literary form of biblical symbolic dreams as evidence of the prestige of deductive oneiromancy and the impact of Mesopotamia.[110] Further support comes from the Bible's use of wordplay as a means of depicting the exegetical methods for interpreting dreams. The story of Joseph's incarceration with Pharaoh's chief cupbearer and baker demonstrates this well. While in prison, the cupbearer dreams of three branches of a vine that budded, blossomed, and bore grape clusters from which the cupbearer pressed juice for Pharaoh's cup. Joseph's interpretation exploits the punning connotations of the objects in the dream. Since the vine can represent a person or people (e.g., Deut. 32:32, Ps. 128:3, and Job 15:33), and the word "budded" (*porhat*) also means "flourish," in the sense of a "restored people" (e.g., Hos. 14:6, Isa. 27:6, Ps. 72:7), and since in the dream the cupbearer performs his former duties, Joseph tells him: "In three days Pharaoh will lift up your head" (*nasa' par'oh et r'ôshka*) (Gen.40:13), that is, "he will exonerate you." Here a pun connects the cupbearer's head (*r'ôsh*) and his former position (*mishpat ha-rishôn*).

Similarly, the baker dreams of three baskets of white bread "upon his head" (*me'al r'ôsh*) from which birds were eating. Several puns link the contents of the baker's dream and Joseph's interpretation. The first is the baker's reference to Pharaoh's "food" as *ma'akal* rather than the more common word *'okel*. In addition to its generic meaning "food," *ma'akal* appears as a dead carcass for birds of prey (e.g., Deut. 28:26, Ps. 79:2), as a simile for suffering people (e.g., Jer. 7:33, 16:4), and as a metaphor for "people under attack" (Hab. 1:16). Nowhere does the more common *'okel* appear in reference to people. Thus, the image of birds devouring *ma'akal* from the baker's head suggests a predatory or scavenger action. Additionally, the baker's mention of "white bread," (*hori*) suggests Pharaoh's "heated anger" (*harah*) by way of a pun.[111] Thus, the words used to describe the baker's dream contain the necessary "ingredients" to suggest Pharaoh's heated response.[112] In addition, Joseph punfully incorporates the baker's description of the birds eating bread "from off of me" (*me'alay*) into his antanaclastic[113] interpretation: "In three days Pharaoh will lift up your head [too], [but] *from off of you* [*nasa' par'oh et r'ôshka me'aleka*]" (40:19). Three days later he was promptly beheaded.

In Gen.41:1–7 Pharaoh has two dreams that Joseph interprets identically (41:25–26). In the first, Pharaoh stood by the Nile, from which seven healthy cows emerged and grazed on reeds. Shortly afterward, seven starving cows arose from the Nile and devoured the healthier animals on the riverbank. In the second, seven ears of healthy grain grew on a single stalk and, like the healthy cows, were eaten by seven heat-scorched ears. Unable to locate a dream interpreter who could interpret his mysterious experience, Pharaoh called upon Joseph who interprets:

> The seven healthy cows are seven [*sheba'*] years, and the seven [*sheba'*] healthy ears are seven [*sheba'*] years; it is the same dream. The seven [*sheba'*] lean and ugly cows that followed are seven [*sheba'*] years, as are also the seven [*sheba'*] empty ears scorched by the east wind; they are seven [*sheba'*] years of famine . . . Immediately ahead are seven [*sheba'*] years of great abundance [*saba'*] in the land of Egypt. After them will come seven [*sheba'*] years of famine, and all the abundance in the land of Egypt will be forgotten. . . . As for Pharaoh having the same dream twice, it means that the matter has been determined by God, and that God will soon carry it out (41:26–32).

Here again Joseph exploits the metaphorical range and multiple meanings of the words in Pharaoh's description. As E. Lowenthal observes, the healthy cows, like the full ears, "are not only metaphors for bounty (as lean cows and ears stand for famine), but are 'scissors symbols' for the annual 'plowing and harvesting' . . ."[114] Seven agricultural cycles, therefore, represent seven years. Similarly, the sequence in which withered ears arose "after" (*'aharêhem*) the full ears (Gen.41:23) suggests a temporal nuance that Joseph espies: "After them (*'aharêhen*) will come seven years of famine . . ." (Gen. 41:30). Note also punning relationship between "abundance" (*saba'*) and "seven" (*sheba'*),[115] a type of play found in later rabbinic dream interpretation.[116] As Joseph states in 41:29: "Immediately ahead are seven (*sheba'*) years of great abundance (*saba'*) in all the land of Egypt."

In Judges 7 Gideon overhears an enemy soldier recount his dream and another interpret: "'Listen,' he was saying, 'I had this dream, [in it] there was a moldy loaf of barley [*tselil lehem she'orim*] whirling through the Midianite camp. It came to the tent and struck it, and it fell; it turned it upside down, and the tent collapsed'" (Judg. 7:13). Immediately afterward, the other soldier interprets: "That can only mean the sword of the Israelite Gideon, son of Joash. God is delivering Midian and the entire camp into his hands" (Judg. 7:14). Several puns in the words used to describe the dream inform the interpreter. First is the word *tselil* which means "moldy, stale," and "tingling sound" as in "terrifying (tingling) news" (e.g., 1 Sam. 3:11, 2 Kings 21:12, Jer. 19:3, Hab. 3:16). Second is the expression "loaf of barley" (*lehem she'orim*), which suggests "fighter in the gates" (*lahem she'arim*) as found just prior (Judg. 5:8).

Edifying the meaning of the dream is Judg. 7:15, which tells us that Gideon derived faith from its interpretation. The rare word used for "interpretation" (*sheber*) fits the dream well since it usually means "grain" (e.g., Gen.42:1) or "battle" (e.g., Jer. 50:22). Moreover, when Gideon raids the Midianite camp, the text describes the battle in a way that recalls the dream. Gideon and his troops smash the jars that contained their concealed torches and shout "A sword for Yahweh and for Gideon!" (7:18–20). Here the verb meaning "smash" (*shabar*) punfully recalls the "interpretation" (*sheber*).

Like Joseph and the savvy soldier, Daniel also shows a talent for dream interpretation. I refer now to Nebuchadnezzar's secret dream in Daniel 2, in which the king sees a bright colossal statue whose head was of gold, breast and arms of silver, belly and thighs of bronze, legs of iron, and feet and toes of iron and clay. All at once, a stone struck the feet of clay and iron, destroying the statue. Apparently none of the king's mantic experts could interpret the dream, because the king refused to tell it to them (Dan. 2:10, 2:27).[117] This does not stop Daniel, however, whom the text calls a "chief magician" (4:6) equipped with "knowledge and skill in all writings and wisdom" and an "understanding of visions and dreams of all kinds" (1:17).

Scholars have long proposed that the Book of Daniel is steeped in ancient Near Eastern mantic traditions.[118] Evidence for this view again comes from the punning hermeneutic employed in the dream's decipherment. The words used to describe the king's dream, especially the head of gold and feet of mixed clay and iron, become crucial to the Daniel's interpretive strategy. Note how Daniel opens his interpretation by equating the "head" (*r'ôsh*) of the statue and the king as "head" (*r'ôsh*) of his kingdom. Daniel also plays on the word *'erab* "mix": "You saw iron mixed [*mé'arab*] with clay; this means they [the nations[shall intermingle [*mit'arbin*] with the offspring of men, but shall not hold together, just as iron does not mix [*mit'arab*] with clay" (2:43).[119] Additional wordplays inform Daniel's interpretation, but I shall conclude with just one more. Daniel interprets the hurling stone that became a "great mountain" (*tûr rab*) (2:35) as God (2:44). The Hebrew reflection of Aramaic "mountain" (*tûr*) is *tsûr* "rock," a frequent metaphor for the divine presence (e.g., Num. 20:8, Deut. 32:4, Ps. 31:3).[120]

It should be clear by now that, despite their obvious cultural and theological differences, Mesopotamia and Israel share a great deal in common with respect to dreams and their interpretations. These parallels, both in details and in conceptual framework, when used with caution, help to clarify the mantological social context of dreams and prophetic speech in ancient Israel. With reference to the ubiquity of puns in symbolic dream texts, both the Mesopotamian and biblical texts demonstrate that the function of punning lies in performative divinatory hermenea rather than rhetoric and style, hermenea that are informed by a religious worldview in which the divine principle of the law of retribution is mediated through the spoken and written word. Whether a mantic social context lies behind the production of biblical texts remains debatable, but the parallels with Mesopotamia are suggestive. M. Fishbane concurs:

> The international character and style of our biblical exegetical materials were undoubtedly due, in large part, to the residency of local experts in mantology in different royal courts, where they both learned new techniques and shared professional information. Indeed, some verification for this hypothesis can be seen in the great formal impact which Mesopotamian oneiromancy had upon Egyptian practices, and in the recorded presence of an Egyptian dream interpreter (*hry tp*) in the Mesopotamian court (called *hardibi*) from the seventh century. Moreover, it should not be overlooked that both Joseph and Daniel performed their oneiromantic services in foreign courts, where they grew up, having been transported to Egypt and Mesopotamia respectively during periods of mass population migrations (drought and exile).[121]

The Mesopotamian parallels also demonstrate that we cannot fully appreciate Israelite references to dreams without examining their ideological contexts. Such a context is especially helpful when examining references to dreams in the Bible's prophetic corpus, to which I now turn. Unlike the stories of Abraham, Jacob, Joseph, Gideon, and Daniel, the Bible's prophetic texts reference historical events and figures, and while not devoid of (sometimes incongruent) ideological agendas, they allow us to situate them more concretely in history. What they tell us about changing Israelite attitudes toward dreams is fascinating

✦ ✦ ✦

With the rise of classical prophecy in the eighth century B.C.E., Israelite attitudes toward dreams as reliable modes of divine discourse begin to divide into two camps: those who view dreams as unreliable or unacceptable methods of divine revelation (as opposed to more direct auditory modes) and those who do not. Encapsulating the formative stage of this development is Num. 12:6–8, an early passage that affirms Moses' role as a paradigmatic prophet. "When a prophet of Yahweh arises among you, I make myself known to him in a vision, I speak with him in a dream. Not so with my servant Moses; he is trusted throughout my household. With him I speak mouth to mouth, plainly and not in riddles . . ."[122] Although the verse sees dreams and visions as a less direct form of divine communication and, thus, as more suspicious, it does not delegitimize them, for they still embody the prophetic call to Yahwism.[123] Sweek comments: "The text elevates the principal representative figure of the theocratic rule associated with the center and with sacerdotal institutions, above the contemporary divining professional."[124]

Coinciding with this development is a changing attitude toward prophecy as a cultural institution, a change that must understood in the light of the growing Assyrian political, military, and presumably cultural dominance of the period. It is during this time that aspirations for political independence are reflected in the nature of Israelite prophecy, specifically in the form of legislation that defines sanctioned (Israelite and direct) forms of access to the divine from unsanctioned (foreign and indirect) forms.

> Let no one be found among you who consigns his son or daughter to fire, or who is an augur, a soothsayer, a diviner, a sorcerer, one who casts spells, or one who consults ghosts or familiar spirits, or who consults the dead . . . Yahweh your God will raise up for you a prophet from among your own people, like myself; him shall you heed (Deut. 18:10–11, 15).

Dream interpretation, though representing an indirect form of divine communication, was not grouped with the other mantic arts, but rather was similarly defined along national borders.

> If there appears among you a prophet or dream-diviner and he gives you a sign or portent, saying "Let us follow and worship another god"—whom you have not known—even if the sign or portent that he named to you comes true, do not heed the words of the prophet or dream diviner. For Yahweh your God is testing you . . . (Deut. 13:2–4)

In the following centuries, the auditory form of prophecy increasingly eclipsed dream interpretation as the legitimate mode of divine access (see, e.g., Isa. 65:3–4),[125] but it did not do so entirely. For, as several biblical passages attest, dream interpretation continued to serve a productive social function in Israel,[126] as it did in times past (e.g., 1 Sam. 28:6), even if the interpreters we hear about were not to be trusted. The prophet

Jeremiah thunders against dream professionals who falsify claims of divine inspiration (Jer. 23:25–32, 27:9–10, 29:8–9), and the later prophet Zechariah harangues dreamers who speak lies and console with allusions (Zech. 10:2). They do not, I underscore, speak against dreams as tools of divine revelation, only against those who use dreams dishonestly. A similar development occurs with regard to attitudes toward "visions," which a few prophets (e.g., Isaiah, Micah, and Ezekiel) view with suspicion when announced by figures whom they do not trust (e.g., Ezek. 13:6–9, 13:23, 21:34, 22:28).

Such pronouncements reflect a growing tension between various competing prophetic groups, each vying for influence and delegitimizing the other, thereby positioning itself as an authoritative mediator of Yahweh's word. Whether this development represents a negative reaction on behalf of the sanctioned authorities to direct or indirect Mesopotamian influence (as asserted in Isa. 2:6) or whether such prophetic indictments against oneiromancy are merely polemical tools of self-identity (as found also in Assyria)[127] we cannot be sure, but one thing is certain—the trend did not last. For when prophecy as a cultural institution went into gradual decline (after the fifth century B.C.E.), especially under Hellenistic influence, positive views toward dreams resurfaced. Hence, the positive and late apocalyptic views in the Book of Daniel and in Joel 3:1: "After that I will pour out my spirit on all flesh, your sons and daughters will prophesy; your old men shall dream dreams, and your young men shall see visions."

This remarkable historical resilience attests to the influence and appeal of ancient Mesopotamian intellectual thought. Its impact was indeed geographically and chronologically pervasive. Not only do we find evidence of Mesopotamian influence in early Greek and Indian sources,[128] but the positive attitude toward mantic dreams appears in apocryphal writings (e.g., 2 Macc. 15:11–16), in the New Testament, and in the works of Philo and Josephus. Eventually Hellenistic oneiromancy, itself heir to Mesopotamian traditions, would play a role, along with the biblical texts and native Mesopotamian practices, in shaping attitudes toward dreams in later Jewish[129] and Islamic communities.[130] Later still, these same sources would come to have a profound impact on the development of modern scientific approaches to dreams.[131] Such is the cultural legacy of ancient Mesopotamia.

Notes

1. Initial research focused on the Bible and Talmud. See, e.g., Kristianpoller (1923); Guillaume (1938); Ehrlich (1953); Resch (1964); Davies (1969); Trachtenberg (1974); Walter (1974); Oppenheim (1956, 1966).
2. Oppenheim (1969, 1974) and more recently Butler (1998).
3. Husser (1999), published originally as "Songe," in *Supplément au dictionnaire de la Bible* XII (Paris: Letouzey et Ané, 1996). See also Caquot (1959); Husser (1994).
4. Representative examples include Cryer (1994); Jeffers (1996); Sweek (1996); Bulkeley (1993).
5. E.g., psychoanalytic approaches. See Gnuse (1984), pp. 57–59; Husser (1999), pp. 96–99; Bulkeley (1993); and the still-valid reservations of Oppenheim (1956), p. 185. Purely literary approaches also have not met with success. See Sweek (1996).
6. Hittite dreams (and those mentioned in other Syro-Canaanite sources) fall outside the scope of this chapter. For these see Oppenheim (1956); Vieyra (1959); Husser (1999); Kammenhuber (1976); Frantz-Szabó (1995).
7. Oppenheim (1956), p. 186. The typology was proposed first by Artemidorus of Daldis (ca. 2nd century C.E.). See Daldianus, *Oneirocritica* (1975); Husser (1999), p. 101.

8. Moreover, the cultural context of the dream accounts makes it difficult to distinguish mantic elements from non-mantic elements. The proposed dichotomy often rests on implicit assumptions about sanctioned and unsanctioned modes of divine communication. Husser (1999), pp. 139–154, e.g., suggests that some of the prophets cultivated different types of oneiric experience than those against which they pronounced judgment.
9. The Akkadian word *ittu*. The Egyptian language similarly employs the word *teyet* for an "alphabetic letter" or a "sculpted image," as does biblical Hebrew, which uses *'ôt* for both "visual omen" and "alphabetic letter."
10. Assyrian kings appear to have preferred Egyptian oneirocritics over native experts. See Oppenheim (1956), p. 238.
11. Sumerian is a non-allied agglutinative language written in cuneiform script that was spoken in southern Mesopotamia beginning about 3300 B.C.E., and kept alive with diminished success in the scribal academies to ca. 1700 B.C.E., after which time Akkadian, an East Semitic language, gradually replaced it. Akkadian is comprised of two major dialects: Babylonian, the southern dialect, and Assyrian, the northern dialect. Some add here a third dialect, Old Akkadian (ca. 2500–2100 B.C.E.) and a fourth, Standard Babylonian, which is a literary dialect used in both Babylon and Assyria.
12. For a translation see Jerrold S. Cooper, *Presargonic Inscriptions,* (Sumerian and Akkadian Royal Inscriptions, 1 [New Haven: American Oriental Society, 1986], pp. 33–39. For a survey of Sumerian dream texts, see Falkenstein (1966).
13. Noegel (1993), especially pp. 50–52.
14. Also in the Greek world, e.g., Agamemnon's dream in *Iliad* 2:6ff.
15. For an accessible treatment of Ningirsu (and other Mesopotamian deities mentioned in this article), see Jeremy Black and Anthony Green, *Gods, Demons and Symbols of Ancient Mesopotamia* (Austin: University of Texas Press, 1992), p. 138.
16. Harriet Crawford, *Sumer and the Sumerians* (Cambridge: Cambridge University Press, 1991), p. 173.
17. For provisional edition and translation of only the relevant portion, see Vanstiphout (1998), pp. 397–412.
18. On this figure see below.
19. Translation by Vanstiphout (1998), p. 399. Italics are original.
20. Vanstiphout (1998), p. 402.
21. Cf., Babylonian Talmud, Berakhot 55a: "A dream that is not interpreted is like a letter that is not read."
22. Translation by J. S. Cooper and W. Heimpel, "The Sumerian Sargon Legend," *Journal of the American Oriental Society* 103 (1983), 67–82.
23. Husser (1999), p. 39, observes that the dream poses difficulties for the message dream typology since it "contains a clear visual message that does not require interpretation."
24. Sweek (1996), p. 86.
25. There also exists a seventh-century B.C.E. account known as the "Vision of Kumma," which I omit for reasons of space. See von Soden (1936); Sweek (1996), pp. 109–111.
26. Oppenheim (1956), pp. 249–250.
27. Ibid.
28. Ibid.
29. See also Penelope's dream in *Odyssey* 19 and the Babylonian Talmud, Berakhot 55b. In a dream ritual text from Assur we also find: "If he saw a dream within a dream, and he interpreted whatever was favorable or able to be interpreted—[The dream] will not [affect him] for good or evil." Butler (1998), p. 115.
30. For an edition and translation, see W. G. Lambert, *Babylonian Wisdom Literature* (Winona Lake, IN: Eisenbrauns, 1996), pp. 21–62.
31. Butler (1998), p. 57, suggests that dreams affect the healing of the dreamer. On the medical dimension of dreams, see below.

32. Benjamin Foster, "On Authorship in Akkadian Literature," *Annali* 51 (1991): 17–32.
33. For an edition and translation, see Luigi Cagni, *L'epopea di Erra* (Istituto di Studi del Vicino Oriente, Roma, 1969); *The Poem of Erra* (SAN. Malibu: Undena, 1977).
34. Sasson (1983), pp. 283–293.
35. Sweek (1996), pp. 139–140.
36. Translation by Oppenheim (1956), p. 250.
37. For a translation see Andrew George, *The Epic of Gilgamesh* (New York: Barnes and Noble, 1999).
38. Hittite is an Indo-European language written in the cuneiform script known primarily from the region of Anatolia. The Hittites ruled that region from the 17th to 13th centuries B.C.E. For a close study of the redactional history of the epic, see Tigay (1982).
39. Oppenheim (1956), p. 207, concurs: "This clearly means that the message of warning . . . was not given in an immediately understandable terms but rather in a 'symbolic' way."
40. For an edition and translation, see E. Jan Wilson, *The Cylinders of Gudea* (*Alter Orient und Altes Testament,* 244) (Neukirchen-Vluyn: Neukirchener Verlag, 1996).
41. A testament to the belief that atmospheric phenomenon can influence dreams.
42. Excerpted translation by Th. Jacobsen, *The Harps That Once . . . Sumerian Poetry in Translation* (New Haven: Yale University Press, 1987), pp. 30–31.
43. Butler (1998), p. 18, opts here for the term "symbolic-message" dreams because "these dreams are really a sub-category of message dreams."
44. Translation by Sasson (1983), pp. 283–293.
45. See J.-R. Kupper, "La Date des *Shakkanakku* de Mari," *Revue d'assuriologie et d'archeologie orientale* 65 (1971), 118, n. 3.
46. There are additional elements of ambiguity, which I omit here for reasons of space.
47. Sasson (1983), p. 289.
48. Ulla Jeyes, *Old Babylonian Extispicy: Omen Texts in the British Museum* (Istanbul: Nederlands Historisch-Archaeologisch Instituut Te Istanbul, 1989), p. 35.
49. I shall limit the discussion to just two examples from the Old Babylonian version (ca. 2000 B.C.E.), although my remarks apply to the Assyrian and Standard Babylonian versions as well. See Noegel (forthcoming). I also will not touch on the dream sequences as found in the Sumerian stories "Gilgamesh and the Land of the Living" and "The Death of Gilgamesh." For a translation, see Pritchard (1950), pp. 47–50.
50. The translation, with some modification, is by Dalley (1989), pp. 136–137. Contra Bulkeley (1993), the text does not clarify these dreams as nightmares.
51. Dalley (1989), p. 126, notes a similar pun on the word *tseri* in Gilg I:iv, 20 when we are told that Enkidu "spread open her [the harlot's] garments, and lay upon (*tseri*) her."
52. Kilmer (1982), p. 128, has shown that *kitsru* can be read as *kezru,* "curly-haired male prostitute," which alludes to the erotic relationship between Enkidu and Gilgamesh, Enkidu's relationship with a "prostitute," and the mention of Enkidu as "hairy" (II:iii,23). The word "axe" (*hatsinnu*) puns on "male servant of Ishtar" (*assinu*). See Kilmer (1982), pp. 128–132. Gilgamesh recalls that he put the axe on his side (*ahu*), a phrase that also can be read "I treated it as my friend (lit. brother)," since *ahu,* means both "side" and "brother." See Dalley (1989), p. 152, n. 4. Gilgamesh later calls Enkidu "the axe of my side (*hatsin ahiya*), the trust of my hand" (VIII:ii,4).
53. Noegel (1991).
54. Carl Frank, "Zu den Wortspeilen *kukku* und *kibāti* in Gilg. Ep. XI," *ZA* 36 (1925), 216; Noegel (1997).
55. Alasdair Livingstone, *Mystical and Mythological Explanatory Works of Assyrian and Babylonian Scholars* (Oxford: Clarendon Press, 1986); Parpola (1993), p. 57.
56. "I will reveal to you, O Gilgamesh, hidden words (*amat nitsirti*), and I will tell you the secrets (*pirishtu*) of the gods" (XI:9, 266); "It was not I who disclosed the secret (*pirishtu*)

of the great gods. I caused Atra-hasis to examine a dream, and he perceived the secret (*pirishtu*) of the gods" (XI:186–187).

57. This connection finds support in the archaeological record, which bolsters the role that practicing priests had through the Mediterranean world in controlling a variety of textual materials including literary, magical, and lexical texts. See Jacques-Claude Courtois, "La maison du prêtre aux modèles de poumon et de foies d'Ugarit," *Ugaritica* 6 (1969): 91–119; D. Arnaud, *Emar. Recherches au pays d'Astarta VI/3: Textes sumériens et accadiens* (Paris: Editions Recherche sur les Civilisations, 1985/87); W. G. Lambert, "The Sultantepe Tablets," *Revue d'assyriologie et d'archeologie orientale* 3 (1959): 121–124; P. Walcot, *Hesiod and the Near East* (Cardiff: University of Wales Press, 1966); Antoine Cavigneaux, "A Scholar's Library in Meturan? With an Edition of the Tablet H 72 (Textes de Tell Haddad VII)," in Abusch and van der Toorn (1998), pp. 251–273. Butler (1998), p. 122, also notes that a tablet of dream omens was found in Assur in the home of an exorcist (O. Pedersén, *Archives and Libraries in the City of Assur: A Survey of the Material from German Excavations, Part 2* [Acta Universitatis Upsaliensis, Studia Semitica Upsaliensia 8] [Stockholm, Sweden: Uppsala University, 1986], n4, p. 530).
58. The text uses the verb *bâru,* a lexeme often connected with the activities of "seers" (*bārû*). James R. Davila, "The Flood Hero as King and Priest," *Journal of Near Eastern Studies* 54 (1995), 204–205, 213, refers to Utnapishtim as a *shā'ilu*. See below for an explanation of these terms.
59. On the *realia* reflected in Utnapishtim's rituals, see Butler (1998), p. 237. Butler (p. 226) also notes the cultic significance of the reed hut (*kikkishu*) through which Ea speaks to Utnapishtim. In the Atrahasis Epic, the flood hero offers a *mashshakku,* which is the typical offering of the "dream interpreter" (*shā'ilu*).
60. An unfortunate misnomer since it was written on clay tablets long before the invention of the book. The Mesopotamians referred to the series as *Zaqīqu*. On this term see below. For an edition and translation see Oppenheim (1956), pp. 256–344. An earlier collection of Babylonian dream omens dating to ca. 1700 B.C.E. also exists, but it is not as complete as the *Dream Book* and does not refer explicitly to dreams, although the apodoses make it clear that dreaming is implied. Like the compendium, it points to the importance of recognizing the religious cosmology in which Mesopotamian divinatory conceptions are rooted. One omen demonstrates: "If a man while he sleeps (dreams that) the town falls again and again upon him, and he groans and no one hears him: the (protective spirits) Lamassu and Shedu are attached to this man's body." Interestingly, it is our only Mesopotamian description of a nightmare, although frightening dreams are referenced elsewhere. See F. Köcher and A. Leo Oppenheim, "The Old-Babylonian Omen Text VAT 7525," *Archiv für Orientforschung* 18 (1957–1958), 62–77, quotation on p. 67.
61. Depending on which Mesopotamian culture one discusses, one finds various terms for describing dreams. In Sumerian we find MA.MÚ "God(dess) Dream," identified sometimes as a male god of dreams and in later scribal traditions as the daughter of the sun god Shamash. Another term is AN.ZA.QAR (sometimes written as AN.ZAG.GAR.RA), which appears to be an Akkadian loan into Sumerian, and whose meaning suggests a tower-like structure, a fact that has led some scholars to link it to the biblical pillar stone known as a *matsebah* (cf. the stone in Genesis 28 erected after a dream. See below.). Like the Sumerian MA.MÚ, the Akkadian *Zaqīqu* is known also as a dream god (as found in the invocation discussed above), perhaps originally a dream demon. The Akkadian root *zâqu* appears in conjunction with "breezes," "winds," and demons who enter homes through wall cracks, and for ghosts of the deceased. Such associations have been compared to ancient Greek conceptions as found in the Homeric epics. See Oppenheim (1956), pp. 225, 232–233, 235–236. In Akkadian we find several other words from "dream," including *shuttu* "sleep," *iltu* also "sleep" (or perhaps "pollution [in a dream]), *munattu* "early morning sleep, day dream," and the more poetic *tabrit mushi* "vision of the night."

62. Two Egyptian dream manuals of different types exist, one dating to ca. 1290 B.C.E. and the other to the Greco-Roman period. The Assyrian compendium more closely resembles the latter (Demotic) dream manual, which led Oppenheim (1956), p. 245, to aver a degree of Mesopotamian influence.
63. The remark by Larsen (1987), pp. 209–212, refers to lexical lists. But see also Sweek (1996), pp. 144–147.
64. Only one dream omen pertains to a king. See Oppenheim (1956), p. 239.
65. Ibid., p. 289.
66. Oppenheim (1956), p. 241, suggests that such punning is rare, but until recently no systematic attempt has been made to study the compendium's employment of hermeneutical punning. The evidence will appear in Noegel (forthcoming).
67. Noegel (1995).
68. Punning is a ubiquitous feature in magic texts generally. See, e.g., Walter Farber, "Associative Magic: Some Rituals, Word Plays, and Philology," *Journal of the American Oriental Society* 106 (1986), 447–449; Piotr Michalowski, "Carminative Magic: Towards an Understanding of Sumerian Poetics," *Zeitschrift fur Assyrologie* 71 (1981), pp. 1–18; Victor Avigdor Hurowitz, "Alliterative Allusions, Rebus Writing, and Paronomastic Punishment: Some Aspects of Word Play in Akkadian Literature," in Noegel (2000), pp. 63–87; Sheldon W. Greaves, "Ominous Homophony and Portentous Puns in Akkadian Omens," in Noegel (2000), pp. 103–113.
69. Sigmund Freud, *The Interpretation of Dreams,* trans. A. A. Brill (London: George Allen & Unwin Ltd., 1927), p. 315.
70. For a recent assessment of the impact of Jewish traditions on Freud, see Frieden (1990), pp. 47–93, 117–119; also Roback (1929), pp. 162–165; Grinstein (1968).
71. Daldianus, *Oneirocritica.* For a connection between rabbinic and Greek dream interpretive techniques, see Saul Lieberman, *Hellenism in Jewish Palestine* (New York: Jewish Theological Seminary of America, [1950]; reprinted 1994), p. 71, who cites Heinrich Lewy, "Zu dem Traumbuche des Artemidoros," *Rheinisches Museum für Philologie, Geschichte und griechische Philosophie* 48 (1893): 398–419.
72. It is a curious footnote of scholarship that in his seminal work on the Demotic *Dream Book,* Aksel Volten, *Demotische Traumdeutung (Pap. Carslberg XIII und XIV Verso),* Analecta Aegyptiaca, 3 (Copenhagen: Einar Munsgaard, 1942), p. 60, n. 2, remarked: "word play is a feature of dream interpretation for all peoples (lit. "Das Wortspiel ist bei allen Völkern ein Charakteristikum für die Traumdeutung"), a remark that Oppenheim (1956), p. 241, appears to have accepted. Nevertheless, this assumption is problematic. Evidence suggests that both the Demotic *Dream Book* and the later rabbinic materials represent Mesopotamian influence. There also are no extant non-Near Eastern dream manuals contemporaneous with the materials we have examined, and thus we have nothing to which we might compare our texts for the presence of punning. Even the Greek dream manual of Aremidorus shows signs of interregional influence. See Noegel (forthcoming). Moreover, later Byzantine sources do not aid comparative analysis since they represent the influence of Greek and Arabic dream manuals (both the legacy of ancient Mesopotamia). Finally, as far as I have been able to determine, the punning strategy is not employed by dream interpreters in traditional societies in modern Africa, where one might look for analogs or survivals of this technique. See, e.g., M. C. Jedrej, and Rosalind Shaw, eds., *Dreaming, Religion and Society in Africa* (Leiden: E. J. Brill, 1992). Thus, Volten's assertion concerning the universality of the punning oneirocritic strategy cannot be supported by the evidence. I suspect (and this brings the topic full circle) that on this point he was influenced by Freud!
73. Stanley J. Tambiah, "The Magical Power of Words," *Man* 3 (1968), 175–208; F. L. Moriarty, "Word as Power in the Ancient Near East," in H. N. Bream et al, eds., *A Light Unto My Path: Old Testament Studies in Honor of J. M. Myers* (Philadelphia: Temple University,

1974), pp. 345–362; I. Rabinowitz, *A Witness Forever: Ancient Israel's Perception of Literature and the Resultant Hebrew Bible* (Bethesda, MD: CDL Press, 1993); Sheldon W. Greaves, *The Power of the Word in the Ancient Near East* (Ph.D. diss., University of California, Berkeley, 1996).

74. Georges Contenau, *Everyday Life in Babylon and Assyria* (London: Edward Arnold, 1955), p. 164.
75. See Butler (1998), p. 36.
76. Francesca Rochberg, "Empiricism in Babylonian Omen Texts and the Classification of Mesopotamian Divination as Science," *Journal of the American Oriental Society* 119 (1999): 559–569.
77. Compare the remark of Shaul Shaked, "The Poetics of Spells: Language and Structure in Aramaic Incantations of Late Antiquity. 1: The Divorce Formula and its Ramifications," in Abusch and van der Toorn (1998), p. 174, with respect to the language of magic: "spells are like legal documents, . . . in that they have the tendency to use formulaic language, and that the language they use creates, by its mere utterance, a new legal situation."
78. Jean Bottéro, *Mesopotamia: Writing, Reasoning, and the Gods* (Chicago: University of Chicago Press, 1992), p. 121.
79. Oneiromancy was practiced at least eight hundred years earlier. See Butler (1998), p. 97. On the complex history of ritual texts, see Oppenheim (1956), pp. 295–307.
80. The gods Gibil, Husku, Shamash, Sin, Ea, or Marduk. See Butler (1998), p. 135.
81. See Oppenheim (1956), p. 239.
82. Ibid., p. 300.
83. At least one medical text even contains a prescription for dream content, and the *Dream Book* itself is mentioned by name in two different catalogs, one belonging to an exorcist and the other to a doctor. See Butler (1998), p. 115. See, also Bottéro (1974), pp. 88–89, 188–190. Daldianus, *Oneirocritica* (1975), p. 195, also notes the connection between dream interpretation and medical prescriptions.
84. Butler (1998), p. 23.
85. da Silva (1993); Butler (1998), pp. 28, 62.
86. As described also in the Epic of Gilgamesh IV.1.4–32'. See Husser (1999), 49.
87. Butler (1998), pp. 123–124. Dreams experienced just before morning appear to have been viewed as more prophetic.
88. The Mesopotamian belief in the medicinal properties of dream interpretation influenced later Talmudic traditions, which, according to Monford Harris, *Studies in Jewish Dream Interpretation* (Northvale, NJ.: Jason Aronson, 1994), especially pp. 29–32, pervaded rabbinic writings well into the 13th century C.E.
89. Parpola (1993), p. 52.
90. Gadd (1966), pp. 21–34; Parpola (1993), pp. 47–59; Nissenen (2000), p. 108. On the relationship between dreams and sacrifice see Bottéro (1974), p. 112; Erle Leichty, "Ritual, 'Sacrifice,' and Divination in Mesopotamia," in Quaegebeur (1993), pp. 237–238. Reiner (1995), pp. 15, 72, cites texts that invoke the power of stars in dream oracles. For these figures in the context of ancient medicine, see Avalos (1995), pp. 157–172; Scurlock (1998); Oppenheim (1956), pp. 225–226; G. Castellino, "Rituals and Prayers against 'Appearing Ghosts,'" *Orientalia* 24 (1955): 240–274; Bottéro (1974), p. 97; Miranda Bayliss, "The Cult of Dead Kin in Assyria and Babylonia," *Iraq* 35 (1973): 115–125. On the relationship between Mesopotamian and Talmudic necromancy, see Irving L. Finkel, "Necromancy in Ancient Mesopotamia," *Archiv für Orientforschung* 29 (1983): 14–15.
91. The difficulty distinguishing prayers from incantations is a case in point. See, e.g., Mark E. Cohen, "The Incantation-Hymn: Incantation or Hymn?" *Journal of the American Oriental Society* 95 (1975), 592–611.
92. Bottéro (1974), p. 129, n. 7.

93. W. G. Lambert, "The Qualifications of Babylonian Diviners," in Stefan M. Maul, ed., *Fesschrift für Rykle Borger zu seinem 65. Geburtstag am 24. Mai 1994,* Cuneiform Monographs, 10 (Gronigen: Styx, 1998), pp. 141–158.
94. Although the connection could be due to the fact that both practices privilege access to liminal space. In the cuneiform archive found at Amarna in central Egypt (ca. 1350 B.C.E.) the *shā'ilu* is a diviner of birds.
95. In fact, the earliest glyptic evidence (ca. 24th century B.C.E.) for dream interpretation depicts a woman. See J. M. Asher-Greve, "The Oldest Female Oneiromancer," in J. -M. Durand, ed., *La femme dans le proche-orient antique,* XXXIIIe rencontre assyriologique internationale (Paris: Recherches sur les civilisations, 1987), pp. 27–32. The only female recipient of a message dream is a Hittite queen. See Oppenheim (1956), p. 197. Others typically are important figures (kings and priests), except at Mari, where there exist no royal message dreams and where nine out of seventeen individuals whose dreams are mentioned are female. Neo-Assyrian dream narratives report only the experiences of men. See Butler (1998), p. 17.
96. Contra Oppenheim (1956), p. 190, whose view is adopted by Husser (1999), pp. 37–38, Butler (1998), p. 19, does not agree that women experienced symbolic dreams more often than men, but rather sees the evidence as roughly equally distributed between men and women. Husser (1999), pp. 170–171, also asserts that the distinction between the *bārû* and the *shā'ilu* rests in the degree of training, i.e., the former is highly trained and familiar with the pertinent scholarly compendia and divinatory lore, whereas the latter relies less on deductive practices and more on intuition. This distinction is difficult to maintain given the paucity of evidence. As Ivan Starr, *The Rituals of the Diviner,* Bibliotheca Mesopotamica, 12 (Malibu, CA: Udena, 1983), p. 7, remarks: "It is interesting to note that both in the literary and popular idiom, the dream interpreter (*shā'ilu/shā'iltu*) and the diviner (*bārû*) often appear side by side."
97. Butler (1998), p. 120.
98. For more than a century, Bible scholarship has proposed a complex redactional history for the biblical text. This source-critical theory, known commonly as the Graf-Wellhausen hypothesis, while once dominant in biblical studies, has largely given way to other methodological approaches, many of which reject the criteria upon which the hypothesis is based and which instead opt to see the text as holistically as possible, regardless of which sources underlie the text as we have it. Thus, for some scholars (e.g., Gnuse [1984], Husser [1999]), to understand biblical dream narratives, one must understand the proposed compositional history of the text as well, whereas for others, including this writer, such an approach is less useful.
99. Husser (1999), pp. 103–104.
100. Whereas a polytheist worships and believes in the existence of many gods, and a monotheist worships and believes in only one, a monolatrist worships one god but believes in the existence of many. Such is the religious system of ancient Israel for much of its history.
101. Husser (1999), p. 102, avers that some biblical passages (e.g., Isa. 29:8, Qoh. 5:2, Job 20:8, Ps. 73:20, 126:1) contextualize some dreams as natural as opposed to supernatural. Thus, this distinction signals an increasing desacralization of the phenomenon, one that comes to the fore under the impact of Hellenism in the second century B.C.E. However, the passages in question do not explicitly deny the divine origin of dreams, only the value or perhaps possibility of interpreting them (accurately) for the dreamer. Perhaps, then, the change testifies to an increasing skepticism with regard to the dream interpretation as a cultic institution.
102. See, e.g., Delbert R. Hillers, "The Effective Simile in Biblical Literature," *Journal of the American Oriental* Society 103 (1983): 181–185; Walter Houston, "What Did the Prophets Think They Were Doing?: Speech Acts and Prophetic Discourse in the Old

Testament," in Robert P. Gordon, ed., *The Place Is Too Small for Us: The Israelite Prophets in Recent Scholarship,* Sources for Biblical and Theological Study, 5 (Winona Lake: Eisenbrauns, 1995), pp. 133–153.

103. See, e.g., Philip J. Nel, "The Talion Principle in Old Testament Narratives," *Journal of Northwest Semitic Languages* 20 (1994), 21–29; Scott B. Noegel, "Drinking Feasts and Deceptive Feats: Jacob and Laban's Double Talk," in Noegel (2000), pp. 163–179.

104. Another conceptual difference is suggested by the Hebrew root for "dream" (*ḥālam*). Cognate evidence shows that the word essentially means "strong," in the sense of "sexually mature" (e.g., Job 39:4, where it is used of beasts). Much has been made of the root's sexual dimension. Husser (1999), p. 88, e.g., sees it deriving more from the notion of penile erection during sleep than from the content of a mature person's dreams. Also used of dreams is "night vision" (*ḥāzôn laylāh*). A third term is "deep sleep" (*tardemāh*) of Yahweh, said, for example, of Adam (Gen. 2:21), Abraham (Gen. 15:12), Jonah (1:5), Daniel (8:8), Saul (1 Sam. 26:12), and Job (4:13, 33:15).

105. For Oppenheim (1956), p. 331, all message dreams derived from incubation rites. Not all scholars agree, and the evidence is often ambiguous. Gnuse (1984), p. 82, summarizes arguments on both sides. Other texts suggested as having origins in incubation practices include: Gen. 15, 28:10–17, 46:1–4; Isa. 65:4, Ps. 3:6, 4:6, 17:5, 63. The oldest clear reference to incubation appears in an early magic incantation from Mari (ca. 2500 B.C.E.). See Bonechi and Durand (1992).

106. The passage presents two difficulties. First, the word usually translated "ladder" (*sullām*) appears only here and must be translated based on cognate evidence. (Akkadian *simmiltu* means "steps of a ziggurat.") The second crux involves why the angels first ascend then descend the steps; one would expect the direction to be just the opposite, since the angels come from the heavens (noted already by Rashi [= Rabbi Shlomo Yitzhaqi], ca. 1040–1105 C.E.).

107. Husser (1999), p. 135, sees this dream as a message dream superimposed by an oneiric vision.

108. See Noegel (1997), pp. 7–17.

109. Some add the sacrifice of Isaac (Genesis 22), based on the Qur'anic parallel (37:100), which states that God commanded Abraham to sacrifice his son in a dream.

110. The relationship between the literary accounts of symbolic dreams and the Assyrian compendium was espied by Richter (1963), who suggested that symbolic dreams derive from the practice of oneiromancy.

111. The idiom meaning "anger" usually requires the use of the word "nose" (*'ap*), and so "nose" is played on the word "baker" (*'oph*), the verb "baked" (*'apāh*), and in the baker's declaration to Joseph in 40:16: "In my dream, similarly (*'ap*), there were three baskets of white bread on my head."

112. This resembles the use of "nose" (*'ap*) in a dream interpretation found in the Babylonian Talmud, Berakhot 56b, in which Bar Kappara reports a dream in which his "nose" (*'ap*) falls off. As Rabbi interprets his dream: "Heated anger (*hārôn 'ap*) has been removed from you."

113. Antanaclasis is a form of wordplay that repeats a word or expression, each time with a different meaning.

114. Eric I. Lowenthal, *The Joseph Narrative in Genesis* (New York: Ktav, 1973), p. 54. Observed already by Ramban (= Rabbi Moses ben Nahman, 1194–1270 C.E.).

115. Noted also by Fishbane (1985), p. 451.

116. The play involves moving the diacritical dot above the Hebrew letter *shin*. Babylonian Talmud, Berachot 57a and Megillah 15b. Found also in Finkel (1963), p. 368.

117. Opinion appears to be divided on whether the king forgot his dream, which, of course, in the Mesopotamian context, would spell disaster. See John J. Collins, *Daniel: A Commentary on the Book of Daniel* (Minneapolis: Fortress Press, 1993), p. 156.

118. Hans-Peter Müller, "Magisch-mantische Weisheit und die Gestalt Daniels," *Vqarit Forschungen* 1 (1969), 79–94; B. A. Mastin, "Wisdom and Daniel," in John Day et al., eds., *Wisdom in Ancient Israel: Essays in Honour of J. A. Emerton* (Cambridge: Cambridge University Press, 1995), p. 166.
119. This root is similarly played on in a dream interpretation, *Yalqut* I, 26a.
120. André LaCoque, *The Book of Daniel,* trans. David Pellauer (Atlanta, GA: John Knox Press, 1979), p. 49.
121. Fishbane (1985), pp. 455–456.
122. Prov. 1:6 states that God's wisdom must be sought in word play and riddles, so perhaps Num. 12:6–8 hints at the punning hermeneutic. Compare Artemidorus' comment that symbolic dreams "are those which disclose their meaning in riddles." See Daldianus (1975), p. 185.
123. Note that, contra Bulkeley (1993), p. 162, no attempt is made to distinguish "the clear dream of the Jews and the 'dark' speech of the Gentile's dreams as a way of illustrating the special relationship of the Jews with God." In fact, the use of divinatory punning in biblical texts suggests that "dark sayings" were quite at home in Israel.
124. Sweek (1996), p 198.
125. Cf., the Septuagint. Isa. 29:7–8 does not, in my view, constitute a negative assessment of dreams, only a poetic metaphor.
126. On suggested social functions, see McDermot (1971), p. 192; Sweek (1996).
127. Nissenen (1996).
128. Gnuse (1984), pp. 42–44; Daldianus (1975); Noegel (forthcoming).
129. Lieberman (1987); Tigay (1983), pp. 169–189; Elman (1998); Geller (2000).
130. E.g., Oberhelman (1991); Lamoreaux (1999).
131. Frieden (1990), pp. 47–93, 117–119.

References

Abusch, T., and Karel van der Toorn, eds., *Mesopotamian Magic: Textual, Historical, and Interpretive Perspectives,* Studies in Ancient Magic and Divination, 1 (Groningen, the Netherlands: Styx, 1998).

Avalos, Hector. *Illness and Health Care in the Ancient Near East: The Role of the Temple in Greece, Mesopotamia, and Israel,* Harvard Semitic Monographs, 54 (Atlanta: Scholars Press, 1995)

Bonechi, M., and J.-M. Durand. "Oniromancie et magie à Mari à l'époque d'Ebla," *Quaderni di Semistica* 18 (1992): 151–159.

Bottéro, Jean. "Symptômes, signes, écritures en Mésopotamie ancienne," in J. P. Vernat et al., eds., *Divination et rationalité* (Paris: Éditions du Seuil, 1974), pp. 70–197.

Bulkeley, Kelly. "The 'Evil' Dream of Gilgamesh: An Interdisciplinary Approach to Dreams in Mythological Texts," in Carol Schreier Rupprecht, ed., *The Dream and the Text: Eassays on Literature and Language* (Albany: State University of New York Press, 1993), pp. 159–177.

Butler, S. A. L. *Mesopotamian Conceptions of Dreams and Dream Rituals,* alter Orient und Altes Testament 258 (Münster: Ugarit-Verlag, 1998).

Caquot, André, "Les songes et leur interprétation selon Canaan et Israël," in *Les songes et leur interpretation,* Sources orientales II (Paris: Editions du Seuil, 1959), pp. 99–124.

Cryer, Frederick. *Divination in Ancient Israel and its Near Eastern Environment: A Socio-Historical Investigation,* Journal for the Study of the Old Testament Sup., 142; (Sheffield: Sheffield Academic Press, 1994).

Daldianus, Artemidorus. *Oneirocritica,* trans. Robert J. White, Noyes Classical Studies (Park Ridge, IL: Noyes Press, 1975).

Dalley, Stephanie. *Myths from Mesopotamia: Creation, the Flood, Gilgamesh, and Others* (Oxford: Oxford University Press, 1989).

Davies, T. Witton. *Magic, Divination, and Demonology among the Hebrews and Their Neighbors* (New York: KTAV, 1969).

Ehrlich, Ernst Ludwig. *Der Traum im Alten Testament,* Beiheft zur Zeitschrift für die Alttestamentliche Wissenschaft, 73 (Berlin: Verlag Alfred Töpelmann, 1953).

Elman, Y. *Dream Interpretation from Classical Jewish Sources by Rabbi Shelomo Almoli* (Hoboken: KTAV Publishing, 1998).

Falkenstein, A. "'Wahrsagung' in der Sumerischen Überlieferung," in D. F. Wendel, ed., *La divination en Mésopotamie ancienne et dans les régions voisines,* XIVe rencontre assyriologique Internationale (Saint-Germain, Paris: Presses Universitaires de France, 1966), pp. 45–68.

Finkel, Asher. "The Pesher of Dreams and Scriptures," *Revue de Qumran* 15 (1963): 357–370.

Fishbane, Michael. *Biblical Interpretation in Ancient Israel* (Oxford: Clarendon Press, 1985).

Frantz-Szabó, Gabriella. "Hittite Witchcraft, Magic, and Divination," in Jack M. Sasson, ed., *Civilizations of the Ancient Near East,* vol. 3 (New York: Scribner, 1995), pp. 2007–2019.

Frieden, Ken. *Freud's Dream of Interpretation* (Albany: State University of New York Press, 1990).

Gadd, C. J. "Some Babylonian Divinatory Methods, and Their Inter-relations," in D. F. Wendel, ed., *La divination en Mésopotamie ancienne et dans les régions voisines,* XIVe rencontre assyriologique internationale (Saint-Germain, Paris: Presses Universitaires de France, 1966), pp. 21–34.

Geller, M. J. "The Survival of Babylonian Wissenschaft in Later Tradition," in Sanno Aro and R. M. Whiting, eds., *The Heirs of Assyria: Proceedings of the Opening Symposium of the Assyrian and Babylonian Intellectual Heritage Project Held in Tvärminne, Finland, October 8–11, 1998,* Melammu Symposia I (Helsinki: Neo-Assyrian Text Corpus Project, 2000), pp. 1–6.

Gnuse, Robert Karl. *The Dream Theophany of Samuel: Its Structure in Relation to Ancient Near Eastern Dreams and Its Theological Significance* (Lanham, MD: University Press of America, 1984).

Grinstein, Alexander. *On Sigmund Freud's Dreams* (Detroit: Wayne State University Press, 1968).

Guillaume, Alfred. *Prophecy and Divination among the Hebrews and Other Semites* (London: Hodder, 1938).

Harris, Monford. *Studies in Jewish Dream Interpretation* (Northvale, NJ: Jason Aronson, 1994).

Husser, Jean-Marie. *Dreams and Dream Narratives in the Biblical World,* Biblical Seminar, 63 (Sheffield, UK: Sheffield Academic Press, 1999).

Husser, Jean-Marie. *Le songe et la parole: Étude sur le rêve et sa fonction dans l'ancien Israël,* Beiheft zur Zeitschrift für die Altestamentliche Wissenschaft, 210 (Berlin: Walter de Gruyter, 1994).

Jedrej, M. C., and Rosalind Shaw, eds. *Dreaming, Religion and Society in Africa* (Leiden: E. J. Brill, 1992).

Jeffers, Ann *Magic and Divination in Ancient Palestine and Syria* (Leiden: E. J. Brill, 1996).

Kammenhuber, Annelies. *Orakelpraxis, Träume, und Vorzeichenschau bei den Hethitern* (Heidelberg: Carl Winter Universitätsverlag, 1976).

Kilmer, Anne Draffkorn. "A Note on an Overlooked Word-Play in the Akkadian Gilgamesh," in G. van Driel et al., eds., *Zikir Shumin: Assyriological Studies Presented to F. R. Kraus on the Occasion of His Seventieth Birthday* (Leiden: E. J. Brill, 1982).

Köcher, F., and A. Leo Oppenheim. "The Old-Babylonian Omen Text VAT 7525," *Archiv für Orientforschung* 18 (1957–1958): 62–77.

Kristianpoller, Alexander. *Monumenta Talmudica. Traum und Traumdeutung* (Wien: Benjamin Harz, 1923).

Lamoreaux, John C. *Dream Interpretation in the Early Medieval Near East* (Ph.D. diss., Duke University, 1999).

Larsen, Mogens Trolle. "The Mesopotamian Lukewarm Mind: Reflections on Science, Divination, and Literacy," in Francesca Rochberg-Halton, ed., *Language, Literature, and History: Philological and Historical Studies Presented to Erica Reiner* (New Haven: American Oriental Society, 1987), pp. 203–225.

Lieberman, Stephen J. "A Mesopotamian Background for the So-Called Aggadic 'Measures' of Biblical Hermeneutics," *Hebrew Union College Annual* 58 (1987): 157–225.

McDermot, Violet. *The Cult of the Seer in the Ancient Middle East* (Berkeley: University of California Press, 1971).

Nissenen, Martti. "Falsche Prophetie in neuassyrischer und deuteronomistischer Darstellung," in Timo Veijola, ed., *Das Deuteronomium und seine Querbeziehungen,* Schriften der Finnischen Exegetischen Gesellschaft, 62 (Göttingen: Vandenhoeck & Ruprecht, 1996), pp. 172–195.

———. "The Socioreligious Role of the Neo-Assyrian Prophets," in Martti Nissenen, ed., *Prophecy in Its Ancient Near Eastern Context: Mesopotamian, Biblical, and Arabian Perspectives,* Society of Biblical Literature Symposium Series, 13 (Atlanta: Society of Biblical Literature, 2000), pp. 235–271.

Noegel, Scott B. "Atbash in Jeremiah and Its Literary Sigificance," *Jewish Biblical Quarterly* 24/2–4 (1996): 82–89, 160–166, 247–250.

———. "Fictional Sumerian Autobiographies," *Journal of the Association of Graduates in Near Eastern Studies* 4 (1993): 46–55.

———. "Fox on the Run: Catch a Lamassu by the Pun," *Nouvelles assyriologiques brèves et utilitaires* 73 (1995): 101–102.

———. "A Janus Parallelism in the Gilgamesh Flood Story," *Acta Sumerologica* 13 (1991): 419–421.

———. *Nocturnal Ciphers: The Allusive Language of Dreams in the Hebrew Bible and Ancient Near Eastern Literature* (forthcoming).

———, ed., *Puns and Pundits: Wordplay in the Hebrew Bible and Ancient Near Eastern Literature* (Bethesda, MD: CDL Press, 2000).

———. "Raining Terror: Another Wordplay Cluster in Gilgamesh Tablet XI (Assyrian Version, ll. 45–47)," *Nouvelles assyriologiques breves et utilitaires* 75 (1997): 39–40.

———. "Sex, Sticks, and the Trickster in Gen. 30:31–43: A New Look at an Old Crux," *Journal of the Ancient Near Eastern Society of Columbia University* 25 (1997): 7–17.

Oberhelman, Steven M. *The Oneirocriticon of Achmet: A Medieval Greek and Arabic Treatise on the Interpretation of Dreams* (Lubbock: Texas Tech University Press, 1991).

Oppenheim, A. Leo "A Babylonian Diviner's Manual," *Journal of the Ancient Near Eastern Society of Columbia University* 33 (1974): 197–220.

———. "New Fragments of the Assyrian Dream-Book," *Iraq* 31 (1969): 153–165.

———. "Perspectives on Mesopotamian Divination," in D. F. Wendel, ed., *La divination en Mésopotamie ancienne et dans les régions voisines,* XIVe rencontre assyriologique internationale (Saint-Germain, Paris: Presses Universitaires de France, 1966), pp. 35–43.

———. *The Interpretation of Dreams in the Ancient Near East: With a Translation of the Assyrian Dream Book,* Transactions of the American Philosophical Society, volume 46/3 (Philadelphia: American Philosophical Society, 1956).

Parpola, Simo. "The Forlorn Scholar," in F. Rochberg-Halton, ed., *Language, Literature, and History: Philological and Historical Studies Presented to Erica Reiner,* American Oriental Series, 67 (New Haven: Yale University Press, 1987), pp. 257–278.

———. "Mesopotamian Astrology and Astronomy as Domains of Mesopotamian 'Wisdom,'" in Hannes D. Galter, ed., *Die Rolle der Astronomie in den Kulteren Mesopotamiens,* Beiträge zum 3, Grazer Morganländischen Symposion (23–27 September 1991) (Graz: GrazCult, 1993), pp. 47–59.

Pritchard, James B. *Ancient Near Eastern Texts Relating to the Old Testament* (Princeton: Princeton University Press, 1950).

Quaegebeur, J., ed., *Ritual and Sacrifice in the Ancient Near East,* Orientalia Lovaniensia Analecta, 55 (Leuven: Uitgeverij Peeters, 1993).

Reiner, Erica. *Astral Magic in Babylonia,* Transactions of the American Philosophical Society, 85/4 (Independence Square, PA: American Philosophical Society, 1995).

Resch, Andreas. *Der Traum im Heilsplan Gottes: Deutung und Bedeutung des Traums im Alten Testament* (Freiburg: Herder, 1964).

Richter, W. "Traum und Traumdeutung im Alten Testament," *Biblische Zeitschrift* 7 (1963): 202–220.

Roback, A. A. *Jewish Influence in Modern Thought* (Cambridge: Sci-Art Publishers, 1929).

Sasson, Jack M. "Mari Dreams," *Journal of the American Oriental Society* 103 (1983): 283–293.

Scurlock, JoAnn. "Physician, Exorcist, Conjurer, Magician: A Tale of Two Healing Professionals," in T. Abusch and Karel van der Toorn, eds., *Mesopotamian Magic: Textual, Historical, and Interpretive Perspectives,* Studies in Ancient Magic and Divination, 1 (Groningen, the Netherlands: Styx, 1998), pp. 69–79.

Silva, A. da. "Dreams as Demonic Experience in Mesopotamia," *Studies on Religion* 22 (1993): 310–310.

Soden, Wolfgang von. "Die Unterweltsvision eines assyrischen Kronprinzen," *Zeitschrift für Assyriologie* 9 (1936): 1–31.

Sweek, Joel. "Dreams of Power from Sumer to Judah: An Essay on the Divinatory Economy of the Ancient Near East," Ph.D. diss., University of Chicago, 1996.

Tigay, Jeffrey H. "An Early Technique of Aggadic Exegesis," in H. Tadmor and M. Weinfeld, eds., *History, Historiography, and Interpretation: Studies in Biblical and Cuneiform Literatures* (Jerusalem: Magnes Press, 1983), pp. 169–189.

———. *The Evolution of the Gilgamesh Epic* (Philadelphia: University of Pennsylvania Press, 1982).

Trachtenberg, Joshua. *Jewish Magic and Superstition: A Study of Folk Religion* (New York: Atheneum, 1974).

Vanstiphout, H. L. J. "Reflections on the Dream of Lugalbanda (A Typological and Interpretive Analysis of LH 332–365)," in Jirí Prosecky, ed., *Intellectual Life in the Ancient Near East: Papers Presented at the 43rd rencontre assyriologique internationale, Prague, July 1–5, 1996* (Prague: Academy of Sciences of the Czech Republic, Oriental Institute, 1998), pp. 397–412.

Vieyra, Maurice. "Les songes et leur interprétation chez les Hittites," in *Les songes et leur interpretation,* Sources orientales II (Paris: Éditions du Seuil, 1959).

Walter, Gerry H. *Dreams in the Literature of the Ancient Near East and the Babylonian Talmud,* (Masters Thesis, Hebrew Union College, 1974).

73-86

4

Dreams and Dreaming in Islam

Marcia Hermansen

Once a Caliph saw his teeth falling out in a dream. The dream interpreter said, "The entire family of my master will perish." The Caliph became upset and he called for another interpreter and recounted the dream to him. The second interpreter replied, "The dream of my master is good, for he shall live the longest among his relatives." Immediately the Caliph embraced the man and rewarded him for his skill and tact.[1]

—*Adapted from Muhammad Akili, Ibn Seerin's Dictionary of Dreams*

In my overview of approaches to dreams and dreaming in Islam, I focus primarily on hermeneutic questions about the practice of dream interpretation. As the passage cited above suggests, the idea that there is a factual meaning or indication to a dream is assumed in the tradition. However, the interpretive process, the contextualization of dream and dreamer, and the relation between them are all factors of successful exegesis. This is foundational in approaching Islamic understandings of dreams and dreaming.

The Islamic oneiracritical tradition emerged at the intersection of ancient Near Eastern, biblical, Greek, and Asian concepts of dreaming, synthesizing and Islamicizing these traditions into its own unique and rich heritage. One aspect of "Islamicizing" this broader tradition was to locate legitimizing references in the authoritative sources, such as the Qur'ān and the Sunna, and to develop theological and philosophical theories that contextualized the dream experience within the developing Islamic sciences and intellectual heritage.

Dreams in the Qur'ān and Sunna

Briefly considering the role dreams have played within the Islamic religious tradition, one finds from the earliest authoritative sources, the Qur'ān and the life and practice of Muhammad, a significant role given to dream content as reflecting both spiritual and real-world truth and in establishing the connection of everyday reality to another dimension often referred to as the *ghaib,* the absent or unseen realm.

The Qur'ān includes and amplifies aspects of the biblical acceptance of the significance of dreams, for example, the story of Joseph (Qur'ān 12:6) and the account of Abraham (37:102), in which God's command to sacrifice Ismā'īl[2] is spoken of as coming in a dream. Several Qur'ānic references indicate that Muhammad received information in dreams. For example, Qur'ān 8:43, "God showed the opponents to be few," has been identified with a prophetic dream preceding the battle of Badr, which showed the enemies to be weak. An additional instance is Qur'ān 48:27, "God has fulfilled your dream,"[3] which refers to a dream confirming that the Prophet would reenter Mecca."[4] This dream was said to anticipate the results of the treaty of Hudaybiyya.[5]

The collected sayings of the Prophet (hadith) preserved a number of the specific dreams of the Prophet. For example, his wife 'Ā'isha related:

> Allah's Apostle said to me, "You were shown to me twice (in my dream) before I married you. I saw an angel carrying you in a silken piece of cloth, and I said to him, 'Uncover (her),' and behold, it was you. I said (to myself), 'If this is from Allah, then it must happen.' Then you were shown to me, the angel carrying you in a silken piece of cloth, and I said (to him), 'Uncover (her), and behold, it was you. I said (to myself), 'If this is from Allah, then it must happen.'"[6]

In the spiritual experience of the Prophet, there is a certain overlap between information conveyed in dreams and the revelatory process. According to some hadith reports, revelation began for Muhammad in the form of true dreams anticipating his Prophetic role.[7] In fact, all his dreams were said to ultimately come true. In addition, the very first revelation of the Qur'ān in the cave of Ḥirā' might have come as a dream.[8] Was the apparition of the angel Gabriel inner or external? Was it a vision or a dream? Even today commentators do not agree, although mainstream orthodoxy has tended to stress the externality of the experience as a means of emphasizing the wholly other and wholly divine provenance of revelation.[9]

The early Muslim writer on dreams, al-Dīnawārī (d. 1020), distinguished earlier dream revelations from the Prophet's encounter with the angel: "Most of the Prophets did not see the angel except for a very few, rather they received revelation while sleeping. It was thus that the Prophet habitually saw dreams for twenty years before he saw the angel; however, what he saw was already prophecy."[10]

The Mi'rāj, or Night Ascension, in which the Prophet felt himself transported first to Jerusalem and then through the seven heavens, is variously interpreted as having been a dream, a vision, or an actual experience of bodily, physical locomotion.[11] Successive Muslim mystics such as Abū Yazīd Bisṭāmī (ca. 875),[12] Rūzbehān al-Baqlī (1209), and Ibn 'Arabī (1240) articulated their own versions of ascension, preserving in many instances the motifs of the Prophet's Mi'rāj.

The most authoritative collection of the sayings of the Prophet, *Ṣaḥīḥ al-Bukhārī,* includes a whole chapter regarding dreams and their significance.[13] The themes of these collected reports, perhaps some sixty of them, include:

- The importance of dreams and their being a form of prophecy. For example the saying, "The good dream is 1/46 of prophecy."[14] Ibn Khaldūn (1406) mentions an interesting explanation for the source of the number forty-six in this report.

He states that the Prophet's official "mission" endured for twenty-three years and that the period during which dreams anticipated revelation was six months, hence it constituted 1/46 of the total Prophetic mission.[15]

Two further traditions on this theme are "(When I am gone) there shall remain nothing of the glad tidings of prophecy except for true dreams. These the Muslim will see or they will be seen for him,"[16] and "The dreams of the Prophets were revelation."[17]

- Particular symbols and their interpretation by the Prophet. It is clear from these reports that Muhammad interpreted both his own dreams and those of his companions. In fact, one hadith states, "When the companions of the Messenger of God saw dreams while he was still alive they would tell him their dreams and he, for his part, would interpret them as God willed."[18]

  An instance of the Prophet's interpretations is a series of dreams that have to do with the person of 'Umar, his close companion who later became the second successor (khalīfa) to Muhammad. 'Umar's preserving knowledge and religion is variously symbolized in the Prophet's dreams by his drinking milk left by the Prophet or by his wearing a long shirt whose ends trailed down. In another hadith the Prophet sees a palace of gold in Paradise, which is said by the angels to belong to 'Umar.[19] A case in which the Prophet interprets his own dream is this:

  > The Prophet said, 'I saw in a dream that I waved a sword and it broke in the middle, and behold, that symbolized the casualties the believers suffered on the Day (of the battle) of Uhud. Then I waved the sword again, and it became better than it had ever been before, and behold, that symbolized the Conquest (of Mecca) which Allah brought about and the gathering of the believers.'[20]

- Statements about the veridical nature of dreams in which the Prophet appears. A hadith affirms that: "Whoever sees me (the Prophet) in dreams will see me in wakefulness (the Hereafter) for Satan can not take my shape."[21] The mystics often quote a related hadith, "Whoever sees me (i. e. the Prophet [in a dream]) then he indeed has seen the truth,"[22] inferring that "the truth" might indicate witnessing the divine theophany itself, rather than a true dream.
- Strategies recommended in order to incubate good dreams. Various hadith reports advise that one should try to go to sleep in a state of ritual purity in order to have good dreams[23] and that a person should habitually sleep on the right side.
- Ways to mitigate any potential harm or distress from bad dreams. The Prophet said, "If anyone of you sees a dream that he likes, then it is from Allah, and he should thank Allah for it and narrate it to others; but if he sees something else, i.e., a dream that he dislikes, then it is from Satan, and he should seek refuge with Allah from its evil, and he should not mention it to anybody, for it will not harm him."[24] Thus, "if someone has a dream which he dislikes, he should not tell it to others, but should get up and offer a prayer."[25] Another report indicates that the dreamer should spit three times on the left side if he sees a bad dream, recite some Qur'ān and give charity to mitigate its effect.[26]
- The possibility of collective dreams and their validating role. A number of the Prophet's companions are said to have dreamed that certain nights near the end of Ramadan were particularly blessed. It was thus declared that the "Night of

Power" would fall somewhere during the last ten days of the month on odd-numbered nights.[27]

- The power of voicing a dream is indicated in a number of reports. For example, the hadith "Whoever claims to have had a dream in which he says he saw something he did not shall be ordered (in Hell) to tie a knot between two barley grains and will not be able to do so,"[28] warns against the disruptive nature of claims on authority and the danger of misrepresentation. The Prophet said, "A dream will take effect according to how it is interpreted," and, "A dream rests on the feathers of a bird and will not take effect unless it is related to someone."[29] Therefore "tell your dreams only to knowledgeable persons and loved ones," not your enemies, children, or impious persons.[30] The example of Joseph telling his dream to his jealous bothers is said to validate this cautious attitude.

Classical Islamic Tradition and Dreams

Worthy of note among the fundamental principles of Islamic dream interpretation are the importance of seeking truthfulness in the interpreter and maintaining caution or secrecy when sharing dream interpretation. The veracity of dreams is also indicated by the type of dream experience, and the specific terminology employed gives some indication of the provenance and character of dreams. For example, "ḥilm" pl. "aḥlām," a very common word for dream(s) in modern Arabic, was derived from the idea of dreams signaling the onset of puberty through sexual content and nocturnal emission. Hence one fragment of a hadith states that the "righteous dream (ru'yā ṣāliḥa) comes from God while the deceptive or impure dream (ḥilm) is from the Devil." [31] Yet another term used for dream in the Qur'ān is "manām." One of the signs of God is said to be one's dreams (manām) in the night and the day (30:23), God's shows things to the Prophet in a dream (manām) (8:43), and dream experiences have some analogy with death (39:42).

"God receives souls at the time of death and those souls that have not yet died in their sleep. He keeps the souls for which He has ordained death and dismisses the rest until an appointed time." Alternatively, death is paralleled to awakening from slumber in the saying "Men are asleep, when they die they awake."[32]

Islamic dream manuals constitute an important subgenre of divinatory literature in Islam. The most common form of these texts is a dictionary of dream images, usually prefaced by the author's introductory comments on methodology and technique.[33]

Contemporary scholarship traces the evolution of these manuals in Arabic and later in other languages of Muslim societies to the translation into Arabic from Greek by Ḥunayn ibn Ishāq (877) of the manual of Artemidorus. While some adaptations had to be made in the symbols and their interpretation for cultural and religious reasons, many of the essential ideas and organizing principles that gave shape to the developing oneiracritic tradition in Islam may be traced to this source.[34]

In most Muslim dream manuals a brief introduction was followed by a catalog of symbols and subjects organized by categories, such as dreams of Prophets, fish, flowers, occupations, and so on.[35] The subjects could evoke positive, negative, or neutral evaluations from the dreamer's perspective. Thus, while one may imagine a concerned individual consulting the printed manual on his or her own, much as a modern would try to divine using the *I Ching*, the divinatory process was ultimately subtle enough that the services of a qualified interpreter would be desirable. Some manuals were teaching tools for would-be interpreters. Evidence of this is that they were composed in rhyming quatrains contrived in order to facilitate memorization, as were other texts in the Islamic curriculum, such as the rules of Arabic grammar and the categories for classifying the Prophetic traditions.[36]

The introductions to dream manuals provide some indication of the methodology of dream interpreters. Ibn Qutayba's (d. 889) manual[37] provides nine methodological principles as follows:

1. Divination by using the etymology of the dreamer's name or the name of the object that figures prominently in the dream. This might provide an auspicious or ominous context to the reading. A further divinatory technique involved calculating the numeral values for names or objects according to the system of Arabic numerology, known as "abjad."
2. Extrapolating from characteristics of the objects seen in the dream. Nabulusī gives the example of breaking this down into subcategories so that

> The fundamental aspects of the dream are the category, the type, and the disposition. The category is like trees, wild animals. or birds, and these usually stand for people. The type is to discern what type of tree, animal or bird it is. Thus, if the tree is a palm this means an Arab man because the growing places of most palms are in the Arab countries. If the bird is a peacock it means a non-Arab and if it is an ostrich it means a Bedouin Arab. The disposition is that you take into account the disposition of that tree and apply it to a person with that characteristic. Thus if the tree is a walnut it will apply to a person who is difficult to deal with and argumentative in a debate. If it is a palm it will be applied as his being a person who benefits with goodness, is productive and easy going since God says in the Qur'ān, "Like a good tree, its roots are firm and its branches reach the sky,"[38] i. e. the palm. If the bird is flying it indicates a person who travels a lot, like the bird.
>
> Then its disposition is considered. If it is a peacock, then it indicates a good-looking, wealthy foreigner. Likewise, if it is an eagle then it indicates is a king and if it is a crow it indicates a corrupt, disloyal, and lying person according to a saying of the Prophet, may the peace and blessings of God be upon him and because Noah, peace be upon him, sent out a crow to know whether the water had receded or not and it found a corpse floating on the water and landed on it and didn't come back. From this the expression was coined for someone who keeps you waiting or leaves without returning, "Noah's crow." If it is a magpie it is an unreliable, forgetful, and irreligious person. The poet said:
>
> Isn't is so that if you dream of something as a magpie
> It means a yearning for those of high status in the lands.
>
> If it is a vulture then he is a warlike, tyrannical, sinful, terrifying Sultan, like the vulture with its talons, body and power over the other birds, and its rending their flesh.[39]

3. The third principle consists of finding correspondences to the pairing of ideas in Qur'anic verses. Ibn Qutayba's illustration of this is that seeing eggs in a

dream may mean something referring to women since there is a Qur'anic verse (37:49) "Where chaste women who restrain their eyes are likened to 'well-guarded eggs,'" that links the two things.[40]

4. Finding correspondences in the text of Prophet's sayings.
5. Finding correspondences in proverbs and poetry.
6. Opposition and inversion (maqlūb),[41] so that seeing something in a dream might actually mean its opposite.
7. Increase and decrease.
8. The time of year.
9. The state of the dreamer.

One section of the Islamic dream manuals' introduction was usually consecrated to the qualities most desirable in an interpreter, which, given the above methodologies, would include knowledge not only of the Islamic canonical sources but of proverbs and poetry as well. Manuals produced in Pakistan and India today often begin by providing a number of charts that facilitate performing subsidiary types of divination along with the symbolic correspondences of the actual dream content.

These additional charts may be astrological, indicating the correspondence of the various planets with certain days and hours.[42] They may indicate the auspiciousness of dreams occurring on various days of the month,[43] or they may be charts for the consultant's carrying out a divination on the spot by randomly pointing at grids containing the names of the various Prophets or certain letters of the alphabet.[44] Even the earlier manuals suggested ways for dream interpreters to come up with something if the client had forgotten the dream or could not articulate it in a coherent manner.[45]

Due to his fame as a dream interpreter, later dream manuals were often circulated under the name of Ibn Sīrīn (d. 728).[46] The two best known are a shorter version, "Ta'bīr al-Ru'yā" (Interpretation of Dreams), and a longer text.[47] "Ibn Sīrīn's" manual is specific about how the status of the dreamer should be taken into account. A true dream interpreter would not try to apply the same symbol equivalently to every person seeing it in a dream. For example, an anecdote tells how while he was in the presence of his pupils, two dreamers came to Ibn Sīrīn within an hour of each other and each had dreamed of being the caller to prayer (muezzin). The first person was told that his dream foretold that he would perform the Muslim pilgrimage to Mecca. The second man, who seemed to be of baser character, was told that he would be accused of a theft. The pupils then questioned how Ibn Sīrīn could come up with two radically different interpretations for the same dream. His response was that the character of each dreamer was evident from his appearance and demeanor. Therefore, the first one's dream evoked the Qur'anic verse "Proclaim to the people a solemn pilgrimage" (20:28) since he was clearly pious. The second man's dream evoked the verse "Then a crier called after them, O company of travelers (Joseph's brothers), you are surely thieves" (12:70).[48]

This anecdote also reveals the intimate connection of dream interpretation to Qur'anic references. Not only do they legitimate the interpretations, but the actual content of the dreams could contain recitations from the Qur'an. This is apparent since common features of manuals are explanations of the symbolism of a dreamer seeing himself reciting any one of the 114 chapters of the Qur'an.[49] Not every derivation from Qur'anic associations is self-evident and intuitive. For example, a man dreamed that he was reciting the chapter "al-Naṣr" (Assistance from God), which would appear to be a highly favorable omen. However, "Ibn Sīrīn bade him repent and prepare for death as this was one of the last chapters of the Qur'an to have been revealed."[50]

Another example of the circumstantial factors that must be weighed in interpretation is said to be the timing of a dream. In one manual a dream of sitting on a road is said to mean good luck if seen at night and divorcing one's spouse if seen during the day.[51] Tiflisī states that according to Ja'far al-Ṣādiq,[52] a dream from early night might take up to twenty years to be fulfilled; one at midnight, six months to a year; and one in the morning, a few days.[53]

Alphabetically indexed symbols to dreams appeared relatively early in the tradition and now generally supplant earlier broader categories for objects seen. One may assume that due to the lack of qualified interpreters, the do-it-yourself aspect now predominates.

Modern academic scholarship has generally neglected these dream manuals and even failed to include them in manuscript catalogs and bibliographies although the number of these manuals rivals that of commentaries on the Qur'ān itself.[54] Occult sciences including astrology, talismans, and dream manuals were quite popular and continue to circulate today in many Muslim societies. In fact, the number of reprints of this sort of text appearing in the Arab world is indicative of a return of interest in the "sciences of the unseen" among the generation of young Muslims influenced by Islamic revival, since this is an aspect of spirituality with a certain legitimacy in the religious tradition.[55] While astrology may have been condemned in the hadith reports, dream interpretation was clearly sanctioned. The use of Islamic symbols such as the Qur'ān and Prophets and the appeal to traditions of recognized hadith scholars such as Ibn Sīrīn and Ibn Qutayba as authorities also Islamicized the discipline.

In her study of Ibn Abī ad-Dunyā's *Book of Dreams,* Leah Kinberg differentiates the oneiracritic works that consist of lists of standard correspondences between dream motifs and their imputed meanings from those Islamic works that recount dreams primarily for purposes of edification.[56] A further way of formulating this distinction is that the manuals or "ta'bīr" (dream interpretation) works present symbolic dreams whereas dreams in the edifying genre tend to be taken literally.[57] Among the best known dream manuals are the two by pseudo-Ibn Sīrīn and 'Abd al-Ghānī Nabulusī's (1731), *Ta'ṭīr al-anām fi ta'bīr al-Manām* (The Perfuming of Humanity in the Interpretation of Dreams).[58]

Certain edificatory texts are "autobiographical" narratives of the dream diary genre. Sufi and Shi'i sources are particularly rich in this aspect.[59] The dreams of the mystics Rūzbehān Baqlī[60] and Ḥākim al-Tirmidhī (ca. 910)[61] formed part of their autobiographical accounts, and some medieval Sufis wrote almost exclusively on their dreams in dream diaries.[62] As Carl Ernst cautions in his study of Rūzbehān Baqlī, these dream diaries are not "autobiographical" in the modern sense. Rather than demonstrating character development in the context of external challenges and events, they demonstrate, probably to an initiated circle, the spiritual status and authority of the dreamer.

Besides satisfying interest in more personal types of divination, dream material could be evoked by Muslim writers to adjudicate the relative merits of the legal schools,[63] to determine which reading of the Qur'an was correct,[64] or to resolve theological questions.[65]

Our attention clearly falls in different ways on the various Muslim dream narratives as it would on our own dreams. It is clear that certain dreams are powerfully symbolic and allegorical, the stuff of Jungian analysis and archetypal motifs,[66] while others are more mundane.[67]

The porousness of the boundary between the world of the living and the world of the dead meant that dreams were also acknowledged as a source of communication between the two realms. For example, al-Ghazzālī's (d. 1111) chapter, "The States of the Dead which have been known through Unveiling (mukāshafa) in Dreams,"[68] presents a collection of reports about people in the afterlife. a sort of confirmation beyond the grave. For example, "On the night that he died, al-Ḥasan al-Baṣrī was seen in a dream. The gates of heaven had been opened and a voice was calling out, 'Al-Ḥasan al-Baṣrī has come to God, and He is well-pleased with him!'"[69] Other dreams recounted by al-Ghazzālī fall more into the category of edification proposed by Kinberg, as they counsel which sins could be avoided, warn against pride, and so on.

A common topos of Sufi or Shi'i dreams is spiritual (ijāza),[70] initiation, or approval from authorities and saints confirming the authority of the living. For example, during encounters with the Prophet in his dreams, the fifteenth century Moroccan Sufi al-Zawāwī saw the Prophet bestowing robes of honor on him and spitting in his mouth, both symbols of spiritual transmission.

Philosophical Psychology of Dreaming and the Idea of the 'Ālam al-Mithāl

Building on the pattern of the famous report in al-Bukhārī attributed to Ibn Sīrīn, dreams are classified as being true, dubious, or definitely false.[71] Sufi interpreters developed this discussion by associating the three categories with processes of pure unveiling, imaginative unveiling, and being patently false.[72] These categories are said to parallel the sources of dreams coming respectively from God, the angels, or Satan. Dreams from God are clear, those from the angels allegorical, and those from the devil confused or misleading.[73] It was also held by most authorities that physiological factors such as overeating or imbalances of the humors could provoke certain types of dreams, generally unworthy of being subjected to interpretation. In fact, the Prophet Muhammad once told a Bedouin inquirer that his dream was jumbled and confused because he had consumed too many dates the previous evening.[74]

As the tradition developed, both philosophers and mystics explored the connection of the content of dreams to the reality of the dreamer. This "reality" of the dream was understood as having to do both with the faculties for perceiving, storing, and working with everyday experience and with the level of the soul or spirit that might connect these individual experiences with a higher level of meaning.

A thirteenth century Sufi text, the "Lamp of Guidance," differentiates between external visions and dreams in the following way:

> The people of seclusion/retreat sometimes experience during dhikr[75] and being overwhelmed with ecstasy that they become absent from sensory effects and see some things of the unseen world are disclosed to them, as for a sleeper while sleeping. The Sufis call these "spiritual events" (waqi'āt).[76] Unveilings (mukāshafāt), on the other hand, occur while they are conscious and present.
>
> In most of the "events" and dreams the lower soul becomes identified with the spirit and in some it remains independent. Truth is an attribute of the spirit and lying is an attribute of the Lower Soul (nafs). A waking vision is always true and an "event" or dream may be either true or false.[77]

In mystical practice, one was said to have need of the "constant direction of a shaykh who could explain the meaning of one's dreams and visions."[78] Ibn Khaldūn explains the difference between true dream visions and false, confused dreams according to the level of the soul implicated. All dreams are pictures in the imagination. However, if these pictures come from the rational soul,[79] then they are true. If they are derived from images preserved in the dreamer's faculty of memory, where they had been deposited while the person was in the waking state, then they are confused imaginings. In Ibn Khaldūn's view, some signs of a dream being true are that the dreamer will awaken quickly as if trying to hold on to the image and that the vision given in the dream will remain clear and be remembered.[80]

In order to explain how dream symbols could bear on real-world truth, various strands of theology were woven together with a neo-Platonic metaphysical model. The main thrust of Islamic theology is predestinarian. Some expressions of this are the hadith statement that, "The pen has run dry" or the Qur'anic assertions that God has measured out destinies. One term for "fate" in Persian is "sar navesht," from the idea of one's destiny already being already written on the forehead. In this sense the Qur'anic reference to a "Preserved Tablet"[81] came to be associated with the idea of an eternal record stored at a higher level of reality of all that would come to be.

Fazlur Rahman has traced the development in Islamic philosophy and mysticism of the idea of this intermediary realm where dream or psychological experiences may anticipate or shape physical reality.[82] Here the Preserved Tablet performed a function similar to the locus of the Platonic forms, where the archetypal realities of things existed in ideal form before coming into physical being. Muslim scholars referred to this intermediary level of reality as the 'ālam al-barzakh, "World of Isthmus," or 'ālam al-mithāl, the "World of Images" or the "Imaginal World." Avicenna (Ibn Sīnā) (d. 1037) used the Imaginal World concept to explain the source of the foreknowledge of the Prophet while al-Ghazzālī drew on it in order to validate religious teachings such as the punishment in the grave. According to al-Ghazzālī, since it is clear that we do not see people being bitten by snakes and scorpions in their graves as the hadith reports indicate, it is necessary to explain the ontological status of this punishment. He concluded that the punishment was real at the level of the World of Images by analogy to the pain that dreamers may believe they are experiencing during a dream.[83] For dreamers this pain is as real as a physical experience, and they may wake up crying out.[84] The Imaginal World concept was further elaborated by the Sufi philosophers al-Suhrawardī (d. 1191), Ibn al-'Arabī (d. 1240), and Mullā Ṣadrā Shīrāzī (d. 1311). According to Fazlur Rahman, "During the later centuries of the Muslim Middle Ages, the 'ālam al-mithāl increases in importance and forms an integral part of Sufi spiritual culture."[85] Although Rahman commented that "The use of reason in the world of imagination is not that easy to understand," the symbols of the world of mithāl, including dream images, were manipulated by Sufis or dream interpreters according to canons of correspondence and analogy within the system of rationality involved in canon building and divinatory practices.[86]

Relationship of Dreams to Memory

In looking at the historical role of dreams and visions within a specific religious tradition, in this case Islam, I would contend that cultural practices such as writing and divination definitely influence interpretive strategies. The unmitigated content of the dream experience is more difficult to assess for, as is the case in the discussion of mystical experience, it is difficult to establish if there is a sort of ground zero of pure experience that is appreciated or understood only once some elements of interpretation have occurred.[87] It is clear that cultural practices or techniques would have a impact on dream experiences as well as on their subsequent interpretation.

Examples would be the dhikr practices of the Sufis and memorizing the Qur'ān and other texts. Dhikr means "remembrance," and the ritual remembrance of God might involve individual or collective rituals of repeated repetition of the divine names or other pious phrases. Memorization of the Qur'ān was an extremely pervasive cultural practice and in fact was the basis of all elementary education until the modern period. In this regard, even non-Sufi Muslims recognize a practice called *istikhāra*—"seeking help in making a choice or decision"—in which, after a ritual prayer, a Muslim asks for a sign or a form of guidance, which is often believed to come in a dream.[88]

The body is cultivated in each of these cases. Dhikr practices might involve isolation, fasting, and a repetition of phrases, possibly hundreds of thousands of times. This would certainly induce a trance-like state that could well persist into dream experiences or meld with them in a hynagogic state.

Ibn Khaldūn provides a formula for incubating and memorizing dreams that he refers to as "special dream words." [89] A person was to recite some cryptic, non-Arabic phrases, rather like a spell, at a critical point when falling asleep while remaining conscious and ask to be shown specific information while dreaming. Ibn Khaldūn himself asserts that "With the help of these words, I have myself had remarkable dream visions, through which I learned things about myself I wanted to know."[90]

Memorizing of extensive material and the art of recollection and repetition of memorized words would also seem to have some parallel qualities to dream experience. Al-Ghazzālī is very explicit about this.

> The metaphor for the heart is a mirror in which images and realities are reflected. Everything that has been decreed by God from the beginning of the world's creation until its close, has been written and maintained in something He created, which at times He calls the Tablet and at others the Clear Book or the Clear Example. All that has passed in the world and all that is to come is inscribed thereon as an inscription invisible to our eyes. The maintenance of the destinies on this tablet is analogous to the maintenance of the words and letters of the Quran on the mind and heart of a man who has committed it to memory . . . When he recites it seems he is looking at it book if you searched his brain you could not find a single letter of script.
>
> The tablet might be compared to a mirror in which images appear, if another mirror is positioned before it the images in the first mirror will be reflected therein. This second mirror is the heart—but desires and sense demands are a veil between the heart and the tablet.[91]

For al-Ghazzālī, dreams are a proof of higher reality as they demonstrate both the fallibility of reliance on sense perception and the possibility of the reality of unseen dimensions.

> Do you not see how when you are asleep you believe things and imagine circumstance, holding them to be stable and enduring, and, so long as you were in the dream condition have no doubts about them? Is it not the case that when you awakened you knew that all you had imagined and believed was unfounded and ineffectual? When then are you confident that all your waking beliefs are genuine?"

> Perhaps in another state such as the ecstasy of the Sufis you will go beyond the intellect. Perhaps the life of this world is like a dream in comparison to the world to come. The Quran says, "We have taken off your covering and your sight today is sharp (50:21)."[92]

In his study of dream manuals as a genre, John Lamoreaux, whose dissertation is the most comprehensive study along these lines, traces the historical and epistemological sources shaping both diverse and homogenizing elements of the Muslim oneiracritic tradition. Among the competing legacies that emerged by the fourth Islamic century were those works that he termed, following Marshall Hodgson's coinage,[93] "sharīʿa minded," that is, those that stress Islamic themes and the tradition of prophetic teachings. Fewer works were produced in a Sufi, mystical mode, and these would tend to be more individualistic and idiosyncratic, like the dream diaries mentioned above. A much rarer, more cosmopolitan strand of dream manual more fully integrated the Hellenistic tradition of Artemidorus, both epistemologically, by honoring the status of royalty and sages as interpreters, and in matching interpretations to specific dream symbols.

An important distinction made by Lamoreaux is that between the theistic orientation of the "sharīʿa-minded" manuals and the emanationist cosmology of the much smaller number written in a Hellenized philosophical tradition. The former focus on dreams as signs of God, revealed through the agency of an angelic being, sometimes named by authors to be "Ṣiddiqūn," the angel of dreams.[94] The more philosophical or Hellenized tradition of dream interpretation in Islam, on the other hand, primarily understood the meaning and value of spiritual or visionary dreams to be a reflection or emanation from the higher realities to the human sphere.

The process of Islamicizing this material, despite its various strands, ultimately resulted in relatively similar assumptions and interpretations pervading the literature and in its acceptance and integration by the custodians of religious legitimacy, the ulema, or religious scholars.[95]

Contemporary Muslim Dreams and Dreamers

Persistent themes arising in the consideration of dreaming among contemporary Muslims are the interaction with modern Western theories of dreaming, the evidence of dreaming for cultural difference, and the persistence of meaningful dreaming as evidence for religious truth.

At the popular level, dream manuals of the traditional sort continue to be produced, translated, and adapted for popular consumption in Muslim societies. New developments are works that recount the dreams of contemporary Muslims as proofs of the validity of religious truth and experience generally, despite the encroachments of modernity and Western education. One of these manuals, for example, explains that Freud's theory of dreaming only takes into account those sorts of dreams that traditional Islamic dream science would classify as arising from physiological factors such as indigestion. Therefore, Freudian theory does not apply to the type of "spiritual" dreams[96] that the author recounts in order to convince others of the reality of the religious dimension, rather than to promote his own saintly stature.

Anthropological studies of contemporary Muslim societies also note the significance they accord to dreams. Katherine P. Ewing working in Pakistan and Michael Gilsenan in Egypt comment on the persistence of meaning associated with dreams in popular Muslim cultures, in particular as associated with the subtraditions of belief in Sufi saints.[97]

The connection of dreams to social action is thought provoking when it occurs on the personal level. Reflecting on the role of dreams in public life, Ewing observes:

> Dreams have the greatest transformative potential in cultures that allow people to experience their dreams as significant. Because we Westerners separate our dreams sharply from waking life, we typically do not regard our dreams as significant, at least in public discourse. When the dreamer remains silent about his dream, it usually slips away and takes on no social significance, so that even highly synthetic, reconstitutive dreams, while they may help the dreamer to assimilate his experiences to existing self representations, may not provide any basis for actually modifying the self representations. But other eras and other cultures have attributed significance to dreams in very different, far more public ways.[98]

Ewing notes the potential of dreams to motivate decisions and real-world actions. She analyzes the dream narratives of modern Pakistanis who are conflicted about the role of Westernization in their lives but may experience dreams much along the pattern of al-Ḥakīm al-Tirmidhī's tenth century dream of initiation by the saints. Some individuals will actualize these dreams by seeking out Sufi masters and reforming their own personal behavior. Others, lacking cultural reinforcement or the confluence of external events sustaining their attempts to integrate dream material with external behavior, may marginalize and forget the dream content.

Gilsenan cites dream material from Egyptian peasant women as one strand of evidence, among many, that the component of enchantment or magical thinking is not absent from the modern world and, furthermore, that disenchantment has less of a hold on postmodernity than most theorists have accepted.[99]

> Opponents in al-Azhar, the professions, and the newspapers denounced all this [dream validation] as an illusion. None the less, dream visions were integral to identity as followers of a sheikh and a modality of discipleship, as they might be to many who had only the most tenuous links to the brotherhoods. In dreams began responsibilities. Judgements were made. Commands issued. Justifications provided. Hope renewed. Conduct was commented on by holy figures, by the Prophet himself, by the founding sheikh who had died some years before but who appeared with his son and successor.
>
> Dreams were public goods, circulated in conversational exchanges, valorizing the person, authoring and authorizing experiences, at once unique and collective visual, verbal epiphanies. Dreams thus constituted a field of force and framed interchanges between the living, and between the living and the only apparently dead.[101]

At the level of public or mass consciousness, Johansen[100] and Gilsenan indicate another theme of Muslim dreaming, both traditional and contemporary, that of the empowerment of women as dreamers. The modern example is the cult of the saints in Egypt. While women's dreams of saints commanding them to attend shrines are disparaged by scripturalist male religious authorities, such dreams allow the women to penetrate more public social spaces.

Another area of contemporary developments in the area of the "Islamicate" dream traditions is the role of dreams in American Sufi movements.[102] Some of these movements place particular emphasis on the role of dreams in spiritual guidance and give significant attention to theories of dream interpretation. One aspect of traditional Sufi practice is said to be submitting one's dreams to the Shaykh for spiritual analysis and guidance. In the modern, Western context, the process of this traditional mode of spiritual direction is not easily accessible from the traditional texts. Western psychotherapeutic models and practices, however, provide bridges and techniques, in particular those derived from Jungian or Gestalt "dream work."

Pir Vilayat Khan, head of the Sufi Order in the West,[103] specifically acknowledges the role of Carl Jung's theories of the self and the interpretations of Islamic spirituality articulated in the works of the scholar Henry Corbin (d. 1978)[104] in formulating his understanding of spiritual transformation and dreaming.[105]

A key Corbinian theme, derived from a Jungian reading of Sufi texts, is the idea of active or creative imagination. Khan connects this to dream work in Sufism. The dreamer who can maintain focus and lucidity is able to work with the symbols of the "World of Images" and participate with awareness in her own process of spiritual development.[106] The spiritual master is one facet of the archetype of the self that may appear in dreams or guided meditations in order to bestow guidance.

The Golden Sufi Center, a movement following the British Naqshbandi-Mujaddidi teacher Irena Tweedie (1999), has significantly incorporated dream work into its practices. Tweedie's successor, Llewellyn Vaughan-Lee, has developed dream workshops and writes on the topic of dreaming.[107] Sara Sviri, a contributor to academic discussions of dreaming and Islamic mysticism, is also involved with the teachings of this group.[108] The practices cultivated in ongoing dream groups among this circle include the sharing and collective interpretation of dreams, as well as the cultivation of lucid dreaming. Lucid dreaming, in particular, is understood among some Western Sufi movements as an effective spiritual technique practiced in diverse esoteric paths.[109]

Among the more "sharīʿa-oriented" Western Sufi movements, dreams play a role in the testimonies of followers of Shaykh Nazim[110] and feature in the advice of a Mevlevi Shaykh to Western aspirants.[111]

The use of dream material on the part of Western Sufi movements constitutes an appropriation of the powerful symbolism and depth of an established tradition that accepts dream material as providing guidance to aspects of the dreamer's being as well as to external reality. While the concepts of person and social relationships unquestionably vary between medieval Muslim societies and the modern West, the ideas of spiritual development are not as radically different as those between the Hindu yogis and modern Westerner dreamers that are commented on by Wendy Doniger.[112]

Conclusion

As a final statement on the interpretation of dreams in the Islamic tradition, I include an interview with a contemporary Muslim interpreter of dreams. Shaykh Muḥammad Afzaluddīn Niẓāmī is a ninety-four-year-old Chishti Sufi from Hyderabad, India, who now resides in Chicago. He is consulted both by disciples and a broader public in search of spiritual guidance or, more often, spiritual cures and solutions to worldly difficulties. Shaykh Niẓāmī has published several dream manuals and has prepared a number of other manuscripts on the interpretation of dreams. An examination of these works discloses that they follow the traditional format of brief introductions accompanied by alphabetically indexed readings for dream symbols.

I conducted an interview with him concerning the science of dream interpretation. Since the interview was informal and conducted in Urdu and English, I summarize the conversation below.

When asked why dreams are important, the Shaykh mentioned the hadith report that they are 1/46th of prophecy. When I commented that the link to the Prophet might be rather beyond the aspirations of ordinary dreamers, the Shaykh commented that ordinary persons would benefit in terms of their character development through having their dreams explained to them.

His methodology seemed largely grounded in Ibn Sīrīn's categories of first applying to the dream any possible associations to the text of the Qur'ān or the hadith. As a second principle the context of the dreamer, the country where he is living and the climate all would be taken into account. The inquirer's personality would have a major impact on the interpretation. For example, dream content is indicative of the person's level of development. Those of baser characters tend to have many violent dreams or dreams of tricking or harming others. Someone of quarrelsome temperament will see fiery things in his dreams. Very spiritual people may be visited by angels, although this is relatively rare.

Following the traditional Sufi texts, Niẓāmī explains how the objects sighted in dreams disclose the level of the soul's development. Seeing base or vicious animals is indicative of the predominance of the lower soul and engagement with worldly desires. Seeing humans in dreams indicates further spiritual development while the appearance of angelic beings reveals that the person is cultivating the angelic level of "Malakūt" and receiving knowledge from the 'Ālam al-Mithāl. The dream or vision of the Prophet represents the next level of spiritual development and the active participation of the dreamer in implementing the divine command. The content of the vision of the Prophet would be shared with the shaykh or master for confirmation. The master, due to his own spiritual powers and the likelihood of shared dream realities, would likely have heard whatever the Prophet said or disclosed to the person or received a report of it, as a control on fabricated dream accounts.

I asked Shaykh Niẓāmī whether his own Sufi master, Khwāja Ḥasan Niẓāmī, of India (d. 1955) had made use of dream interpretation. He answered yes, but not so much to inform people about the outcome of their dreams. His Shaykh would rather listen to the dream and then give guidance that seemed to be based more on the science of recognizing the traits and destiny of a person as derived from their appearance (qiyāfa shanāsī). Shaykh Niẓāmī also remarked on the commonality of results obtained by dream interpretation as employed by both Hindu and Muslim practitioners in India.

Despite the category-based nature of his own writings, he believes that the highest form of dream interpretation is the development of immediate insight into the mind of the person reporting a dream. Like many other types of divinations, the symbols and calculations are more of a springboard or prop sustaining the interpreter's immediate intuition.

When asked whether the role of dream interpretation has changed in modern times, Shaykh Niẓāmī replied that the mind-set of the human being has significantly altered today so that people see many more terrifying dreams of world cataclysms, plane crashes, and so on. In previous eras people were more simple and receptive, and thus they received more inspiration (ilqā') from God in dreams. Today people are arrogant about their own knowledge and capabilities so that they consider their own dreams to be useless and trivial; therefore, less inspiration is received.

Notes

1. An early interpretation of a dream of teeth falling out meaning the death of relatives is also reported in Ibn Sa'd, *Ṭabaqāt* V (Beirut: Dār al-Kutub al-'Ilmiyya, 1990), p. 93.
2. Islamic commentators usually consider Ismā'īl to have been the son who was nearly sacrificed, although the Qur'ān does not state this explicitly.
3. The Arabic word "ru'yā" can mean either "dream" or "vision." Al-Bukhārī cites this verse of the Qur'ān as evidence for the confirmation of the dreams of the righteous. *Ṣaḥīḥ al-Bukhārī,* vol. 9, book 87, chapter 2, heading. Trans. M. M. Khan (Beirut: Maktaba al-Arabiyya, 1985), and online at www.usc.edu/dept/MSA/reference/searchhadith.html.
4. John C. Lamoreaux, "Dream Interpretation in the Early Medieval Near East," Ph.D. diss., Duke University, 1999, p. 186.
5. Toufic Fahd, *La divination arabe: Etudes religieuses, sociologiques et folkloriques sur le milieu natif de l'Islam* (Leiden: E. J. Brill, 1966), p. 271.
6. *Ṣaḥīḥ al-Bukhārī,* vol. 9, book 87, no. 140.
7. Ibid., no. 111.
8. Ibn Ishāq, *The Life of Muhammad (Sīrat rasūl Allāh),* trans. A. Guillaume (Karachi: Oxford University Press, 1980), p. 106.
9. Fazlur Rahman, *Islam* (Chicago: University of Chicago, 1979), pp. 13–14.
10. Toufy Fahd, "Les songes er leur interpretation selon l'islam" in *Les Songes et leur Interpretation* (Paris: Editions du Seuil, 1959), p. 137.
11. Rahman, *Islam,* p. 14.
12. The Arabic text of Bisṭāmī's dream, "An Early Arabic Version of the Mi'rāj of Abū Yazīd Bistāmī," was published by R. A. Nicholson in *Islamica* 2, no. 3 (1926): 403–408. It is translated by Michael A. Sells in *Early Islamic Mysticism* (Mahwah, NJ: Paulist Press, 1996), pp. 242–250.
13. *Ṣaḥīḥ al-Bukhārī,* vol. 9, book 87.
14 Ibid., 9, 87, 117, and 144. Some reports vary the number from 46 to 70.
15. Ibn Khaldun, *Muqaddimah* III, trans. Franz Rosenthal (New York: Pantheon, 1958), p. 209.
16. *Ṣaḥīḥ Al-Bukhārī,* vol. 9, book 87, no. 119.
17. Ibid., vol. 1, book 4, no. 140, and vol. 1, book 12, no. 818.
18. Ibid., vol. 9, book 87, no. 155.
19. Ibid., no. 150. Narrated by Abu Huraira. Toufic Fahd speculates as to whether this series of dreams involving 'Umar reveals the Prophet's sense that 'Umar would be the strongest successor.
20. Ibid., vol. 9, book 87, no. 164.
21. Ibid., no. 126. This report and the role of dreaming of the Prophet in Islam are discussed in Ignaz Goldziher, "The Appearance of the Prophet in Dreams," *Journal of the Royal Asiatic Society* 33 (1912): 503–506. Methods for incubating dreams in which the Prophet will appear are given by al-Jīlī and discussed in Valerie J. Hoffman, "Annihilation in the Messenger of God: The Development of a Sufi Practice" *International Journal of Middle East Studies* 31, no. 3 (August 1999): 351–369. The fact that the concept of seeing the Prophet in dreams remains important in certain contemporary interpretations of Islam may be verified by consulting *Sīrat al-nabī ba'd az wiṣāl al-nabī* (Biography of the Prophet after the Death of the Prophet) by Muḥammad 'Abd al-Majīd Ṣiddiqī (Lahore: Marḥabā Publications, 1979). The major topic of the book is the continuous and important sighting of the Prophet in dreams as reported in Islamic religious and biographical literature until the present time.
22. *Ṣaḥīḥ Al-Bukhārī,* vol. 9, book 87, no. 125.
23. Ibid., no. 168.

24. Ibid., no. 114.
25. Ibid., no. 144.
26. Ibid., nos. 115, 133.
27. Ibid., no. 120, p. 100.
28. Ibid., no. 165.
29. Reported in al-Dārimī's and other hadith collections.
30. Afzaluddin Nizami, *A Comprehensive Interpretation of Dreams* (Lahore: Mavra, 1993), p. x.
31. Cited in Fahd, *La divination arabe,* p. 271.
32. Attributed variously to the Prophet or to 'Alī, *The Remembrance of Death and the Afterlife,* book XL of *The Revival of the Religious Sciences,* trans. T. J. Winter (Cambridge: Islamic Texts Society, 1995), p. 124.
33. Lamoreaux, "Dream Interpretation," p. 5.
34. For a discussion of this transmission, see Fahd, *La divination arabe,* pp. 326–328; Lamoreaux, "Dream Interpretation," pp. 14–15, 78–86.
35. N. Bland translates eighty titles of the chapters from the dream manual of Ibn Shahīn in "On the Muhammedan Science of Ta'bīr, or the Interpretation of Dreams," *Journal of the Royal Asiatic Society* 16 (1856): 118–171.
36. Toufic Fahd, "Ru'yā," *Encyclopedia of Islam,* second ed. (Leiden: E. J. Brill), pp. 645–649.
37. Ibn Qutayba's manual, "'Ibārat al-ru'yā" appears only in two manuscripts, which have not been edited or printed. I owe the following material to Lamoreaux's study, especially pp. 50–53. See also M. J. Kister, "The Interpretation of Dreams: An Unknown Manuscript of Ibn Qutayba's "Ibārat al-Ru'yā'" *Israel Oriental Studies* (1974): 67–103.
38. Qur'ān 14:24.
39. Al-Dārī, *Muntakhab al-kalām* (Cairo: Maktaba Muḥammad 'Alī Ṣubaiḥ, 1963), pp. 13–14. Similar but less eloquent formulations in Nabulusī, *Ta'ṭīr al-anam,* p. 8 and pseudo-Ibn Sīrīn, *Kitāb ta'bīr al-ru'yā* (Beirut: Maktaba al-Tawfīq, n.d.), pp. 4–5.
40. Lamoreaux, "Dream Interpretation," p. 51.
41. Muhammed Akili translates this concept as "contraposition," in *Ibn Seerin's Dictionary of Dreams* (Philadelphia: Pearl Publishing, 1992), p. xxx.
42. One such Urdu manual is *Mukammal khwābnāmā-i Haḍrat Yūṣuf* (The Complete Dream Manual of Prophet Joseph) ed. 'Abd al-Raḥmān Shauq (Srinagar, India, 1992), featuring astrological charts on pp. 31–32. Nizami, *Comprehensive Interpretation,* p. xx.
43. Nizami, *Comprehensive Interpretation,* p. xvii.
44. Ibid. Such a letter and number based divination chart is found in the popular *Ta'bīr al-ru'yā* attributed (by the editors) to Imām Muḥammad Baqr al-Majlisī, ed. a committee (Lahore: Maktaba Hamdānī, 1976), p. 30. Nizami, *Comprehensive Interpretation,* p. xviii.
45. Abū al-Faḍl Ḥubaysh ibn Ibrāhīm al-Tiflisī, *Ta'bīr-i khwāb-i Ibn Sīrīn-o-Dāniyāl* (Tehran: Maṭbū'ātī Ḥusaynī, 1988), pp. 15–17.
46. Toufic Fahd, "Ibn Sīrīn," *Encyclopedia of Islam* III, pp. 947–948.
47. *Muntakhab al-Kalām fī ta'bīr al-manām,* ed. 'Abd al-Raḥmān al-Jūzū (Beirut: Dār Maktaba al-Ḥayāt, n.d.), the longer text, was actually written by al-Dārī (ca. 1009–1237). See also John Lamoreaux, "Some Notes on the Dream Manual of al-Dārī," *Rivista degli studi orientali* 70 (1996): 47–52.
48. al-Tiflisī, *Ta'bīr-i khwāb,* 13. Also cited by N. Bland, "On the Muhammedan Science," p. 133.
49. These interpretations could be quite extensive. Ibn Shāhīn's material on the chapters of the Qur'ān in dreams fills thirty pages as he gives three readings for each chapter, his own, al-Kirmānī's, and Ja'far al-Ṣādiq's. Ibn Shāhīn, *Tafsīr al-aḥlām: al-ishārāt fī 'ilm al-'ibārāt* (Cairo: Maṭba'a al-Madanī, 1991), pp. 57–87.
50. Bland, "On the Muhammedan Science," p. 143, citing Ibn Shahīn.
51. Nizami, *Comprehensive Interpretation,* xvi.

52. Ja'far al-Ṣādiq, a scholar considered to be the fifth Imam for the Shi'a Muslims, was also associated with mastery over the occult sciences and aspects of oneiracritic lore were often ascribed to him.
53. Tiflisī, pp. 13–14. Also mentioned in Nizami, *Comprehensive Interpretation,* with some alterations, p. xvii.
54. Lamoreaux, p. 9.
55. Leah Kinberg, *Ibn Abī al-Dunyā Morality in the Guise of Dreams: A Critical Edition of Kitāb al-Manām* (Leiden: E. J. Brill, 1994), p. 44. Marcia Hermansen, review of Leah Kinberg, *Morality in the Guise of Dreams, Oxford Journal of Islamic Studies* 8, 1 (1997): 91–92.
56. Kinberg, *Ibn Abī al-Dunyā Morality in the Guise of Dreams.*
57. Ibid., pp. 44–45.
58. Cairo, al-Bābī al-Ḥalabī, 1972. See also G. E. von Grunebaum, "The Cultural Function of the Dream as Illustrated by Classical Islam," in *The Dream in Human Societies,* eds. G. E. von Grunebaum and Roger Caillois (Berkeley: University of California Press, 1966), 3–21.
59. Hossein Ziai, "Dreams and Dream Interpretation," *Encyclopaedia Iranica* VII (Costa Mesa, CA: Mazda, 1989-), pp. 549–551. Online at www.iranica.com/articles/v7f5/v7f569.html.
60. Carl Ernst, *Rūzbihān Baqlī, Mysticism and the Rhetoric of Sainthood in Persian Sufism* (Richmond, Surrey: Curzon Press, 1996).
61. Bernd Radtke, *The Concept of Sainthood in Early Islamic Mysticism: Two Works by al-Hakim al-Tirmidhi* (Richmond, Surrey: Curzon Press, 1996). Tirmidhī's dreams are commented on by Sara Sviri, "Dreaming Analyzed and Recorded: Dreams in the World of Medieval Islam," in *Dream Cultures: Toward a Comparative History of Dreaming,* eds. Guy G. Stroumsa and David Shulman (New York: Oxford University Press, 1999), pp. 252–273. Sviri discusses al-Tirmidhī specifically pp. 261–268.
62. Jonathan Katz, *Dreams, Sufism, and Sainthood: the Visionary Career of Muhammad al-Zawāwī* (Leiden: E. J. Brill, 1996).
63. Leah Kinberg, "The Legitimation of the Madhāhib through Dreams," *Arabica* 32 (1985): 47–79.
64. Leah Kinberg, "The Standardization of Qur'ān Readings: The Testimonial Value of Dreams," in *Proceedings of the Colloquium on Arabic Grammar,* ed. K. Devenyi (Budapest: Eotvos Lorand University, 1991), pp. 223–238.
65. See Kinberg, *Ibn Abī ad-Dunyā,* and Marcia K. Hermansen, "Mystical Visions as 'Good to Think': Examples from Pre-Modern South Asian Sufi Thought," *Religion* 27 (January 1997): 25–43.
66. Louis Massignon, "Themes archetypiques en onirocritique musulmane," *Eranos Jahrbuch* 12 (1945): 241–251. Henry Corbin, "The Visionary Dream in Islamic Spirituality," *The Dream in Human Societies,* pp. 381–408.
67. Jonathan Katz, *The Visionary Career of al-Zawāwī*, xvi.
68. al-Ghazzālī, *The Remembrance of Death and the Afterlife,* book XL of *The Revival of the Religious Sciences,* trans. T. J. Winter (Cambridge: Islamic Texts Society, 1995), pp. 149–169.
69. Ibid., 164.
70. The "ijāza" was the formal permission to teach or transmit knowledge or spiritual authority.
71. Al-Bukhārī, vol. 9, book 87, no. 144.
72. Maḥmūd ibn 'Alī al-Kāshānī, *Kitāb miṣbāḥ al-hidāya wa miftāḥ al-kifāya* (Tehran: Kitābkhāne-i Sanā'ī, 1946), pp. 171–179.
73. Ibn Khaldūn, *Muqaddimah* I, p. 212.
74. Reported in al-Tiflisī, *Ta'bīr-i Khwāb,* p. 10.
75. Ritual practice of reciting some of the divine names or other pious phrases.

76. An "incident" (wāqi'a) is a true dream or vision. 'Ibn al-'Arabī says that "incidents come from inside, since they derive from the essence of man. Some people see them in a state of sleep, some in a state of annihilation (fanā) and others in the state of wakefulness. They do not veil man from the objects of his sense perception at that time" (*Futūḥāt* II.491.6). William C. Chittick, *The Sufi Path of Knowledge* (Albany: State University of New York Press, 1989), p. 404, note 24.
77. Maḥmūd ibn 'Alī al-Kāshānī, *Kitāb miṣbāḥ al-hidāya,* p. 171.
78. Annemarie Schimmel, *Mystical Dimensions of Islam* (Chapel Hill: University of North Carolina Press, 1975), p. 225, quoting Najmuddīn Kubrā (1220).
79. Al-nafs al-nāṭiqa. In this tradition the meaning is more than "rational" since this level of the soul bestows the individual identity and connects the person to the higher level of the spirit.
80. Ibn Khaldūn, *Muqaddimah* III: 105.
81. Qur'ān 85:22.
82. Fazlur Rahman, "Dreams, Imagination and the 'Ālam al-Mithāl," in *The Dream in Human Societies,* pp. 409–419.
83. Based on al-Ghazzālī, *Remembrance of Death and the Afterlife,* pp. 139–140.
84. Rahman, "Dreams, Imagination and the 'Ālam al-Mithāl," p. 411.
85. Ibid., 419.
86. On divination and canon formation as forms of rationality see Jonathan Z. Smith, "Sacred Persistence: Towards a Redescription of Canon," in *Imagining Religion* (Chicago: University of Chicago Press, 1983), pp. 36–52, and Hermansen, "Mystical Visions as 'Good to Think.'"
87. Vide the ongoing discussion in the study of mysticism between the constructivists, who hold that all experience is mediated by thinking in cultural symbols and the advocates of pure ineffable unitive consciousness.
88. Fahd, "Istikhāra," *Encyclopedia of Islam IV,* pp. 259–260.
89. Ibn Khaldūn, *Muqaddimah,* 1: 231.
90. Ibid., 3: 213.
91. Al-Ghazzali, *Ihya,* book 40, trans. T. J. Winter, pp. 151–152.
92. Al-Ghazzālī, *Deliverance from Error,* trans. Watt (Oxford: One World, 1998), p. 23.
93. Marshall Hodgson, *The Venture of Islam* (Chicago: University of Chicago, 1974).
94. Lamoreaux, "Dream Interpretation," 135.
95. Ibid., pp. 128–227.
96. Sayyid Muḥammad Rezā, *Ufaq-i Mustabil* (Horizons of the Future) (Karachi: Idāra-'Ulūm-si Āl-i Muḥammad, 1989), p. 6.
97. Katherine P. Ewing. "The Dream of Spiritual Initiation and the Organization of Self-Representations among Pakistani Sufis," *American Ethnologist* 17 (1990): 56–74.
98. Ibid., 57–58.
99. Michael Gilsenan, "Signs of Truth: Enchantment, Modernity, and the Dreams of Peasant Women," *Journal of the Royal Anthropological Society* (December 2000): 597–615.
100. J. Johansen, *Sufism and Islamic Reform in Egypt* (Oxford: Clarendon Press, 1996), p. 138.
101. Ibid., p. 611.
102. An introduction to a range of these movements is Marcia K. Hermansen, "In the Garden of American Sufi Movements: Hybrids and Perennials," in *New Trends and Developments in the World of Islam,* ed. Peter Clarke (London: Luzac Oriental Press, 1997), pp. 155–178.
103. Academic articles surveying the history and teachings of this movement are: James Jervis, "The Sufi Order in the West and Pir Vilayat Khan," in *New Trends and Developments in the World of Islam,* ed. Peter B. Clarke (London: Luzac, 1998), pp. 211–260 and Michael M. Koszegi, "The Sufi Order in the West: Sufism's Encounter with the New

Age," in *Islam in North America: A Sourcebook,* ed. Michael A. Koszegi and J. Gordon Melton (New York: Garden Publishing, 1992), pp. 211–222.

104. On Corbin and Jungian thought see Steven M. Wasserstrom, *Religion after Religion: Gershom Scholem, Mircea Eliade, and Henry Corbin at Eranos* (Princeton: Princeton University Press, 1999).
105. Pir Vilayat Khan, "C. G. Jung and Sufism," in *Sufism, Islam and Jungian Psychology,* ed. J. Marvin Spiegelman (Scottsdale, AZ: New Falcon Publications, 1991), pp. 35–53.
106. Ibid., p. 48.
107. Llewellyn Vaughan-Lee, "Dream-Work within a Sufi Tradition," in *Sufism, Islam and Jungian Psychology,* ed. Spiegelman, pp. 131–146, and *The Lover and the Serpent: Dreamwork within a Sufi Tradition* (Rockport, MA: Element, 1990).
108. Online at www.goldensufi.org/4.1aSSbio.html.
109. For example, in Hindu and Buddhist yogas, as discussed in the present volume.
110. Andrew Vidich, "A Living Sufi Saint: Shaykh Muhaamad Adil al-Haqqani and the Naqshbandiyya Method of Self-Transformation," Ph.D. diss., Berne University, New Hampshire, 2000, pp. 189, 500.
111. Refik Algan, "The Dream of the Sleeper: Dream Interpretation and Meaning in Sufism," *Gnosis* 22 (winter 1992), online at http://www.webcom.com/threshld/society/articles/dreams.html.
112. Chapter 14 in this volume.

5

Sending a Voice, Seeking a Place

Visionary Traditions among Native Women of the Plains

Lee Irwin

According to the Lakota holy man Nicholas Black Elk, *hambleyapi,* or "crying for a vision," predates even the use of the sacred pipe and is the center of Plains Indian spirituality. This emphasis on dreams and visions acquired either spontaneously or through a vision quest is one of the central and unifying factors among many Native American religious traditions. The very earliest historical records all bear eloquent witness to the long-standing importance of the vision quest experience and the close attention given to their contents, enactment, and the ways in which dreaming contributed to cultural transformation and personal achievement. It is these historical sources that I wish to explore, particularly as they relate to women dreamers and visionaries, in order to provide a summary overview of the value and importance of dreams and visions for traditional Plains women.[1]

Among the many native communities of the Great Plains, the experience of a "dream" or "vision" was not usually marked by distinctive native terms or in accordance to the particular conditions or circumstances under which it was received. For example, the Lakota term *ihan'bla* or *hanble* (interpreted by Lakota as either "dreams" or "visions") is defined as follows by the nineteenth-century Lakota holy man George Sword:

> *Hanble* is a communication from *Wakan Tanka* [Great Mystery] or a spirit to one of mankind. It may come at any time, or in any manner, to anyone. It may be relative to the one who receives it, or to another. It may be communicated in Lakota or *hanbloglaka* (language of the spirits). Or it may be only by sight or sounds not of language. It may come directly from the one giving it, or it may be sent by an akicita (messenger). It may come unsought or it may come by seeking it.

Notable in this turn-of-the-century definition is the fact that no distinction is made between either sleeping or waking ("it may come in any manner") and that the dream may have an aural rather than visual content as well as occur spontaneously or through fasting.[2] What matters in the native context is the consequence of the vision experience and not the physiological state of the visionary. Further, what is called a vision or dream may occur while wide awake, as noted by a contemporary elder Lakota woman who reported, speaking in English of her visionary Thunder dream, "I had a dream, a vision. I was wide awake when I had it; I saw it during the day."[3]

The state of the dreamer, either waking or sleeping, is rarely mentioned in the ethnography, and many of the greatest visions occurred in states difficult if not impossible to define, such as Black Elk's great vision at nine years old that came spontaneously while he lay sick and unmoving in his parent's tipi. The Gros Ventre and the Arapaho agree that visions occur both in waking and sleeping circumstances, and among the Oto the distinction was drawn between the power-bestowing vision and the nonpower dream. It is this last distinction that I will use in this chapter, where the terms "dream," "vision" or "visionary dream" refer to receiving a gift of unusual or extraordinary ability in a heightened state of awareness, usually from a humanlike dream spirit or ancestor (while either awake or sleeping) and usually accompanied by specific directions for actions, dress, or songs.[4] This power, when enacted and demonstrated successfully to others, confirms and validates the experience, regardless of the state of the dreamer in which the power was first revealed.

Dreams and visions of power have long been tied to deeply held religious values as primary sources of guidance and affirmation of the sacred quality of the religious world for native peoples.[5] In order to understand women's visionary experience, it is first necessary to cultivate an appreciation for the sensitivity of the subject among Native American peoples today. Many Native American women pay close attention to their dreams and interpret their dream experiences in a cultural or religious context that is alien to most nonnative researchers. Thus there is, first, a need to understand the important *historical* role of dreams and visions in Native American traditional cultures; and second, there is a need to learn respect and appreciate the importance of dreams in *contemporary* native spiritual life. However, because of the sensitivity of the subject for most contemporary native women, there are very few contemporary examples. Dreams are not discussed freely even within a circle of relatives, let alone with nonrelatives and nonnatives. It would be a considerable breech of good manners and politeness to ask native women about their dreamers unless such information is freely volunteered. This is particularly true for men while speaking with native women. Many native people feel that most Anglo-Americans lack the appropriate respect or belief in the sacred character of dreaming because Anglo-Americans have largely ignored or denied dreaming in their own cultures. Because secular dream theories have denied or subverted the sacred meaning of these dreams, most contemporary visionary experiences have remained private and largely confined to those with a more traditional spiritual orientation.

A third problem is the gender problem of the male-dominant paradigms that have functioned so strongly in the gathering of much of the traditional dream materials. This bias is pervasive, as the majority of historical ethnography collected is primarily written by male ethnographers interested in subjects other than women's dreams and visions. Nonnative male ethnographers have generally dismissed the dream experiences of women as marginal to native spirituality—a false and misleading conclusion. Recently however, thanks to the efforts of Mark St. Pierre and his Oglala Lakota wife Tilda Long Soldier (1995), we are able to see both how contemporary dreaming practices still exist among Plains women today and the important role they have played in traditional culture. Their work is exceptional and certainly overcomes the bias of an entrenched nonnative male view of dreaming. Through cooperative and meaningful dialogue, native women's voices emerge with a genuine sense of authenticity and accurate representation long needed to help give a more balanced view of women's role in visionary spirituality.

Most older historical visionary narratives are scattered in the diverse complexity of written sources and are rarely visible in materials of a more general ethnographic nature. To date, few single works have been dedicated exclusively to the subject of Native American dreams and visions.[6] The dream ethnography, of which there is a considerable amount, is tucked into paragraphs and short citations often as an aside or peripheral concern of the ethnographers. Many nonnative dream researchers have marginalized dreaming as epiphenomenal—that is, as an unimportant byproduct of biological processing constructed out of the "bits and pieces" of everyday life. Other researchers have assimilated dreaming into a Euro-American pathological model of psychology, regarding dreams as a disturbed and complex imaging of emotional problems and psychosocial imbalances.[7] A third model is the "culture pattern" model that interprets dreams as nothing other than shared social imagery reinforcing existing, and therefore static, communal structures.[8] None of these models provides an adequate, accurate, or fruitful perspective for understanding the religious or spiritual role that dreams and visions have played as a creative and transformative medium in the maintenance of personal and collective religious identity for First Nation peoples. From the distant past to the immediate present, dreams and visions have been primary and widespread sources of personal empowerment among many Native American communities, particularly on the Great Plains.

Women's Visionary Traditions

Within the existing historical ethnography, recorded among Plains peoples over the last hundred years (over 350 dreams from mostly nineteenth and early to mid-twentieth century sources), I have found approximately 10–15 percent of these narratives are *about* women, while an even smaller percentage are *by* women. There are also frequent comments about female dreaming and visionary practices, usually made by men (and occasionally by women) who acted as knowledgeable interpreters of their shared religious worldviews. What emerges, in a highly fragmentary fashion, is a fascinating picture of the importance that Plains women, like men, gave to their dreams, primarily in the context of a traditional religious orientation of the late nineteenth and early to mid-twentieth centuries. Unlike men, who usually sought dreams in a structured vision quest, the majority of dream narratives clearly show that women did not seek dreams in a ritually structured way.[9] In fact, a majority of narratives about female visionary experiences are based on the sudden and *spontaneous* arising, either in sleep or while awake, of very intense, vivid visionary dreams without the dreamer necessarily making any attempt to seek such a vision. As noted recently by Orville Mesteth in talking about his Lakota grandmother Blue Earring, a respected holy woman: "For women it is different from how it is for men. A woman's calling is in her dreams: it is usually powerful, spontaneous. She does not always need to be trained in the way that a holy man would."[10]

In some traditional cases, young women might have visionary dreams at the onset of first menstruation (age ten to sixteen years), when they could choose to actively seek a vision, such as among the Plains Cree, Lakota, and Gros Ventre. Among the Sioux, George Sword, a Lakota holy man recorded, "A girl may seek a vision by wrapping her first menstrual flow and placing it in a tree. Visions frequently come without seeking to the very old men or women and to shamans."[11] There was no compulsion or even expectation that a woman must seek a vision. The transition from child to woman (the capacity for childbearing) was considered an opportune time for visionary experience, as many different Plains peoples believed that dream-spirits would appear to give guidance and new abilities for future adult life. Also, at the onset of menses, or "moon-time," young women normally went, as other women did, into a special lodge for a traditional number of days (thereby being liberated from all familial obligation and cared for usually by postmenopausal relatives).[12] This period of seclusion was a favored time for visionary experiences, and isolation in the menstrual lodge, coupled with the altered mental and emotional condition attributed by Plains women to this special time, often resulted in visionary experiences. The power of women during this time was considered extraordinary, and while threatening to male spiritual power, it heightened female visionary abilities.[13]

awesome

Young women of certain tribes of the southern Plains, such as Comanche, Apache, Shoshoni and Kiowa, would have been exposed to only minimal recitations of dream narratives by relatives or by a healer who prepared them for their first visionary fast.[14] Such a narrative, for young girls, might have been the first such narrative ever heard, as dreams were rarely recited in public or in private. Further, kinship and gender roles often inhibited communication of dreams between men and women, although postmenopausal healers did prepare female (and sometimes male) candidates for fasting in some tribes.[15] Nevertheless, on the Plains, there was a widespread belief that talking about dreams could lead to losing the power of the dream (this is an additional reason why so few dream narratives exist). Thus young women were not exposed to dream narratives usually until after they had significant visionary experience and began to question elder (usually female) relatives about the meaning of their experiences.[16]

Among some traditional communities, a structured fasting for visions by young adolescent women occurred only during the premarital stage of life. For example, among the Mandan, adolescent women fasted on the top of the corn scaffolds, usually rather large, sturdy racks of several layers made for drying corn and squash next to the earth lodge dwelling—where they were safe from enemy raids and exposed to the spiritual powers of the natural world. The fact that corn was primarily a female power to the Mandan made the corn scaffolds especially potent for women.[17] Among the Kansa, young women also undertook an informal vision quest, but significantly, "women frequently dreamed of the accomplishments and powers of their brothers, aptly illustrating the dominant male structure of the social order."[18] Among the Lakota, the *Tapa Wankayeyapi,* or Throwing of the Ball Rite, was associated with a visionary woman whose behavior was imitated by young girls who were specially initiated into the rite.[19]

However, by far the most pervasive pattern for women dreamers is the spontaneous vision arising under circumstances of stress, loss, or isolation. As Boy told Father John Cooper with regard to the Gros Ventre, "A woman does not ask for power. Power comes to her. When mourning for relatives and sleeping out and suffering without food, somebody might take pity on her and give her power without her asking."[20] For the Absarokee (Crow), Robert Lowie writes: "Young girls did not seek visions, but when older they might and did. Usually this happened when a relative had been killed or died a natural death."[21] While mourning for a loved one, relative, husband, or friend, or by joining other women in mourning for their newly dead relatives, women frequently had visionary experiences. For women throughout the northern Plains tribes, mourning was a time of profound emotional expression—they cut their hair short, wore old cast-off clothing, and often slashed their arms or legs to express their feelings of loss and grief. Men rarely had this kind of sanctioned emotional outlet. Male sorrow and pain was often channeled into aggressive warfare patterns or reserved for the prayerful crying during the structured vision quest. For women, the death of a relative or child often resulted in wandering away from camp, usually alone or with another relative, weeping and mourning. In this condition, a vision might occur in which a dream-spirit would appear and give the woman new power and direction for her life.

A uniquely detailed example of this type of experience is illustrated by the Absarokee medicine woman Pretty Shield, who mourned for more than two months due to the death of her beautiful infant daughter, staying away from the camp and wandering in the hills, day after day:[22]

> I had slept little, sometimes lying down alone in the hills at night, and always on hard places. I ate only enough to keep me alive, hoping for a medicine-dream, a vision that would help me to live and to help others. One morning . . . I saw a woman ahead of me. She was walking fast . . . but suddenly she stopped and stood still, looking at the ground. I thought I knew her, thought that she was a woman who had died four years before. I felt afraid. I stopped, my heart beating fast. "Come here, daughter." Her words seemed to draw me toward her against my will.
>
> Walking a few steps, I saw that she was not a real woman, but that she was a [sacred] Person, and that she was standing beside an ant hill. "Come here, daughter." Again I walked toward her when I did not wish to move. Stopping by her side, I did not try to look into her face. My heart was nearly choking me. "Rake up the side of this ant hill and ask for the things that you wish, daughter," the Person said, then she was gone.
>
> Now in this medicine-dream, I entered a beautiful white lodge, with a war-eagle at the head. He did not speak to me, and yet I have often seen him since that day. And even now the ants help me. I listen to them always. They are my medicine, these busy, powerful little people, the ants.

It is significant to note here that the search for power through visionary experience is often motivated by a desire among female dreamers to *share* the power received for the welfare of the community. This is much less true for Plains male visionaries, who tended to seek dreams in terms of personal, individual empowerment. Further, the power of her vision is not transmitted by the woman who appears but by the ants and a war eagle. The dead woman acts as an intermediary, leading the woman to a more potent source of instruction and power, a common occurrence in many dream narratives for both women and men.

During other periods of stress, in camp as well as away from it, women experienced powerful, meaningful visions that helped to guide them through difficulties in their personal conflicts or that might show them how to respond in family quarrels.[23] Faced with difficulties, frustration, or anger, they would wander away from camp and expose themselves to the spiritual powers regarded as intrinsic to the natural world. For example, one Mandan woman was guided by a wolf spirit who appeared in a vision to help her cope with an abusive husband.[24]

> My mother's mother, Coyote Woman, lived with her [abusive] husband. . . . He sent her out every morning at daylight to see if there were any animals in their pits. One day there was a large wolf in one of the pits. The wolf said, "Take me out, and I will give you power to do anything you ask." Coyote Woman did not know what to do because she was afraid of her husband. The wolf knew her thoughts. He coughed up a blue stone. "Take that stone and use it among your people." . . . She took the stone and let the wolf go. . . . The wolf had told her, "If anybody in your tribe is mean to you and you want to get rid of him, cut out an image of him in leather, put the stone beside the image, and cover both with hot ashes. Then the person will die."

Coyote Woman tells her husband, who then uses the power of the blue stone to kill her first husband, but the wolves tell her in further dreams to send him hunting with great promises of success and he is then killed by a wolf pack.

Another condition of extreme stress was being abducted (and possibly raped) by enemy warriors. An Absalooke woman who was captured by the Piegan (Blackfeet) managed to escape her captors and in the process to steal an otter medicine bundle. While fleeing south to rejoin her people, she was overtaken by a snowstorm and, seeking shelter, fell asleep with the otter bundle clasped tightly in her arms: "The otter gave her a dream and told her that if they got home in safety, they should join the Tobacco [society] and take the lead in going to the garden."[25] While stealing the bundle and escaping from the Piegan would bring her recognition, her vision also sanctioned her participation in an important and central tobacco ceremony and gave her a position of prominence in the religious life of her people. A Kiowa woman who was captured by the Pawnee and then escaped was caught in a huge thunderstorm during her return flight to her people. Taking refuge from the thunder, lightning, and driving hailstones, she crawled under the dried carcass of a dead buffalo laying on the open plains. Subsequently she had a vision in which the buffalo appeared to her and gave her the power to heal wounds received in battle as well as the knowledge of how to handle certain objects sacred to the buffalo. Later, after her safe return to the Kiowa, she passed her knowledge to the members of the Buffalo Society.[26]

Another typical circumstance for visions and remarkable dreams of power was illness. Out-of-body experiences and various types of life-after-death narratives are relatively common in the visionary ethnography, for both men and women. For example, a Cheyenne woman by the name of Picking-Bones Woman had an experience of floating out of her body, out of the lodge where she lay ill and, after running across the ground, entering an earthen butte where she was given visionary instructions by a group of elders. She then returned to her lodge, saw her body lying ill to the point of death, and then suddenly awoke to find her illness gone.[27]

Many women visionaries had experience of meeting or interacting with ancestors or recently departed dead. While on the southern Plains dreams of ghosts were usually taken to be a dangerous sign of enchantment to be avoided, in the northern Plains such dreams were common and indicated a strong tie between the community of the living and the departed, particularly for women. The Lakota woman Mary Buck, or Walks Holy Woman, was saved from a blinding snow storm by a spirit ghost who showed her where to walk and who sang as they walked through the storm. This was the spirit of a man believed to have died but who used to walk the railroad tracks singing as he went.[28] The Lakota singer Madonna Swan told of a visionary dream she had while in the tuberculosis sanitarium in 1973 in which she found herself in a log hall where there was dancing and singing, with many of her dead relatives present. When she followed one relative outside, he led her down a path to a stream: "When I got down there, I thought to myself, 'You know, this man is dead, and I'm talking to him. Now he is trying to get me through that water. I'd better not go through that water, or I'll die.'"[29] She followed him partway into the water but then turned back, only to wake in the hospital sweating and short of breath with the nurse hovering over her exclaiming how she had almost died.

Visionary Power

What exactly did these women receive in their visionary experience? This brings us to the profound and difficult question of female visionary power, another area relatively unexplored in either current or past ethnography. As noted, the power associated with menstruation is characteristic of a distinction often made between male and female power. Ella Deloria, a full-blood Lakota woman writing in the 1930s, referred to women's menstrual power as *Wakan*—mysterious, sacred, and, as clashing with male sacred power, it was *ohayaka,* "causing a block or entanglement."[30] The concept of "power" as attained in a visionary experience or as a consequence of sexual differences had a competitive quality to it. Joseph Rockboy, a Sigangu Sioux elder, told Mark St. Pierre:[31] "When a woman is having her time, her blood is flowing, and this blood is full of mysterious powers that are related to child bearing. At this time she is particularly powerful. To bring a child into world is the most powerful thing in creation. A man's power is nothing compared to this and he can do nothing compared to it. We respect that power."

Women's power and men's power were not the same and, on some occasions, actually worked against each other, a belief that resulted in the creation of various female and male societies, each with their own secret rites. Because of the widespread belief in the contrary qualities of gender-specific power, many women did not actualize the capacities given to them in dreams or visions until *after* they became postmenopausal. And here we have to be careful not to let gender issues obscure the fact that *both* men and women often had a very long period of latency between the vision experience and its actualization—a wait of twenty or thirty years to use visionary power was not uncommon for either gender. One Lakota holy man compared women's power to medicine plants gathered in the fall: "They are like women, these plants are like women you see. It's when all that life-producing stuff is over, then all the wisdom is in the root. That's when they work with medicine the right way."[32]

An example of women's visionary power is that of the elder Blackfoot healer Spear Woman, who would prepare herbs and then, while singing buffalo songs, would kneel by the couch of a sick person and imitate the actions of her dream buffalo "pawing the ground, hooking with her head, and making sounds like a buffalo bull."[33] A more elaborate and complex example is that of Sanapia, a famous Comanche woman healer who spent years learning from her mother the use of eagle power. Her training required four years of careful effort, under strict supervision, the culmination of which was the transfer of visionary power from mother to daughter after a four-day fast. She notes the invocation of that power as recorded by David Jones as follows: "When the eagle came to her, everything around her disappeared with the resultant image of an eagle against a murky gray background. . . . While the eagle was present, Sanapia trembled violently and perspired freely. She states that her heart beat very rapidly and she felt as if she was going to faint."[34] The mastery of this power took many years and required special training and effort. After fully acquiring this power, she was able to heal illness successfully and had other dreams in which she was given further instructions by a dream figure representing her eagle power. This type of complete identification of the dreamer with the dream-spirit during healing and ritual enactment was not uncommon and frequently occurred in ceremonies and dances.[35]

The power given in these dreams and visions was often accompanied by restrictive prohibitions. Rarely did it come without some specific obligations that required special personal discipline and certain restrictions in behavior or normative social habits. For example, a Stoney woman given bear power refused to eat bear meat, a delicacy among the Stoney. When she broke this prohibition once, she felt that she had to struggle against being overwhelmed by her bear spirit. Significantly, her mother also was a bear dreamer who had her husband bring her a bear cub that she "nursed together with her own child, one at each breast."[36] To accept bear power meant forming an intense personal relationship with that power, a relationship that could protect and guide through dreams but also could overwhelm the visionary if prohibitions were ignored. Primarily, the proscription against eating or killing the animal functioned to maintain a relationship of respect for the power of that animal and to protect the individual from an overabundance or excess of visionary power—excess in any form was considered dangerous and threatening for many traditional Plains peoples. The reciprocity between the dreamer and the dream-spirit was balanced through careful attention to everyday behaviors that might in any way distort or obscure the dream power. Other prohibitions included such instructions as not accepting payment for healing, various types of self-discipline and self-control (not behaving in loud or disruptive fashion, not gossiping, and so on), and not misusing or abusing the gift of power.

Not all visionary power was accepted. A woman might reject any power that came to her in a vision or a dream if she felt that is was incongruent or dangerous for her. An Arapaho woman rejected bear power that came to her spontaneously because she did not wish to become a bear doctor, which she regarded as extremely dangerous.[37] Among the Gros Ventre, it was believed that power would shorten the lifespan of the individual, and such beliefs were propagated through exhortations given by the village criers. There are a number of examples recorded of the rejection of visionary power by Gros Ventre women who received spontaneous visions but rejected the power out of dread or because they did not wish to follow the prohibitions involved.[38] On the other hand, rejecting power could be dangerous: A woman (or man) who dreamed of thunder power and rejected it among the Siouan peoples was in danger of being struck by lightning as punishment for refusing to accept the power and its responsibilities.[39]

Among the Tsistsistas (Cheyenne), power was often *shared* between husband and wife. Women married to a healer or visionary might assist and participate in the use of those special mysterious abilities. George Grinnell wrote, "A [Tsistsista] man cannot become a doctor by himself; when he receives the power, his wife—who afterwards is his assistant—must also be taught and receive certain secrets."[40] The use of the imperative here is significant. The man *must* have the assistance of a woman. This sharing of knowledge by the husband and the necessary assistance of the wife is expressive of a recognition on the part of some Plains men of the uniqueness of female power and its important contribution to the healing process. Among the some northern Plains groups, there was a shared belief that husband and wife could or should work together. Dream-spirits frequently appear as a couple throughout the ethnography, and many visionaries were taken to places of power where they are received by a man and woman, *both* of whom give the visionary a gift of power. The dual symbolism of this shared power, in the Tsistsista healing context, reflects the intimacy between husband and wife, strengthening the spiritual bonds between them. The healing context thus emulated the sacred powers that also appeared as husband and wife. This co-operative healing was particularly true among the Cheyenne, Blackfeet, Comanche, Gros Ventre and Crow. Data is scanty on the subject, but there are examples of women continuing as healers on their own at the death of their husbands.[41]

Other power gained by women through dreams includes highly complex and divergent traditions in the area of crafts and artistic ability, and particularly discovering specific motifs: Women received visionary dreams for making special bead and porcupine quill designs on clothing and other articles.[42] Among the Lakota Sioux, skill in crafts was a power given by dreaming of Double-Woman, a spiritual being who was credited with the discovery of quill working and its associated arts. Women who dreamed of her became members of the *Wipata Okolakiciye*' society and shared their dreams and techniques with each other. Nellie Two Bulls, a Lakota elder, had a series of dreams involving the appearance of three spirits that she continually saw during the day when she was eleven or twelve years old. After a number of such appearances, she had the following experience:

> I woke up from my sleep and opened my eyes to see three women standing before me . . . They said, "We want you to see this. We brought all our work and we are going to display it." And they each got a bundle of their work and put it on the table before me. The first tall one, had all bead work, and the middle one, all quill work, and the third one didn't display her work. "Do you want this?" she said, "I am Blue Bird Woman and this bag is full of songs. I am going to give you a voice."[43]

Her mother interpreted this dream as a Double-Woman dream investing her daughter with special craft ability, and her grandfather put her on a hill to fast and pray. The dream, although unwanted and unexpected, nevertheless became a source of power for making beautiful and complex quill and bead designs.

Another representative example of dreams sanctioning clothing designs for protective power is the well-known Ghost Dance dress or shirt, which was made by women as a result of their visionary experience during the Ghost Dance movement in the early 1890s.[44] William Whitman recorded the following among the Ponca: "Vision frequently validated techniques in the arts. A woman went fasting. She was daubed with mud. She was going along a creek when she saw a little bush covered with yarn in pretty designs. That was how she learned those designs."[45] Often these spontaneous visions were attributed to Spider Woman, who appeared to Plains women visionaries and whose complex and intricate creations served as models for symbolic designs on clothing and other articles. Face painting was another sacred visionary context; for example, among the Blackfeet, a medicine woman, after receiving a special vision, could paint her face in such a way as to control the weather.[46]

On a wider social basis, a woman visionary could receive dreams that acted as a means of validating her entry into a visionary society. For example, among the Lakota, a woman might dream of the Thunder Being and become a *Heyoka,* or "Thunder Dreamer," who was specifically empowered to perform special rituals or to act in a somewhat eccentric, humorous, or "backward" manner.[47] This was regarded as particularly powerful and mysterious by many groups, particularly as a *Heyoka* often challenged social norms and leadership roles in the community. Another example comes from the Absalooke woman dreamer Magpie On Earth who fasted while mourning the death of her elder husband:

> The Evening Star came toward me in human form. It was wrapped in a red blanket and its face was painted with red parallel lines. It told me that I would marry again. This time it would be young man of the tribe. . . . The Evening Star disappeared. I heard a voice speaking to me from the sky, "You are called over there." I looked up and saw a chickadee flying overhead. It repeated those words. I stood up and followed the bird. I came to a place where four men were building four sweat lodges. They were jack rabbits, the servants of Morning Star. I was told to build four similar sweat lodges. . . ."If you do this, " I was told, "and you desire something, it will come to you easily."[48]

Among the traditional Pawnee, Yellow Corn Woman, during a meeting of the Bear medicine society, told of her recent vision:

> I had a vision. I saw Bear Chief wearing the bear robe over his shoulders and the bearclaw neck piece around his neck. . . . He said, "My sister, Father [Bear] and Mother [Cedar Tree] have not had any smoke for many years. We (dead people) are watching for our people to have the ceremony. The people think the ceremony is lost. It is not, for one of the Bear men who knows the secret ceremony is still with you. I ask that you tell the people so they can have the ceremony, for it is time." I woke up and the last few days I have been crying to think that I should be the one to tell you. I have a cow which you can have so you can have the ceremony. Then she began to cry."[49]

Thus female visions could sanction sponsorship for many ritual activities. A woman dreamer might receive an injunction to sponsor a ceremony or to revive an old practice or rites. Equally significant are records of women dreamers given foundational ceremonies in *male* ritual activities, such as in the building of the Sun Dance lodge among the Blackfeet initiated by the female visionary Mink-Woman, who wandered away from camp in the winter desperate for food for her children and who heard singing in the distance:

> She went under a big tree that had shed the snow, and found that the singing was under a big log there . . . she could hear the words of the song, which were: "Woman, come and take me. I am strong with Sun's power." . . . She conquered her fear, and, kneeling, lifted some bark that had slipped down from the log, and found under it, and resting upon a mat of buffalo hair, a small reddish-colored stone that had the shape of a buffalo. . . . Mink-Woman carried the buffalo stone concealed in her bosom, slept with it close under her pillow. . . . Then, on the fourth night, while she slept, the stone said to her: "Poor woman, I pity you and your poor starving people, and am going to help you. Now, listen carefully; I am going to tell you what you must do to save your people." And with that, the stone talked to her for some time.[50]

The visionary powers of dreams also gave a sanction for switching gender identity and roles among women (and men). Such women as the Pawnee Woman-Who-Goes-As-A-Warrior show clearly that women could have visions that allowed them to participate fully in male-dominant activities.[51] Among the Piegan (Blackfeet), this resulted in a special social category called "Manly-Hearted Women" who might, as a result of dreams or visions, live a life modeled on male behavior.[52] Such women might take up the life of a male as warrior and provider and actually marry another woman based on her visionary experiences. Other dreams or visions could sanction a later return to more conventional social roles. Women also might receive dreams that gave them knowledge of contraceptives or how to unite women with unfaithful husbands.[53]

In a more advanced sense, women dreamers and visionaries could become medicine women and spiritual leaders depending on a continued pattern of dreaming over many years. Based on her dreams, Martha Bad Warrior became the first woman keeper of the Lakota Sacred Calf Pipe bundle just as the Cheyenne woman dreamer Josie Limpy became the keeper of the Sacred Hat Bundle.[54] A Lakota woman could become a *Winyan Wakan,* or "holy woman," based on her many dreams and the successful demonstration of her abilities acquired in them, and would be generally known in terms of the specific power or ability she had received in visions. For example, she might be known as a bear dreamer or an eagle healer (*Wambli Wapiye*). Usually a crisis preceded her ability to integrate and use the power successfully, followed by a period of learning and continued dream instruction from the spirit world and from other advanced dreamers. The Lakota healer Yellow Bird Woman describes her visionary healing:

> It's getting a little bit stronger and stronger every time I go into a sweat lodge. If I take somebody in there, there are spirits in there, and I see them. Little lights, little blue lights. There are two of them—one is red inside and white around the edge, the other one blue and white around the edge. They come on each side of me and sit there. . . . And when I pray for someone they go across and sit beside them. . . . I doctor people for all sorts of things, mostly women for alcohol, spouse problems and even witchcraft.[55]

Conclusion

In the dreaming ethnography, dreams and visions of power among Native American women in the context of their traditional religious orientation was an important and even crucial aspect of social identity and personal, spiritual empowerment. Dreams sanctioned roles of religious leadership, participation in healing rites, ceremonies, dances, warfare expeditions, gender identity, and social activism. These visionary dreams resulted in the ability to perform healings, to acquire special knowledge of herbs, to lead gender-specific rites, and to attain an ability to resolve conflict and provide sound and meaningful leadership both in annual rituals and in times of crisis or severe need. Elder women frequently were regarded as fully empowered religious specialists with unique and sometimes even frightening abilities. However, while witchcraft and sorcery might be practiced by any empowered dreamer, the visionary ethnography is remarkably lacking in instances of the negative or destructive use of visionary power by women. The majority of the ethnography shows women acting primarily as healers and adjudicators of conflict in communal circumstances, sharing their power and seeking power for the benefit of others.

The question then arises: What are Native American Plains women dreamers dreaming today? As noted, this is a subject of great sensitivity among many Plains peoples. Further, these traditions have undergone rapid transformation into the present. There are still native oral traditions, distinct from the somewhat oblique nonnative written traditions, that fully affirm the value and importance of women's dreams as sources of spiritual empowerment. There is no doubt that among many contemporary native women, the dreaming tradition is still an "underground" tradition for evaluating and synthesizing issues of personal relatedness, identity, and social transformation. Among the Lakota, the *Sina Wakan Okolakiciye,* or Sacred Shawl Society, was founded in 1979 on the basis of a woman's visionary dream. This society is dedicated to contemporary concerns, such as providing shelter and support for battered women and helping to rebuild the Lakota family.[56]

Among Plains women the capacity to dream, to have powerful, meaningful visions, functions as an expression of their relatedness to both the social and natural world—as a sacred relationship to unseen and mysterious dimensions and powers. The reality of the visionary dream is an opening into greater empowerment and identity and as such is still an important and provocative activity. Contemporary dreams or visions still come to women in an unplanned and at times unwanted series of experiences that culminate in the acquisition of spiritual power and understanding. Dreaming for women is not so much a function of an active search as it is a discovery of *deep potential,* regardless of the conditions of the individual. This is particularly illustrated by the dreaming path of a contemporary Lakota healer and mother of five, Good Lifeways Woman (her sacred name). In 1975 she began to have a long series of visionary experiences completely spontaneously. They became particularly vivid during certain healing ceremonies she attended. Later she fasted on Bear Butte and had the following vision:

> I was facing north, and fell asleep. In that state I saw a large shape approaching me. I assumed it was an eagle. It was so big that it almost covered the sky. When it got closer I could see that it was an owl. It looked at me with those same yellow eyes. Soon that owl took on the shape of a man. . . . The man drew a circle in the dirt. In the dirt appeared an owl's face and an eagle's face. The blue light [which she had seen several times before this] was also present. It marched up my pipe stem. The blue light asked, "Are you ready? When you are ready I will help you," and that blue light traveled all around me.[57]

After this experience it still took many more years of dreaming for her to begin to use the power of her dreams correctly and in a healing manner. She dreamed of an altar with three flags and discovered the meaning only in subsequent dreams. Along with owl and eagle power she also acquired bear power and had to learn how to use it with the assistance and guidance of other spiritual teachers among the Lakota. Other such contemporary examples of woman dreamers can be found, including dreams foretelling death, warning dreams, medicine dreams, and many dreams of the recently dead.[58]

The capacity to enter into visionary worlds, to open the inner person to sacred potential and a focused, creative content that gives a sense of not only direction and purpose but an enhanced sense of personal empowerment is *crucial* in a largely secular world suffering from the contractions and unnecessary failures of the spiritual imagination. If we as human beings wish to attain to our full inner potential, we must, like the courageous women visionaries of the Plains, believe in our capacity to enter deeper visionary realms. As responsible members of a healthy world community, we need to search within the depths of the human heart and find there a voice speaking mythically, magically, and powerfully to guide us toward a greater realization of what we may fully become as human beings.[59] Native women dreamers certainly epitomize a tradition of dreaming in the face of great challenge and frequent hardship, which resulted in an enhancement of their individual capacity and their social ability. The continuation of that tradition in the present (and future) certainly represents a spiritual activity that unites many central issues of women's spiritual identity. It also provides an example for further assessment of the importance of women's visions in relating to many other religious worldviews. Perhaps this cannot be said better than by the following dream of the Lakota, Good Lifeways Woman:

> Once I dreamed I was in a room like a Gymnasium; it was broad daylight. I was called to the corner of the room, where I found a peculiar light. It was in the form of a medicine wheel. From one quadrant of the wheel came a red light. It represented the Red Man. It came to me that the Red Man's contribution to the whole was spiritual insight. From another quadrant came a dark light; it represented the Black Man and it came to me that his gift was the expression of emotions, expressed physically in things like music and dance. In another corner was the white light, it represented the White Man. It came to me that the White Man's gift was in bringing ideas into physical reality. In another quadrant was a yellow light; it represented the Yellow Man. It came to me that his gift was in mental powers such as meditation and ancient wisdom that produced acupuncture. Each has a gift to share with the whole, none can exist without the other; all people must have balance in themselves. Neither should one be too powerful and ignore the importance of the other, in this way all things will be balanced.[60]

Notes

See Joseph Epes Brown (1973: 44). This chapter is written in honor of Joseph Epes Brown and his many years of work in the field of Native American religions. I also want to take this opportunity to express my thanks to his wife Elenita Brown and to their daughter, Emily, who both read and commented on this chapter and made significant contributions to its contents.

1. Contemporary research has only begun to unpack the intricacies and complexity of dreaming among North American indigenous religions. For a summary, see Erika Bourguignon (1972), Richard Applegate (1978), William Powers (1982), Barbara Tedlock (1987), Robert Ruby (1989), Lee Irwin (1994), and David Shulman and Guy Stroumsa (1999, containing articles on native dreaming by Barbara and Dennis Tedlock). Native American authors writing on the subject have been very few; see John Fire and Richard Erdoes (1972), Garter Snake (1980), Arthur Amiotte (1982), Ed McGaa (1990), Heather Valencia (1991) and more recently, Mark St. Pierre and Tilda Long Soldier (1995).
2. James R. Walker (1980: 79) gives the quote on George Sword. Among other tribes, little or no distinction is made linguistically between dreams or visions as most groups have only one term for both, for example traditional Absarokee used *Bacire* for dreams in sleep and for waking visions. Among the old Iroquois, the term *ondinoc* was often used for waking and sleeping dreams and interpreted as "a desire inspired by a spirit." Among ethnographers over the last hundred years the terms "dreams" and "visions" are used interchangeably. Contemporary native people have also confirmed that a sharp distinction between waking or sleeping is not necessary today (personal communication).
3. St. Pierre and Long Soldier (1995: 122, 132).
4. See Lee Irwin (1994: 90, 129, 257, note 1, and 263–264, note 8).
5. For more on essential religious values among Native American communities, see Joseph Epes Brown (1982: 57ff).
6. The early work of the pioneer ethnographer Ruth Benedict (1922, 1923) has been a primary reference for all studies in Native American dreams and vision. Significantly,

early Native American dream ethnography has been discussed by women authors with more frequency and depth than many other early areas of ethnographic concern. Few other early works exist. Some of the primary ones include the following, arranged chronologically: Barbara Freire-Marreco (1912); William Morgan (1932); Jackson Lincoln (1935); Gertrude Toffelmier and Katherine Luomala (1936); and Dorothy Eggan (1949, 1966).

7. Dream theory in cognitive psychology is a dominant trend in academically oriented dream research and epiphenomenal models are pervasive. See, for example, David Foulkes (1985); for a more historical overview and critique, see R. E. Haskel (1986) and Harry Hunt (1986). Pathological models of dreaming can be traced from Freud and have been pursued in the Native American context; see Clyde Kluckhohn and William Morgan (1951) and George Devereux (1951, 1956, 1957).
8. The "culture pattern" theory in dreaming originated in the Franz Boas school of anthropology (Columbia University) and is strongly present in Native American dream analysis through the 1960s. Moderated by behavioral psychological theory in dreaming, it has emphasized dreaming as a reinforcement of existing cultural norms; see Roy D'Andrade (1961). This trend was carried out particularly in the writings of Anthony Wallace (1958) and modified with much greater sensitivity by Morris Opler (1959) and particularly by A. Irving Hallowell (1966); see also Patricia Albers and Seymour Parker (1971).
9. The male vision-quest pattern was highly diverse and heterogeneous and did not follow a rigidly conventionalized form, although many of the elements of the practice overlapped. Men primarily went a significant distance from the camp and often stripped of everything except a robe and a pipe, then fasted without water or food for up to ten days and nights. Such a vision quest practice among nineteenth-century Plains women was rare, as it made them far too vulnerable to predatory males from enemy tribes. For the formal, supervised male vision quest, see: James Walker (1980: 151); Clark Wissler (1912: 104); Ernest Wallace and E. Adamson Hoebel (1952: 157); Irwin (1994); passim. However, more recently women have begun to engage in a structured vision quest; see Mark St. Pierre and Tilda Long Soldier (1995: 55, 135–136).
10. St. Pierre and Long Soldier (1995:126); also personal communication.
11. James Walker (1980: 79); John Cooper (1957: 273–74); Jennifer Brown and Robert Brightman (1988: 140); concerning the Plains Cree, D. G. Mandelbaum (1940: 252) writes:

> "The typical age of the faster showed some regional variations, ranging from the age of ten, through fourteen to sixteen. Girls sometimes underwent an isolated fast as well. More typically, however, they acquired spirit guardians during their first menstrual isolation or during dreams or trances not purposely induced."

12. For good Lakota examples, see Walker (1980: 242) and Brown (1973: 117) where the close association between menstrual rites and the vision power of the buffalo is mentioned.
13. See Patricia Albers and Bea Medicine (1981), passim; also St. Pierre and Long Soldier (1995: 67–71).
14. Elsie C. Parsons (1929: xix).
15. One example of a Lakota medicine woman, Lucille Kills Enemy, preparing males for vision questing is found in St. Pierre and Long Soldier (1995: 198–199).
16. For a contemporary example of how a mother waited for her daughter to explain her unsual behavior based on visions, see ibid., 55.
17. Alfred Bowers (1950: 174).
18. Alanson Skinner (1915: 769); a similar account in found in William Wildschut and John Ewers (1960: 79, 83).

19. Brown (1973: 134–35).
20. Cooper (1957: 293).
21. Robert H. Lowie (1947: 332); Willaim Wildschut (Nabokov, 1974: 69) claimed that Crow women "rarely sought visions before the age of 30."
22. Frank Linderman (1932: 166); for another example see Nabokov (1974: 72–78).
23. Nabokov (1974: 70) gives a good example of a woman fasting because her husband had left her for another woman. After her fasting she predicted correctly his return to her. Wildschut and Ewers (1960: 105) record a woman's experience based on her finding spiritual aid after being ignored by her husband because of her status as second wife.
24. Bowers (1950: 175).
25. Robert H. Lowie (1919: 182); "going to the garden" refers to leading the ceremonial march during the Tobacco Planting ceremony.
26. Wilbur Nye (1962: 47).
27. George Grinnell (1923, II: 92–93).
28. St. Pierre and Long Soldier (1995: 107–108).
29. Ibid., 100–102.
30. Patricia Albers and Bea Medicine (1981: 257).
31. St. Pierre and Long Soldier (1995: 74–75).
32. Ibid., 88.
33. Walter McClintock (1941: 83).
34. David Jones (1972: 31–39).
35. See Kenneth M. Stewart (1946).
36. Lowie (1909: 47).
37. Alfred Kroeber (1904: 434); Cooper (1957: 266–67).
38. Cooper (1957: 265–267).
39. James O. Dorsey (1890: 471); Francis Densmore (1918: 159).
40. Grinnell (1923, 2: 128–129).
41. For cooperative medicine relationships among the Comanche, see Wallace and Hoebel (1952: 168); for the Blackfeet, McClintock (1941: 83); for the Gros Ventre as represented by First Woman and First Man, see Cooper (1957: 451–54). The high frequency of male and female dream-spirits appearing as dual helpers suggests the Crow attitude, see Lowie (1947: 329).
42. For an interesting and important discussion of indigenous visual art, and women's roles in craft making, see Brown, 1982: 76–77.
43. St. Pierre and Long Soldier (1995: 54–55); see also Clark Wissler (1916: 92).
44. Clark Wissler (1907: 32).
45. William Whitman (1937: 88).
46. Wissler (1912: 72–7, 82).
47. Densmore (1918: 159); Wissler (1916: 83).
48. Nabokov (1974: 82).
49. John R. Murie and Douglas R. Parks (1981: 319).
50. For the Blackfoot story of Mink-Woman see, James Schultz (1923: 170–176); for women founders of rites among the Cheyenne, see E. Adamson Hoebel (1978: 91); for the Ponca, see, Skinner (1915: 784); and for the Gros Ventre, see Cooper (1957: 323).
51. Murie and Parks (1981: 156); see also Kohl (1985: 126).
52. Oscar Lewis (1941).
53. Nabokov (1974: 69).
54. St. Pierre and Long Soldier (1995: 126–128).
55. Ibid., 150.
56. Ibid., 208.
57. Ibid., 130–148.
58. Ibid., passim.

59. For a good summary of the importance of the vision in Plains life, see Brown (1982: 78–81).
60. St. Pierre and Long Soldier (1995: 49).

References

Albers, Patrica and Bea Medicine (eds.). 1981. *The Hidden Half: Studies of Plains Indian Women.* Washington D.C.: University Press of America.

Albers, Patrica and Seymour Parker. 1971. "The Plains Vision Experience." *Southwestern Journal of Anthropology,* vol. 27: 203–33.

Amiotte, Authur. 1981. "Our Other Selves: The Lakota Dream Experience." *Parabola,* Vol 6: 26–32.

Applegate, Richard. B. 1978. *'Atishwin: The Dream Helper in Southern California.* Albequerque: Ballena Press.

Benedict, Ruth F. 1922. "The Vision in Plains Culture." *American Anthropologist,* vol. 24: 1–23.

———. 1923. *The Concept of the Guardian Spirit in North America.* American Anthropological Association Memoirs, No. 29. Menasha: Banta Publishing Company.

Bourguignon, Erika. 1972. "Dreams and Altered States of Consciousness in Anthropological Research." In Francis Hsu (ed.), *Psychological Anthropology,* second ed. Cambridge: Schenkman.

Bowers, Alfred W. 1950. *Mandan Social and Ceremonial Organization.* Chicago: University of Chicago Press.

Brown, Jennifer S. and Robert Brightman. 1988. *The Orders of the Dreamed: George Nelson on Cree & Northern Ojibwa Religion & Myth, 1823.* St. Paul: Minnesota Historical Society Press.

Brown, Joseph Epes. 1973. *The Sacred Pipe: Black Elk's Account of the Seven Rites of the Oglala Sioux.* New York: Penguin Books.

———. 1982. *The Spiritual Legacy of the American Indian.* New York: Crossroads Publishing Company.

Cooper, John M. 1957. *The Gros Ventres of Montana: Religion and Ritual.* Washington, D.C.: The Catholic University of America Press.

D'Andrade, Roy G. 1961. "Anthropological Studies in Dreams." In Francis Hsu (ed.), *Psychological Anthropology.* Homewood: Dorsey Press.

Densmore, Francis. 1918. *Teton Sioux Music.* Bureau of American Ethnology, bulletin no. 61. Washington, D.C.: Smithsonian Institution.

Devereux, George. 1951. *Dream and Reality: The Psychotherapy of a Plains Indian.* New York: New York University Press. (2nd ed.,1969.)

———. 1956. "Mohave Dreams of Omen and Power." *Tomorrow: Quarterly Review of Psychical Research,* vol. 4: 17–24.

———. 1957. "Dream Learning and Individual Ritual Differences in Mohave Shamanism." *American Anthropologist,* vol. 59: 1036–1045.

Dorsey, James O. 1890. A Study of Siouan Cults. *Bureau of American Ethnology, Annual Report,* No. 11. Washington, D.C.: Smithsonian Institution.

Eggan, Dorothy. 1949. "The Significance of Dreams for Anthropological Research." *American Anthropologist,* vol. 51: 171–98.

———. 1966. "Hopi Dreams in Cultural Perspective." In G. E. Von Grunebaum and R. Caillois (eds.), *The Dream and Human Societies,* pp. 237–265. Berkeley: University of California Press.

Fire, John and Richard Erdoes. 1972. *Lame Deer: Seeker of Visions.* New York: Simon & Schuster.

Foulkes, David. 1985. *Dreaming: A Cognitive-Psychological Approach.* New York: Lawrence Erlbaum Associates.

Freire-Marreco, Barbara. 1912. "The 'Dreamers' of the Mohave-Apache Tribe." *Folklore,* vol. 23: 172–174.

Garter Snake. 1980. *The Seven Visions of Bull Lodge as Told by His Daughter, Garter Snake.* Edited by George Horse Capture. Lincoln: University of Nebraska Press.

Grinnell, George Bird. 1923. *The Cheyenne Indians: Their History and Ways of Life.* 2 vols. Lincoln: University of Nebraska Press.

Hallowell, A. Irving. 1966. "The Role of Dreams in Ojibwa Culture." In G. E. Von Grunebaum and R. Caillois (eds.), *The Dream and Human Societies,* pp. 267–292. Berkeley: University of California Press.

Haskel, R. E. 1983. "Cognitive Psychology and Dream Research: Historical, Conceptual, and Epistemological Considerations." *Journal of Mind and Behavior,* vol. 7: 131–159.

Hoebel, E. Adamson. 1978. *The Cheyennes: Indians of the Great Plains.* New York: Holt, Rinehart and Winston.

Hunt, H. 1984. "Some Relations Between the Cognitive Psychology of Dreams and Dream Phenomenology." *Journal of Mind and Behavior,* vol. 7: 213–228.

Irwin, Lee. 1994. *The Dream-Seekers: Native American Visionary Traditions of the Great Plains.* Norman: University of Oklahoma.

Jones, David E. 1972. *Sanapia: Comanche Medicine Woman.* New York: Holt, Rinehart and Winston.

Kluckhohn, Clyde and William Morgan. 1951. "Some Notes on Navaho Dreams." In George B. Wilbur and Warner Muensterberger (eds.), *Psychoanalysis and Culture: Essays in Honor of Geza Roheim,* pp. 120–131. New York: International Universities Press.

Kohl, Johann Georg. 1985. *Kitchi-Gami: Life Among the Lake Superior Ojibway.* St. Paul: Historical Society Press.

Kroeber, Alfred L. 1904. *The Arapaho.* New York: Anthropological Papers of the American Museum of Natural History, vol. 18.

Lewis, Oscar. 1941. "Manly-Hearted Women Among the North Piegan." *American Anthropologist,* vol. 43: 173–187.

Lincoln, Jackson S. 1935. *The Dream in Primitive Cultures.* Baltimore: Williams & Wilkins.

Linderman, Frank B. 1932. *Pretty-Shield: Medicine Woman of the Crow.* Lincoln: University of Nebraska Press.

Lowie, Robert H. 1909. "The Assiniboine." *Anthropological Papers of the American Museum of Natural History,* vol. 4.

———. 1919. "The Tobacco Society of the Crow Indians." Anthropological Papers of the American Museum of Natural History, vol. 21, Part II.

———. 1947. "The Religion of the Crow Indians." *Anthropological Papers of the American Museum of Natural History,* vol. 25: 309–444.

Mandelbaum, D. G. 1940 "The Plains Cree." *Anthropological Papers of the American Museum of Natural History,* vol. 37.

McGaa, Ed (Eagle Man). 1990. *Mother Earth Spirituality: Native American Paths to Healing Ourselves and Our World.* San Franscisco: HarperCollins Publishing.

McClintock, Walter. 1941. "Saitsiko, the Blackfoot Doctor." *The Masterkey,* vol. 15: 80–86.

Morgan, William. 1932. "Navaho Dreams." *American Anthropologist,* vol. 390–405.

Murie, John R. and Douglas R. Parks (eds.). 1981. *Ceremonies of the Pawnee.* Part 1 and 2. Smithsonian Contributions to Anthropology, num. 27. Washington, D.C.: Smithsonian Institution.

Nabokov, Peter. 1974. "Vision Quests of Crow Women." *Indian Notes,* vol. 10: 66–83.

Nye, Wilbur S. 1962. *Bad Medicine & Good: Tales of the Kiowas.* Norman: University of Oklahoma Press.

Opler, Marvin K. 1959. "Dream Analysis in Ute Indian Therapy." In Morris K. Opler (ed.), *Culture and Mental Health,* pp. 97–117. New York: Macmillan.

Parsons, Elsie C. 1929. *Kiowa Tales.* New York: American Folklore Society.

Powers, William. 1982. *Yuwipi: Vision and Experience in Oglala Religion.* Lincoln: University of Nebraska Press.

Ruby, Robert H. 1989. *Dreamer-Prophets of the Columbia Plateau: Smohalla and Skolaskin.* Norman: University of Oklahoma Press.

Schultz, James W. 1923. *Friends of My Life as an Indian*. New York: Houghton Mifflin.

Shulman, David, and Guy G. Strouman (eds.). 1999. *Dream Cultures: Explorations in the Comparative History of Dreaming.* Oxford: Oxford University Press.

Skinner, Alanson. 1915. "Societies of the Iowa, Kansa, and Ponca Indians." *Anthropological Papers of the American Museum of Natural History,* vol. 11: 681–801.

St. Pierre, Mark, and Tilda Long Soldier. 1995. *Walking in a Sacred Manner: Healers, Dreamers and Pipe Carriers—Medicine Women of the Plains Indians.* New York: Simon & Schuster.

Stewart, Kenneth M. 1946. "Spirit Possession in Native America." *Southwestern Journal of Anthropology,* vol. 2: 323–339.

Tedlock, Barabra. 1981. *Dreaming: Anthropological and Psychological Interpretations.* Cambridge: Cambridge University Press.

Toffelmier, Gertrude and Katherine Luomala. 1936. "Dreams and Dream Interpretation of the Dieguenо Indians of Southern California." *Psychoanalytic Quarterly,* vol. 5: 195–225.

Valencia, Heather. 1991. *Queen of Dreams: The Story of a Yaqui Dreaming Woman.* New York: Simon & Schuster.

Walker, James R. 1980 (originally published 1914). *Lakota Belief and Ritual.* Ed. R. DeMallie and E. Jahner. Lincoln: University of Nebraska Press.

Wallace, Anthony. 1958. "Dreams and the Wishes of the Soul: A Type of Psychoanalytic Theory Among the Seventeenth Century Iroquois." *American Anthropologist,* vol. 60: 234–248.

Wallace, Ernest, and E. Adamson Hoebel. 1952. *The Comanches: Lords of the Southern Plains.* Norman: University of Oklahoma Press.

Whitman, William. 1937. *The Oto.* New York: Columbia University Press.

Wildschut, William and John Ewers. 1960. *Crow Indian Medicine Bundles.* New York: Museum of the American Indian Foundation.

Wissler, Clark. 1907. "Some Protective Designs of the Dakota." *Anthropological Papers of the American Museum of Natural History,* vol. 1: 21–53.

———. 1912. "Ceremonial Bundles of the Blackfoot Indians." *Anthropological Papers of the American Museum of Natural History,* vol. 7: 65–298.

———. 1916. "Societies and Ceremonial Associations in the Oglala Division of the Teton-Dakota." *Anthropological Papers of the American Museum of Natural History,* vol. 9: 1–100.

6

The Role of Dreams in Religious Enculturation among the Asabano of Papua New Guinea

Roger Ivar Lohmann

In the early morning in Yakob village, all is fresh and renewed from the rains that fall almost every night. The sun beams warmly upon the drenched land, and the Fu River can be heard rushing far below. The rain forest-covered mountains begin to poke through the mists that envelop them, while smoke from morning fires sifts through the leaf thatching of houses. Gentle murmurs grow into conversations, babies cry, and sleepy dogs occasionally yelp, slapped to get out of the way. Asabano people awaken to such a scene each day, with their dreams still fresh in their minds.

On such a morning, after the mists had cleared away and the sun was shining intensely to the accompaniment of the songs of a dozen species of birds, a young woman named Lin, after finishing her breakfast of sweet potatoes baked in the ashes of the hearth, was deep in thought. She proceeded up Samlai hill, which rises above the village, to the house of the *dablesebobu:* the white man from America who had come to live with her people and learn about their culture. I was interested in religion, but I was not a Christian, which made me anomalous in Asabano eyes. Lin had promised the day before to come and talk with me about her religious beliefs. We sat on the floor with cups of coffee, and I asked her if she thought the Holy Spirit and angels truly exist. "In my dreams, angels come and sleep with me at night," she answered. She then continued:

> Last night was my first time to see an angel; he was a man, and he said, "Do you know my name?" I said, "No." And he said, "My name is Isaac." He was a white man. He came down and said, "Let's go up." I said, "I'm afraid my faith isn't strong enough, and that God will reject me." He replied, "No, don't worry, let's go." We flew like birds without wings and came to a big door. The angel knocked on the door,[1] and the Lord opened it, saying to the angel "Come inside." The angel entered and asked the Lord, "May this woman come inside and see your house?" The Lord said, "All right, you call to her to come inside." The angel called me inside, and the Lord got a big book and put it on a table. He wrote and

> said to the angel, "Take her around so she can see inside my house." In the house I saw pictures of men and pretty flowers. The Lord is a very handsome young white man.
>
> After we went around, the Lord said to the angel, "Show her the book I'm writing in." I stood next to him. The Lord said to me, "I won't take everyone, only a few will come to me." He said the names of all the important men and women at Duranmin, Onai, Wani, Mandi, Diyos [all active in the church]; and said those whose names he hadn't called he will throw into the fire. Then he said, "That's all." The angel said, "I wanted to show you these things." The Lord said to the angel, "Take this woman back to her own place now." So the angel took me to the door and pushed me out, saying "Go back." I protested, "We came a long way, how do I get back?" I then fell down, and I hit Semi, Walen's little girl who had come to sleep with me. She cried, and then I woke up.
>
> So this story the angel gave me. I thought, "I have to come tell you this." I dreamed it only last night. I had agreed to come and interview today, so this morning I dreamed a lot. This is the first time I had this kind of dream. Now this afternoon I'll tell others this dream in church. Now that I've seen this I know the Lord is there and it's changed my belief a little. Having seen this, I think I must truly believe in this now.

Narratives such as this one were told to me very frequently during the year and a half of my fieldwork among the Asabano, in 1994–95. My research focused on religious change. I extensively interviewed virtually all adults and older children about their religious beliefs to document belief patterns remembered from precontact days, the conversion process, and current beliefs.

I concentrated my inquiries on transmission patterns and on local forms of evidence invoked in accepting and rejecting beliefs. When I asked people to describe their religious beliefs and the reasons why they found them compelling, very often dreams were given as an explanation. Asabano attribute a high degree of experiential reality to the dream (*aluma*). Elders and missionaries assert the existence of certain mythological beings, and when Asabano in turn have dream encounters with these beings, it is easy for them to believe that they in fact exist: Seeing is believing. Dreaming is, therefore, a catalyst for cultural transmission, providing personal experiential verification of incoming information.

To the Asabano, dreams represent the wanderings and adventures of one's disembodied soul. As real experiences, dreams are a valued source of information. Asabano describe dreams either as actual events directly witnessed or as symbolic messages displayed by other beings. Dreamers learn characteristic forms of information from interactions with the dead, with benevolent forest beings, with malevolent place spirits, and with characters from recently introduced Christian mythology. The beings encountered can impart knowledge to dreamers by telling them in words, or by showing them images.

The use of dreams to communicate with powerful beings has not changed through the conversion to Baptist Christianity in the 1970s. In fact, dreams played a major role in the initial acceptance of Christianity, and remain important in the maintenance of faith and in the enculturation of the next generation. In Asabano thinking, dream encounters with angels, Jesus, the Holy Spirit and God provide direct evidence for the existence and power of these supernatural beings.

The Asabano

The Asabano are a small, ethnolinguistic group numbering about 200.[2] They are swiddeners and small-scale pig raisers, living on the fringe of the highlands of Papua New

Guinea, at Duranmin in Sandaun Province. They are culturally part of the Mountain Ok or Min sphere,[3] centered to the south at Telefomin, but linguistically are tied to the Sepik-Ramu language groups to the north.[4]

Asabano traditional religion revolved around male initiations into secret myths and magicoreligious practices that were marked by progressive presentations of formerly tabooed foods. Offerings for hunting and gardening success were made to wild humanlike beings called *wobuno*[5] and to ancestors, whose bones were kept in sacred houses or rock shelters. Vindictive spirits of stones, trees, and waters could be persuaded through offerings to cease causing sickness.

Stephen (1995: 131) observes that through understanding dream theories, local notions of self—its partitions, propensities, abilities and place, in the cosmos—are revealed. Indeed, my understanding of the Asabano conception of personal existence in life and death became clear only when I investigated ideas about sleep.

According to traditional and contemporary Asabano religious belief, each person has two souls, the *alomo kamalanedu* (little soul) and the *alomo kamayadu* (big soul), each of which plays an important role in life as well as after death. Sesi, a vivacious, hardworking young mother, explained what happens when a person is dreaming:

> The big soul goes around at night and shows us good dreams while we are alive. When we sleep, the little soul watches the body, and the big one goes around. So dreams are what the big soul sees when it's traveling around. What we see in dreams will happen later. When I have a bad dream I wake up afraid, and then I pray and the Lord shows me a good dream.

Analogously, at death the two souls part ways. The little soul remains a potentially dangerous presence at the gravesite, while the benevolent big soul travels to one of several villages of the dead, located in tabooed sections of forest.

Local beliefs have been influenced by a cascade of events in the past half century. During the 1940s, Asabano heard stories of the arrival of white people in nearby areas. Shortly afterward they heard aircraft overhead, and neighboring groups brought the first steel axes to trade. In about 1951, two men, Bledalo and Sumole, walked through the mountain passes to Telefomin, where the nearest government station had been established, and made first contact. The first official contact was made by an Australian colonial patrol to their territory in 1963 (Marks 1963).

The Asabano were converted to Baptist Christianity by Papua New Guinean missionaries from Telefomin. The mission was led by a well-educated and charismatic pastor named Diyos, who arrived in 1974. In 1977 a "revival" movement involving revelatory dreams, visions, and Holy Spirit possession began at the Asabano mission and Bible college at Duranmin. It soon spread throughout the region (Brumbaugh 1980: 16–19; Brutti 1997; Gardner 1981: 32–34; Hyndman 1994: 131–142; Jorgensen 1981; Morren 1986: 300–301; Robbins 1995, 1997a, 1997b, 1998. For a discussion of dreams in African churches, see Charsley 1992). As a consequence, traditional sacred houses and relics were destroyed, and virtually all Asabano embraced a charismatic form of Christianity.

I argue that because individual Asabano often cited their dreams as sources of reliable supplementary information on newly learned religious matters, dreams played a significant part in their religious enculturation before, during, and after the conversion process. As such, dreams are a significant factor in cultural transmission—or, more specifically, in cultural *reception*.

Enculturation and Cultural Transmission

A word of explanation is necessary regarding my generalized use of the terms "enculturation" and "cultural transmission." Many of the religious beliefs that I describe moving between individuals initially came from a source external to Asabano society. Therefore, some readers could object to my use of the term "enculturation" to describe this process. Likewise, in some quarters, "transmission" is used to refer only to cultural learning between generations, while "diffusion" is reserved for the horizontal movement of information. Indeed all of these distinctions could be made in the examples that I present here. However, because I wish to emphasize a similar process common to all these variant forms, I use "cultural transmission" and "enculturation" for all cases of individuals adopting beliefs that are new to them.

As Boyer (1994: 22) has noted, the nature of cultural transmission is frequently glossed over rather than being explicitly considered in anthropology. That cultural learning happens is often taken for granted, and therefore the focus of interest becomes the source of the cultural information: insider or outsider, elder or junior. To be sure, a young mind that has not previously received cultural information faces somewhat different challenges from an older mind attempting to incorporate incongruous new ideas. However, the situations are similar enough to be grouped together for the purpose of demonstrating common underlying processes. It is also clear that beliefs transmitted from elders to juniors within a society have a different aura from beliefs diffusing to an individual in the acculturative process. "Tradition" may have connotations of legitimacy, venerability, and respectability (or old-fashioned insignificance) while beliefs exotic to one's parents may be laced with a sense of danger, excitement, and progressivity (or absurdity and incomprehensibility). While distinguishing the sources of cultural information is necessary, my data indicate that for the Asabano, dreams served a similar catalytic role in accepting novel propositions regardless of the source of those ideas.

When I say "cultural transmission," I mean the process of moving information between any two individuals through social learning. By "enculturation," I mean learning how to think and behave according to whatever source is currently relevant and authoritative. Thus, cultural transmission leads to enculturation.

Dream Perception and Cultural Transmission: Producing Faith

It is widely known that dreams vary cross-culturally in the way they are experienced, in the imagery and symbolism that they contain, in their manner of disclosure and concealment, and in their interpretation and meanings.[6] A number of authors that I refer to below have pointed out that in many societies, dreams are attributed a special sense of reality. Under these circumstances, dreams can also be a means of acquiring information, verifying dubious statements, and filling gaps left in messages from others. They are relevant in this regard in cultural exchanges both within and across societal boundaries. I wish to call attention to two generalized implications of these observations. First, as epistemological devices, dreams act as catalysts in cultural transmission, in particular of religious beliefs. Under certain commonly occurring cultural conditions, namely the presence of notions that dreams are in some way valid, real experiences, dreams have an especially great impact on the believability of religious ideas. The second implication is that in all likelihood, this fact may be easily overlooked by ethnographers, and therefore underreported. As they are private experiences, dreams are not always shared. While they might be very important in enculturation, the people we study may not themselves outwardly emphasize this. If they do believe that dreams are important in social learning, they may not discuss this among themselves or with a researcher. Dreams are experiences hidden from public life; they become social only in the telling. The Asabano provide a good case in which to observe how dreams serve the process of cultural transmission because they do share their dreams widely, especially their religious dreams. Also, the Asabano believe that dreams are more than mere fantasy.

Clearly, among the Asabano, dreams are very important for the transmission of religious beliefs between individuals. Simply being told that something is true is often insufficient for the recipient of cultural information to believe. Some form of evidence or personal experience is usually required for transmission to be successful.

Dreams provide Asabano with evidence for the factuality of religious statements because they provide a virtually tangible indication of truth, according to their epistemology. Asabano myths are always told on the premise that there is some piece of evidence for their veracity. Mythical episodes are considered likely to be true if the teller is somehow connected to the events described or refers to external objects that figure in the story or came about as a result of the story's events. For example, stories of ancestral exploits were bolstered by displaying the bones of the protagonist to wide-eyed boys in the initiation house. Genealogies that included ancestors who were not true human beings but enchanted animals or *wobuno* are backed up by pointing to living descendants. Many traditional stories are paired with songs, which are supposed to have been sung by protagonists in a distant time. The song itself is evidence that the story behind it is true. Since the introduction of Christianity, Asabano see the presence of physical Bibles as evidential of the truth of Christian myths. In these ways, Asabano listeners judge the veracity of the myths they are told.

The common feature of all these examples is that to be believable, words must be backed up with sensory evidence to bring to mind some of the conditions of consciousness experienced by the myth's characters. In other words, listeners expect some kind of emulation of direct experience, allowing them to, in a sense, make the mythical scenarios real. In life, one knows one has encountered a supernatural being by, for example, seeing the figure of a person one knows to be dead walking in the forest. Lacking such apparently unambiguous indications, to take another example, one becomes certain a cannibal witch is nearby if one experiences spontaneous feelings of fear or observes animals behaving unnaturally. Asabano consider all of these phenomena strong evidence, and trust the word of those who say they have experienced or witnessed such things because of the storyteller's physical connection with them.

As Boyer (1994) has argued, religious ideas have qualities of intuitive unnaturalness in all cultures, which accounts for their fascination. For such accounts to be believable, stronger forms of evidence, as locally construed, are required. This is especially true for the primary transmission of beliefs that are exotic to the listener.

Asabano frequently cited having witnessed a dream in which mythological characters appeared as evidence for their existence. This same pattern has been documented in many other places, including among the Ilahita Arapesh. "In discussing aspects of ghost belief, Arapesh informants cite their appearance in dreams as evidence in support of certain standard ideas about them" (Tuzin 1975: 566). In Tahiti, many dreams represent "the wanderings of one's own soul" and are "a window opening on the supernatural world"

(Levy 1973: 374–77). Among the Rarámuri of Mexico, souls are believed to wander outside the body during dreams, where they can gather valuable cosmological information (Merrell 1988: 60, 104–105). This understanding of dreams is so common cross-culturally that Stephen refers to it as "classic" (1979: 5). Attributing varying degrees of reality to dream experiences (as opposed to writing them off as fantasy) is in fact more the rule than the exception among human societies.

This way of perceiving dreaming is itself cultural information that needs to be transmitted before dreams can serve as catalysts for accepting other religious beliefs. This occurs when one hears a plausible explanation of what dreaming is from a reputable source, which colors one's perception and interpretation of subsequent dreams. The local system of dream interpretation, writes Tuzin, "appears to have an inordinately large part in constructing the dream's manifest content. The individual is struck by the poignant accuracy of the diviner's interpretation, not realizing that the dream content was itself a partial artifact of his [the dreamer's] prior knowledge of the interpretational system" (1975: 560–61).

In the "classic" view, dreams are elevated sources of knowledge because, as D'Andrade found in his survey of anthropological dream research, there is a "persistent association found between dreams and beliefs about supernaturals, including other souls. Dreams have been shown to be one of the chief means of communication with supernaturals, and supernaturals have been found to have certain similarities to figures which typically appear in dreams" (1961: 298–299).

For this reason, and because in dreams one seems able to transcend boundaries of space, time, and death, dreams stand out as significant. Shamans in some native North American tribes, for example, gained otherwise inaccessible knowledge of healing magic through dream initiations at the hands of dead shamans (Eliade 1964: 101–2; Kilborne 1981: 173; Wallace 1947: 252). In Melanesia, Wagner observes that among Daribi craftsmen, "real talent . . . can only represent something additional to ordinary effort, and must be obtained through a dream" (1972: 74).

In many cultural settings, dreams are considered a source of special knowledge and insight, a kind of inside information or wisdom on cosmological, religious, and magical subjects that is not otherwise available. As Lindstrom has observed regarding Melanesia, "dreaming is a widespread means of inspiration that regulates the formulation of authentic knowledge . . . Dreaming authorizes the production of truth. In dreams, people receive (that is, overhear or observe) knowledge from authoritative sources. Those who dream well thereby qualify themselves to talk seriously" (1990: 87). Lindstrom makes the point here that the transmitter of cultural information, the talker, has greater credibility in Melanesian societies if what he or she has to say derives from dream experiences. I would add the observation that, if the listener then also experiences a similar dream that validates what the speaker said, the information will be accepted as proven by personal direct sensory evidence. This is especially true in the case of the transmission of assertions and beliefs for which ready physical evidence—that is, perceivable by the five senses in waking consciousness—is lacking. Much of the cultural content of religious traditions is information of this nature.

While dreams are private, they are always affected by incoming cultural information. Nevertheless, Lincoln draws a distinction between "individual" and "culture pattern" dreams (1970 [1935]: 22–23). Kilborne (1981: 170) rightly criticizes this dichotomy for its vagueness: Indeed, such pure forms do not exist, and as ideal types they are misleading. As dreams affirm beliefs of external origin, they do so in ways that suit idiosyncratic needs of individual dreamers. For example, Hollan (1989) demonstrates that among the Toraja, individuals develop personalized theories of dream experience and interpretation, allowing them to use dreams for their own psychological purposes. All dreams influenced by surrounding culture, and any cultural motif has its individual manifestations and variations in the dreaming minds of persons. Culture resides, after all, in the minds of individuals, and in dreams the expectations of others and the desires of the self are reconciled.

The dream is among the most private and personal of human experiences. "No observer can directly share in another person's dream visions and sensations" (Stewart 1997: 877). Yet, within this individual, experiential realm socially important processes take place. Stewart points out the importance of the experiential aspect of dreams of myths. "Placing a story within the framework of dreaming . . . grounds the narrative as the report of a direct, individual experience, and it simultaneously brackets the story as extraordinary knowledge (revelatory, transcendental) that demands a different appreciation from ordinary stories, whether factual or fictional" (1997: 878).

Direct experience provides the most compelling evidence for belief. Seeing a quality image, such as that in a dream, or even a video or photograph, can be powerful experiential evidence, especially among people only marginally familiar with the nature of such images. Seeing pictures or videos depicting characters from Christian mythology had a similar impact as dreams, but one much less powerful. A sixteen-year-old girl named Malina, for instance, said: "We saw a picture of angels in a magazine. They were standing holding flowers, and they showed us a video at the Bible College, and we saw it. Jesus went to church and the angels followed him. I believed it because I saw the pictures."

Magic lantern images of Jesus displayed by a missionary in Kgalagadi villages in Botswana had a similarly powerful impact on African converts (Landau 1994). The rhetorical power of direct witnessing combined with the mystical atmosphere of dreams as experiential yet fantastic makes them a potent catalyst for the transmission and reception of religious cultural information.

Dreams can display visual images corresponding to ideas expressed verbally by others, lending them greater credibility (Stewart 1997: 885). Tuzin (1989: 196) notes that among the Ilahita Arapesh, the visual imagery used in sermons had a powerful impact on dream content. One message I frequently heard in church at Duranmin was that the way to heaven is hard, and only a few will have strong enough beliefs and good enough behavior to make it. It is frequently expressed with verbal imagery: "The road to heaven is small, while that to the fire is wide and well traveled." Some Asabano told me of dream experiences in which, by witnessing this verbal description visually, they became convinced of its truth.

Isaguo, a kind and deeply religious woman of about fifty described one such dream:

> Once I wanted to go to Sumwari, and the night before I left I saw a dream, and a man said, "The Holy Spirit is a witness of you." I came to a junction in the road, and the man said, "If you take the big road you will certainly go to hell. If you see a cross and a small road, then you know that's the road to heaven. If you take the small, narrow road it is very hard, hard work to find that road and follow it. If you don't work hard you won't get there." That's the dream. So I thought God showed me a very good dream. This was in 1988. I didn't tell everybody, just a few, I just thought about it. This was a challenge to me and I changed.

By translating verbal messages from others into visual images witnessed by the soul, dreams serve the religious life by "clothing these conceptions with such an aura of factuality that the moods and motivations seem uniquely realistic" (Geertz 1973: 90).

Types of Asabano Dreams and the Information They Contain

Asabano described dreams either as actual events directly witnessed, or as symbolic messages displayed by other beings. In each case, dreams have a reality to them that many Westerners would find uncanny. They are also seen as bearing valuable information that can be exploited in waking life.

Fugod, a powerfully built man in his fifties with a deep voice, described dreams he had of the first type:

> The Holy Spirit and angels exist. The men who can read in the Bible see them mentioned, and I believe them. I myself had a dream, the Spirit of God appeared like a pigeon (*madibenedu*), and I thought, the Bible says the Holy Spirit is like a bird. I saw many birds: They were angels. Some had broken bones. In the Bible there are pictures of these birds, the Spirit of God can turn into them and fly. I thought I was awake, but it was a dream. When I woke up I remembered that Pastor Wani had told me that if you don't look after your spirit and your spirit has sins and burdens it will be bad, so I thought this must be what the dream referred to. I also dreamed of hell, so I believe it must be true. I was walking on a path and red fire came behind me! I was surprised. I woke up and thought God was showing me the fire of hell.

In this narrative, one can discern the place of dreaming in Asabano epistemology: The dream represents direct contact with and perception of reality. Fugod places emphasis on forms of reliable evidence that support his belief in the Holy Spirit and angels. Written references and pictures, which are understood to be a kind of residue of events in themselves, were seen in the Bible by people he knows. In this way a type of substantial connection was established between himself and the mythical beings. His dreams then visually confirmed what he had been told. They also bore certain valuable lessons, which come through in many of the Christian dreams I collected: Human beings are living in a precarious relationship with God. While he offers fabulous rewards, his demands are high and difficult to understand. To fail to meet his demands invites a very unpleasant fate indeed: A fate that most people will ultimately fall into. Therefore, the dreamer is motivated to make renewed efforts at achieving a Christian lifestyle.

Belok, a dependable and well-liked man in his mid-thirties, described dreams of the second, symbolic type: "When you dream and see a picture, sometimes it will come true. For me, when I dream of men cutting sago, a man will die. If I see women processing sago, a woman will die. So we think some dreams predict the future and others don't."

People do not claim always to understand the symbolism of a given dream, which allows them to explain cases of dreams that seem nonsensical or make false predictions.

Belok explained that standard dream symbols are recognized and interpreted according to convention or individual experience. "If I dream of having sex with a woman or getting money from a man, I know the next day I'll kill animals," Belok said on another occasion. Asabano look for patterns in their dreams when something has happened. After the fact, they may notice having had certain types of dreams preceding the events, and can then formulate rules of dream symbolism. One day I told

Wani, the local pastor, about a dream I had had the night before, in which my laptop computer was in a fire. I had interpreted this as simple anxiety about losing my hard-earned data, but he said that both before contact and today, dreams are often interpreted as showing what will happen in the future. He interpreted my dream much more literally than I did, and recommended that I be careful a fire does not burn down my house.

As foreigners and their things have appeared on the scene over the past half century, exotic beings have also come to populate Asabano dreams. Their visitations upon sleepers' souls enlighten dreamers on various concerns ranging from the age-old need for hunting success to new worries on how to attain salvation in heaven. Local dream theory itself has not altered significantly in this process. However, there have been some shifts in the kinds of information that dreamers receive. I will presently demonstrate this by describing the beings that Asabano dreamers encountered before contact in the mid-twentieth century, the role of dreams in the conversion of the 1970s, and dream themes at the time of my fieldwork in 1994–95. Asabano dreamers learn different forms of information depending on what type of being they encounter. Not all of the example dreams occurred during the periods I seek to describe, but each illustrates characteristics of the time's genre.

Traditional Dreaming

Before any Western influences presented themselves to the Asabano, the task of religious transmission from generation to generation was aided by receivers' dream experiences. Consider how Sansib, a literate woman in her thirties, describes her coming to believe that the dead truly appear in dreams:

> I heard my father tell stories that if you walk alone or when you sleep souls of the dead will scare you or chase you. That's all I heard, and I believed it because sometimes at night I would wake up and feel afraid, and I would remember what he said. I have seen spirits of the dead in dreams. Last night I was praying. I closed my eyes and prayed because Walen [my husband] is sick, and I saw Sgane [an old woman who recently died] come in all wrapped in a sheet with only her face exposed, and she went to play with Walen, saying "Walen, are you sick?" as he was sleeping. I was surprised and opened my eyes, and she wasn't there! I feel it's true, her spirit must have come near. I was afraid—I'm not used to seeing this kind of thing.

In this case, Sansib's father told her that the dead visit in dreams, and she was willing to truly believe it because she saw the dead in her dreams and remembered her father's words regarding how to interpret this appearance. This is much like the process of "interpretive drift" that Luhrmann (1989) describes among Londoners who are drawn to witchcraft. These individuals come to believe in magic through changing their habits of perception and interpretation based on principles taught by leaders.

According to older Asabano informants, during the years before contact and missionization, religious dreams were populated by the dead; benevolent *wobuno;* and malevolent tree, stone, and water spirits. Each imparted its own characteristic forms of data, so to speak. In addition to verifying religious beliefs received from others, they were a valued source of information on hunting, defense, and life after death.

Messages of Doom from the Dead. Traditionally, seeing the dead in a dream was a bad omen—an indication that they were near and perhaps preparing to claim some of the living. Belok described a dream in which he saw what the dead were up to. This suggested an impending death.

> On Saturday I saw a dream of my mother [Sgane] before she died, and her dead cousins Aisoibi and Pita. They came to perform a drum dance and put on the *wosaw* [big feather headdress]. While I was dreaming I thought, "I think she's about to die, and her dead relatives are happy to get her so they're singing and dancing." I told my father, and then on Sunday night at 12:00 she died, so I thought it was true. If I dream of a drum dance, it means someone will die. The first time I heard of this was when my father Bledalo told me, "If you see a dead man or the dead show you a drum dance, someone will die." I believed it, because he said it and I saw it come true.

Pigs and Cassowaries from the Wobuno. Before contact, Asabano had regular dealings with *wobuno* to secure hunting success. Then and now, people believe that the wild areas of the forest are filled with numerous *wobuno,* which are generally benevolent anthropomorphic beings who possess fabulous powers. *Wobuno* are believed to look after wild pigs, and therefore successful hunts were preceded by making offerings and entreaties to *wobuno* in a kind of trading relationship. *Wobuno* encountered in dreams told where to find game in response to an offering.

One day I asked Yalowad, a respected former *tultul,* or Australian colonial village headman, if he used to believe in *wobuno,* and why he believed. "Yes," he answered, and continued:

> They certainly exist, even now. My uncles told me they are in the bush. They are just like us: they have houses and villages, but we don't see them. They are in the forest and gave us meat. The ancestors and fathers told us, and I think it's true. When the Holy Spirit hadn't come down yet [during the Christian revival], I used to dream of them when I was in the forest. They would tell me, "You go to this place and I'll give you meat." Then I'd go and it was true.

Yakob village, where I lived, is named after a certain stone brought from the Kienu River area when the Asabano moved to their present location in 1972. This stone has a *wobudu*[7] inside. Its shape is reminiscent of the neck and head of a brontosaurus, about 0.3 meters tall. "Our ancestors said that he will help with hunting if you give him presents of tobacco, sago, and so on," Sumole, a warm, middle-age father, told me.

> Women made offerings to him as well as men. He works by appearing in a dream as a man—I have dreamt of him often—and he tells the dreamer where to go hunting.[8] And it works! If you go there you'll see animals. Yakob appears while hunting as a cassowary who plays with you—no matter how many arrows you shoot, you won't be able to hit him. The offerings left for Yakob didn't just rot there—they disappeared.

Unlike the undesirable dreams of the dead, which bore frightening portents, hunters actively sought dream encounters with *wobuno* as a method of obtaining fat game. Sumole said the *wobuno* also identified malevolent beings responsible for sickness: "We saw *wobuno* in dreams, and they would tell us which *nambeno* [tree spirits] were harming a particular person."

The Antics of Malevolent Beings. At midcentury as today, Asabano felt vulnerable to the heartless whim of a host of malevolent beings, which they believed to be responsible for almost all deaths. Lurking in the forest, *nambeno* (tree spirits), *kabiambeno* (stone spirits), and *nomombeno* (water spirits) could capture the soul of a passerby, resulting in sickness or death. Although negatively disposed toward people, traditionally these demons could be dealt with economically through offerings when they have made a person sick. Enemies from within also threatened. *Sanemono* (cannibal witches) and the little souls of the dead were less controllable and greatly feared.

When people became ill, they tried to recall where they had been in the recent past when they first became afraid or felt ill. This provided a clue as to which being was responsible for their condition and what must be done. Dreamers could also obtain information about the source of illnesses by witnessing the attack. If dreamers saw that a tree, stone, or water spirit was responsible, they made a magico-economic exchange with it. It was vital to know the offending spirit's gender, for, as Omahu, an elderly Towale man living with the Asabano (the two groups are close and intermarry freely), explained, "The Asabano and Towale had the same custom. If a female spirit was causing the trouble, the women had to deal with it; if a male spirit was doing it, the men had to. They found out the sex by seeing a dream."

"People used to dream that a tree spirit or other thing had hurt a certain man, so when we had these dreams we would know," Yalowad said. "I also had dreams about the *nambeno*. The *nambeno* have white skin. The *nambeno* can also give you animals. I have also dreamed when someone was sick that the *nambeno* made him sick."

When cannibal witches were identified, they were killed. Informants told me of several executions that took place. Dying people sometimes named their killers, leading survivors to seek additional evidence to support the accusations. If the accused behaved suspiciously, was known to have had a quarrel with the deceased, and especially if others were dying in his or her sphere, suspicions were confirmed. Dreams depicting the suspected witch's deed constituted strong evidence of guilt. A pious young woman named Maria told me she witnessed in a dream how cannibal witches had killed an older man. "I dreamed that witches killed Abueli," she said.

> Before he died he told me he had visited a certain place where witches got him. I dreamed two men followed the river. We always heard stories that witches like to hide in rivers. The grandfather wanted to harvest sweet potatoes and they shot him in the chest with a bamboo-tipped arrow. If you get shot like that you'll die in a hurry. I dreamed this when he was sick, before he died.

In precontact times, if such a dream revealed the identity of the "witches," and if there was further substantiating evidence, the bereaved would execute the accused.

It must be noted that by giving substance to circulating thoughts and suspicions, dreams frequently lent a sense of certainty to otherwise vague suspicions of witchcraft. In this way, dreams enhanced fragmentary observations and incomplete or even half-baked ideas by solidifying them into a virtually tangible form of evidence. Recurrent propositions that certain individuals were witches were in fact very specific religious beliefs. Like more general beliefs taught by elders or imported from exotic sources, they needed to be substantiated with an acceptable form of evidence.

Dreaming and the Conversion to Christianity

In his study of Madang area cargo cults, Burridge (1960: 28) demonstrated that dreams can serve as a basis for altering religious convictions in the face of foreign influences. The founders of these movements dreamed ritual solutions to the problem of unmet desires to share in Western wealth. The appealing idea that Melanesians could magically gain access to cargo was a religious suspicion that lacked sufficient evidence to be believed with conviction. Leaders' dream images echoed the suspicions that were on people's minds but recast them as factual apprehensions.

With the introduction of Christianity to the Asabano, dreams operated similarly, but backed up the missionaries' message rather than inciting a counter-movement. Conversion dreams expressed and solidified religious suspicions, based on fragmentary evidence, that Christianity was true.

In 1974 the missionary Diyos followed what he believed to be God's command to leave his home in Telefomin and set up a mission and Bible college at Duranmin, several days' walk away. He has published an account of his visions and his mission (Wapnok 1990). Having heard of a revival movement in the Solomon Islands from one of his classmates, he hoped to preside over a revival of his own. In his visions he felt that God offered cryptic indications that this would indeed happen. Toward that end he concentrated prayer, sermons, and the work of organizing the construction of an airstrip and college buildings.

The Asabano people welcomed his efforts and were intrigued by his promises of a heaven where there is plenty of food and European-style houses. Some were concerned, however. Older initiated men were cautious of abandoning their traditional practices, which ensured garden fertility and success in hunting. To allay their fears, converts set out to procure evidence by planting experimental gardens. During preparations, they ignored traditional religious procedures but offered fervent prayers to Jesus. Some old men feared the worst, that this blasphemy would render their gardens forever barren, but the Christian gardens were exceptionally productive, and the mission cleared a major hurdle.

By 1977 many Asabano had accepted Christianity in theory but also continued to practice traditional religion. At this point, the revival that Diyos had been praying for occurred, spurred on by the prophetic dream of one of his Bible college students from Mianmin. The dream indicated that the time was nigh. As Diyos preached with great power one evening, many people fell to the ground, spoke in tongues, and saw visions of the Holy Spirit, Jesus, angels, and other characters from Christian mythology. This experience was profoundly convincing to many who had doubted. In the months that followed, a few women experienced possession by the Holy Spirit, known as *spirit wok* (spirit work). During these episodes, or afterward in dreams, they received messages regarding the activities of local "sinners," including men who were continuing to practice traditional religion. Their apparently divinely inspired admonitions resulted in tremendous social pressure to abandon indigenous religious institutions.

These were very exciting times, and the obvious and dramatic events of the day were taken as clear evidence of a greater power, but making the internal adjustment to the new way of thinking required more personalized evidence. Just as the visions of those who collapsed during that fateful sermon precipitated a cascade of acceptance, dreams convinced the rank and file of the literal truth of the new religion. Dreamers actually saw God, the Holy Spirit, Jesus, and angels; they heard messages, witnessed scenarios, and visited heaven. The deities issued warnings of hell and reminders to believe and behave in order to receive what is needed in life and secure a place in paradise after death.

Smiling broadly, Wosono, an easygoing older woman, told how she flew to heaven in a dream:

> God's talk is true. I am a woman who likes to chew betelnut and smoke, but when Diyos preached I started spirit work and I left all these old ways. Diyos and Wani talked, and my spirit also talked. The Holy Spirit told me, "Whatever custom your father taught you, it was a lie. You must follow God's word." He showed me in a dream—it was his thoughts, not mine. I was asleep and I saw fire, and heard it said, "If you are stubborn you will go to the fire." I saw the ocean, and he said, "On the last day the ocean will come and cover everyone. If you believe you will turn into birds and fly to heaven." I was afraid and so I left my old customs. I saw this after the revival. Then a second time I dreamt the earth was changing, and I wanted to run away, but I turned into a butterfly and flew up. Then I was happy and clapped my hands. I thought it was real, but then I woke up. After this I just wanted to think about the new things and the Bible all the time.

It is significant that Wosono is shown bits of physical evidence to accompany the Christian assertions in her dream. She sees the fire of hell and an apocalyptic deluge with her own eyes. Living in the interior of New Guinea, the Asabano only discovered the ocean's existence in 1963, when a group of men were sent to the coast to stand trial for involvement in a tribal fight. The limitless water they described upon their return must have been a powerful and threatening image. Asabano face the vast and incomprehensible dangers of the outside world by relying on the Christian god: a similarly expansive power that comes from that same world. Wosono's dreams, typical of Asabano conversion dreams, incorporated the new into her imagination of reality—the last day and heaven became real and, therefore, believable.

Men's fears were relieved when, having abandoned traditional food taboos and codes of mythical secrecy, hunting and gardening remained successful. Although they abandoned their relationships with *wobuno,* their dreams confirmed the missionary's rhetoric that God made everything and that prayer to him would bear results. Men sought answers to prayers for a good hunt in dreams. In that realm, encounters with the Holy Spirit served the same purposes and provided the same kinds of information as was formerly provided by *wobuno* and *nambeno.*

Like the *wobuno,* Christian beings directed hunters where to search for animals and provided meat in response to entreaty. Like many men, Onai, a church leader in his late thirties, had a hunting dream to share:

> At the time of the revival in 1977, for the first time I went to the forest and prayed. I said, "God, you made everything; the Bible says if you pray you'll give to us." Then I slept and dreamed. In the dream, I went to the forest with Sinea. We slept, and the next day I killed a young pig. He killed a young cassowary and a big pig. The next morning I told him my dream. We went to the bush and I killed a pig and he killed a pig and a cassowary, just like in the dream. So I know God is truly there and gave me these things.

Just as the Asabano turned traditional dream practices to the task of learning about and from the Holy Spirit, the Christianized Foi, observed by James Weiner, adapted traditional fasting and dreaming to communicate with spirits in the new religion.

"The local Foi representatives of the Christian mission have used the dream quest in their search for divine revelation" (Weiner 1986: 122).

A number of authors have written on dreaming and its role in the incorporation of new cultural material. A brief digression into this literature demonstrates that this principle is frequently important to understanding religious transmission.

Religiously acculturative situations are highly stressful, as long-held beliefs and attitudes face startling challenges. What Watson and Watson-Franke described for Guajiro women facing a stressful adjustment to urban life holds true for Asabano considering conversion as well. "The dream is a particularly significant guide to action and hence a potential solution to a problem for the very reason that the message it contains is a command issued by a higher authority and therefore compulsive in its effects on behavior" (1977: 396).

Stephen has also commented on the importance of dreams through periods of rapid social change, as illustrated by the Mekeo, whose attitude toward dreams is very similar to that of the Asabano. Reminiscent of Wosono's dream is Stephen's description of a Mekeo man who saw heaven and hell in a dream tour given by his dead father. "This dream experience convinced the dreamer that the mission's teachings concerning the fate of the soul in the after life were indeed true" (Stephen 1982: 112).

Even when people are already convinced of the truth of what missionaries are saying, in the face of confusion over newly introduced religious beliefs, dreams help clarify the details in the minds of the converts. In his discussion of the role of dreaming in medieval Muslim culture, Grunebaum points out that "Dreams elucidate theological doctrine" and that "Dreams that clarify the position of the deceased in the Hereafter at the same time frequently instruct on the correct solution of controversial theological issues" (1966: 14–15).

Clearly dreams can serve to incorporate the incongruencies of European-derived culture with Melanesian understandings. As I alluded above, Burridge (1960: 28) shows how dreams speak to contemporary, local concerns but are shrouded in an air of revelation. By sharing these oneiric clarifications with others, dreamers can have great impact on their society because of the resonance of the dream's message with people's deepest, half-articulated suspicions.

Not only widely shared social factors are involved in the content of religiously transforming dreams. Tuzin (1989) demonstrates how factors of individual psychological makeup combine in the making of religious dreams and visions. He effectively argues that dependency needs and guilt feelings shaped a dreamlike conversion experience that thrust a relatively ineffectual Christian man into a leadership position in the revival movement of the Ilahita Arapesh. Imagery associated with exogenous Christianity and its bearers were important components in the manifest content.

Tuzin (1997) further develops this discussion of dreams in relationship to desire, expectation, and myth in his recent book. Dreams were a significant source of knowledge in the Ilahita revival as well. Attending charismatic services well past midnight, revivalists' dreams had remarkably similar content.

> [T]he people took [this] as proof that they were all glimpsing the same spiritual reality, [but this] was in fact the predictable consequence of the feverish reporting and comparing of visionary experiences among members of the Revival community. They were indeed drawing from a common reality, but it was a reality that existed neither "out there" nor "in there," in some profound spiritual sense: it was a reality emergent from the in-

> tense, even obsessional communicating and mutual emulating of personal fantasies within the tightly knit community of believers. [Tuzin 1997: 151]

No doubt, even in societies lacking classic dream beliefs, intense religious movements are bound to produce a spate of similar dreams. In such situations, it is very tempting for believers to find the co-occurrence more than coincidental. Where classic dream beliefs are current, numerous people having similar dreams emulates group verification of an event seen by many witnesses in waking life. Under these circumstances, acceptance of the belief is even more certain.

Tuzin's observations of the role of dreams in Ilahita revival serve also to illuminate the situation during the 1977 revival at Duranmin. The experience of similar dreams and visions by numerous people provided not only personally satisfying evidence and need fulfillment, it also provided a strong sense of verification through common experience. For Asabano converts, dream encounters with angels, Jesus, the Holy Spirit, and God provided direct evidence for their existence and power.

Religious Dream Evidence of the 1990s

I arrived in the field twenty years after Diyos began his mission among the Asabano. I was very impressed with the seriousness and frequency of Christian worship, with prayer meetings at sunrise and sunset of every day and long services on Sundays. However, it gradually became clear to me that people had suffered a declining religious enthusiasm and that they were concerned about this. People cited continued deaths and witchcraft suspicions as responsible for the vague spiritual malaise. They were also regretful that a scandal had resulted in the removal of the Bible college to another area shortly before I arrived. The college put Duranmin on the map of modern Papua New Guinea, and although very few Asabano had studied or graduated at their local school, they were very proud of hosting it.

While this was the situation at the time of my work there, I was nonetheless certain that Christianity was firmly planted in the hearts and minds of these people. Any undertaking called for a prayer, and Christian concepts thoroughly colored their descriptions of the world, their past, and their future.

In the Christian dream world, the dead, while still potentially threatening, often visited to reassure the bereaved that they were in heaven. The *wobuno* were banished to the forest, but the Holy Spirit behaved very similarly to them and was able to fill their role in Asabano dreams. Malevolent nature spirits and cannibal witches remained a threat, to put it mildly, and have been reenvisioned as unambiguously aligned with Satan. Christian spirit work is engaged against these monsters as people wait for the last day. After praying over a sick person, dreams credited to the Holy Spirit often reveal the source of their illness. Rather than seeking to bargain with the offending spirit or to kill the offending witch, women and men offer prayers of redoubled fervor for their own protection and for witches to desist and repent.

Warnings and Messages of Hope from the Dead. A bright-eyed young man named Folen told me what kind of information dreamers received from the dead:

> I heard that the dead come and talk in dreams. Sianso [a young mother] at Daksil village told us she dreamed of her little son who had just died. He appeared to his mother in

> her dream, and said, "If father comes, tell him that his suspicion that I died from cannibal witchcraft isn't true—I just died." He was talking about the fact that there is a man who Salowa wanted Solsi to marry, but she didn't want to. So both men were mad about this, and then Salowa's boy died, so Salowa thought there might be a connection.

In this example, the dead child is perceived to diffuse a conflict-derived witchcraft suspicion. Before colonial pacification in 1963, a conflict like this could easily have lead to feuding or warfare. Execution of witches is no longer carried out, because of the Christian rhetoric that taking vengeance endangers salvation and should be left to God. In this dream, the spirit of the deceased behaved in a very Christian manner, diffusing the danger of vengeful feelings. This is a striking contrast to the traditional practice, in which the dying named their supposed killers. The dream smoothly reaffirmed the still-new Christian ideas in a time of tragedy, when old patterns can surface.

"Sianso then had a second dream," Folen went on, "in which her dead son said, 'There is water on my grave. You must come dig a ditch around it.' But they didn't dig a ditch: They just built a house on top."

Asabano formerly disposed of the dead on exposure platforms and collected the bones for use in offerings and magic. The custom of burial, mandated by the government, is accepted as a good way of handling corpses now that their bones are no longer needed. It is certainly possible that discomfort over the idea of a body in the muddy soil could have inspired Sianso's second dream.

Before the arrival of Christianity, to be approached by a ghost in a dream would have been interpreted as at least dangerous and quite possibly a death sentence. Asabano still speak of this possibility, reasoning that like the living, the dead are also bereaved by the separation from their loved ones. They are capable of capturing the spirit of a living person, resulting in sickness and death. In spite of this, a new genre of dreams of the dead has appeared. In Christian dreams of the dead, the deceased approaches the dreamer to provide solace and assurances that heaven exists and they will one day be reunited. Kanau, a thin, middle-age man, told me, between puffs on his cigarette, the power that such a dream had for him:

> If you see a dead person in a dream, you know she is all right. And she can talk to you and give you advice. She can say, "I'm alive, in the hand of the Lord and well, so you look after your children." I had a dream of my late wife Fodimin. She told me, "You mustn't worry or think a lot or be sad. You must look after the children and relax. You see my body and think that I'm dead, but I'm alive with God. You mustn't worry about death. God made a contract with us, and there's only one road, and we will meet again in heaven." I slept and saw her face and she was with me and told me these things. When I got up, I was happy, and thought, "If I believe, later I'll see her again."
>
> When she died I didn't sleep, I just cried and worried. She died in June last year [1993], and I buried her, and in November I had the dream. I thought about her a lot; she looked after everyone, and we had always talked together. She said in the dream, "I haven't died and left you, I'm walking with you. You have to talk with God and believe, and look after our five children. When our children have grown up, you will come here. We will meet in Paradise. I came here and have a good house, good food, and a good village. The place where we were on Earth is no good—it's just a contract. Our true place is here." I thought, "Diyos's telling us about all this was true." Later, at the end of time when Jesus comes down, all of us who believe will go to heaven, and those who don't will be lost and go to the fire. Then I talked with Wani and Diyos, who read the Bible, and I thought, "It's true."

> When I dreamed of my wife, I saw her skin was good and pretty, and she spoke clearly, so she must be all right. I had thought she died and I won't be able to see her, but then I saw her, so I thought, "It's only her body that's lost, she herself is still alive and well." I believe I saw her in the dream, and she said, "I'm here, I just left my body."

Several people told me dreams similar to Kanau's. In addition to providing comfort and hope, these and other Christian dreams also carry a warning: The comfortable afterlife is reachable but easily lost. One must continue to follow God very carefully, for a few careless steps can land one in the fires of hell. Pastors' descriptions of myth and dogma found in the Pidgin Bible can be difficult for their congregations to imagine. Dreams of the dead provide further information about the nature of God and the afterlife and what one must do to maintain a good relationship with Jesus.

Dreams of Wobuno. The church forbids continued interaction with *wobuno* and labels them as "Satan's line." My impression is that virtually all Asabano obey this rule, and no longer make offerings to *wobuno* or expect them to provide information in dreams because Christian mythological beings can serve the same purposes and require no offerings. However, Asabano attitudes toward the *wobuno* are currently mixed and ambivalent because their encounters with them were generally beneficial. While many youngsters describe them as demons, Bledalo, who is the oldest of the Asabano, feels they must be angels.

One cannot, of course, forbid someone to dream of a particular person or thing, and no one at Duranmin is denying that the *wobuno* exist; they continue to hide in the forest and can be glimpsed when walking or dreaming. "Some are white, some are black, and some of the women wear grass skirts," Yalowad said. "We didn't see white ones until the white people came." Yalowad told me the *wobudu* Yakob is his ancestor, and he has seen him in dreams many times. He named his daughter Omsimin after Yakob's daughter. He not only helped with hunting but with looking after pigs and gardening as well. "The *wobudu* is still there. He appears in dreams or when walking in the forest. The Holy Spirit behaves similarly. He appears as a man, sometimes white, sometimes black; in many forms, in dreams or while walking. I myself have seen the Holy Spirit." It seems clear from this description that some older men use the behavior of *wobuno* as a model for interacting with the Holy Spirit. Dreams can, in this way, graft exogenous religious concepts onto living cosmologies, leaving only a thin scar. Judging by the attitudes of younger people, however, it seems likely that within a generation, *wobuno* will be completely banished to the forest, branded, without reservations, as demons.

Dreams of the Holy Spirit and Malevolent Beings. At the time of my fieldwork, evil spirits and cannibal witches remained a major concern. Sickness and death are believed to result from their activities, and they must be confronted, but now people do this by praying for God's intercession. In a dream or vision the Holy Spirit reveals the evil spirit's identity. The people then prepare a cross bearing a Bible verse, carry it to the site where the offending spirits live, and plant the cross there, blocking their path. Omahu said: "The people will do spirit work to get a vision or dream and say where to plant a cross. We don't kill pigs anymore, but it's the same kind of thing. Now they will get good food, tinned fish and rice, and pray, eat, feel happy, and plant a cross: and the person will get better. It's just like before."

It was during a spirit working session that Mandi, Diyos's wife and fellow missionary to the Asabano, received the method of planting crosses to close the path taken by malevolent spirits. This method, while accepting as fact that such beings are responsible for illness, provides a means of controlling them without dealing with them directly. The Asabano believe that, in effect, Jesus stands where the cross is placed, protecting his believers from the lurking spirit.

Dreams are closely associated with spirit work and often follow prayer sessions, providing information that allows appropriate action to be taken. Young people grow up seeing this use of dreaming, and when they have Christian dreams themselves, they accept the messages they contain.

Dreaming and the Enculturation of Natives and Anthropologists

In cultures that embrace the classic belief that dreams are true experiences of the soul, evidence from dreams can be a necessary factor in the cultural transmission of religious beliefs that lack direct physical perceptive verification. Even in stable societies where foreign ideas scarcely intrude, dreams work to establish as fact the strange ideas about supernatural beings that adults teach children. Although children are relatively credulous in their primary religious enculturation, religious ideas, no doubt, become more real to them through their dream experiences. For example, Lonika, a girl of twelve, told me a frightening dream she had that convinced her that the adults' stories about evil spirits were true. In her dream, while washing clothes with her mother, a stone spirit grabbed her by the neck and pulled her underwater. She struggled with it and was able to escape. In Western societies, a parent might comfort the child by denying the nightmare's reality: "It was just a dream." Asabano parents would have a different reaction, which would tend to reinforce the interpretation that the dream provided reliable intelligence about a spiritually dangerous environment.

Dreaming as an influence on primary enculturation is substantial and yet easy to underestimate. Its role in secondary transmissions or acculturative situations is perhaps even greater. As I have shown, the relatively sudden and complete Asabano conversion to Christianity was greatly facilitated by dreaming.

Unless people have some kind of direct, personal experience with strange new deities, the words of missionaries may seem to be little more than interesting stories. The incongruity of their myths with local assumptions is a major challenge missionaries face in trying to transmit their religions.

Anthropologists at times face similar problems. How many ethnographers, trying to dispel odd ideas circulating about them, meet with doubt or even a condescending glance? To take one example, Lepowsky (1993: 25) was at pains to convince older Vanatinai Islanders that she was not the ghost of a woman who had recently died. Some Asabano were convinced that I had an underground road to America, which explained my plentiful supply of food. We deny these things, because to us they are not only wrong, they are ridiculous—as is the nature of religious beliefs that are not our own. In just the same way our friends from other backgrounds find our denials and explanations absurd.

Religious beliefs are hard to transmit, especially across cultural boundaries, when an entire cosmological system must be altered to accommodate ideas that do not fit. Dreams provide a venue in which these adjustments can be made. Indeed it could be that without the influence of dreams, it would not have been possible for the Asabano to absorb and internalize exotic Christian beliefs. Dreams play a causal role in cultural transmission and enculturation that can be easily overlooked.

Even in societies in which dreams are believed to be fantasies, they are personal, emotionally powerful, and perceived as happening to the dreamer rather than created by the dreamer through the "autonomous imagination" (Stephen 1989). They are important in establishing a comfort level when new cultural information is flowing in from others. Dreams make foreign information our own. "Beliefs," as Stephen writes, "are not something simply imprinted upon the individual by his society and accepted without question, but rather . . . each man and woman, through the creative process of his or her own dreaming, constructs a private symbolic universe" (1989: 120).

In his famous essay "Grief and a Headhunter's Rage," Rosaldo (1993) vividly underscored the importance of personal emotional experience in understanding the explanations of our informants. It is often said that fluency is nigh when one begins to dream in a foreign language; one is learning. Likewise, when one begins to experience dreams in a way that is current in the foreign culture that one is studying, it is a milestone in understanding (Luhrmann 1989: 80).

Ethnographers are professionally engaged in the business of cultural transmission, so it is only to be expected that our own dreams reflect the enculturation (or acculturation?) we receive among our hosts (Tedlock 1994: 288–290). One night, under my mosquito net and to the accompanying din of thousands of forest insects, I dreamed that my sister Sue had just died and we were burying her. (In fact she was accidentally shot and killed in 1971, when I was a child.) In my dream, though, I was grown up. Sue's ghost was appearing and harassing me. When I woke up shortly before dawn, I found myself cowering under the blanket for fear that a malicious ghost should really appear. I thought to myself, "I don't believe in ghosts!" Still, in the darkness I felt afraid and ready in case a ghost actually materialized. I had come to think, if only for a moment, as Asabano do about the dangerous little soul that hovers about the grave. This made me think a lot about belief. No matter what our waking sensibilities may tell us, seeing is believing.

Notes

My primary period of fieldwork in 1994–95 was made possible by a generous Fulbright grant. I wish mainly to thank those dreamers at Duranmin who contributed their words for this article. Eytan Bercovitch kindly shared his fieldnotes and photographs with me from a brief visit he made to the Asabano in 1982. I am grateful to Joel Robbins, who encouraged me to write about dreams for his session on Charismatic and Pentecostal Christianity in Oceania at the 1998 meeting of the Association for Social Anthropology in Oceania. The result is this chapter, which was greatly strengthened by helpful comments from the session participants and observers, especially John Barker, Fred Errington, Deborah Gewertz, Maurice Godelier, Pamela Stewart, and Andrew Strathern. I presented an informal version of this chapter at the Department of Anthropology, University of Wisconsin-Madison, where Maria Lepowsky and Ted Mayer offered particularly valuable suggestions. I wish to acknowledge Kirin Narayan's wonderful influence on my writing style. My thanks to Anne Lewinson, Joel Stocker, and Don Wesolowski for reading and commenting on a draft of the manuscript. Bob Tonkinson, Donald Tuzin, and an anonymous reviewer offered very valuable advice, which I have followed to the best of my ability.

1. Knocking on doors is not an indigenous practice—one simply enters, perhaps speaking a greeting before crossing the threshold.

2. Bercovitch (1982) collected preliminary information on Asabano mythology in conjunction with his fieldwork among the neighboring Atbalmin (1989). MacKenzie (1991) also made a brief visit to Duranmin as part of her research on Telefol net bags.
3. The Min group of cultures are united by their common descent (culturally or physically) from an "Old Woman" known in Telefol as Afek and in Asaba as Semodu, who is said to have wandered through the area (Craig and Hyndman 1990). "Mountain Ok" and "Min" are alternate terms for the group of culturally similar societies found in this region. The former term was coined by Healey to refer to a number of related languages in which the term *ok* means water (Healey 1964). Min is used locally, from the Telefol for "People."
4. *Asaba amole,* or "Asabano talk," has been mentioned by the Telefol designation *Duranmin* in the linguistics literature (Wurm 1982: 218–219).
5. Asaba terms are italicized, while Melanesian Pidgin terms are underlined.
6. For a recent review of the history of anthropological wrangling with the dream, see Tedlock (1994).
7. *Wobudu* is singular, while *wobuno* is plural or collective.
8. An interesting comparison can be made with the role of dreaming for Rock Cree hunters in Manitoba. Here one's "dream image," a kind of spirit helper in the form of an animal or any other object, "may be talked about as essential to foraging success, communicating with its human dependent in dreams, facilitating dreams about individual animals, serving as a conduit for information about animal numbers and movements, and imparting 'power' deployed in hunting" (Brightman 1993: 77).

References

Bercovitch, Eytan. 1982. *Two Sacred Narratives of the Duranmin, Telefomin District, Papua New Guinea.* Unpublished: Department of Anthropology, Stanford University.

———. 1989. "Disclosure and Concealment: A Study of Secrecy among the Nalumin People of Papua New Guinea." Ph.D. diss., Stanford University.

Boyer, Pascal. 1994. *The Naturalness of Religious Ideas: A Cognitive Theory of Religion.* Berkeley: University of California Press.

Brightman, Robert. 1993. *Grateful Prey.* Berkeley: University of California Press

Brumbaugh, Robert C. 1980. "A Secret Cult in the West Sepik Highlands." Ph.D. diss., State University of New York at Stonybrook.

Brutti, Lorenzo. 1997. "Waiting for God: Ecocosmological Transformations among the Oksapmin (Sandaun Province - PNG)." In *Millennial Markers.* P. J. Stewart and A. Strathern, eds. Pp. 87–131. Townsville, QLD Australia: Centre for Pacific Studies, James Cook University of North Queensland.

Burridge, Kenelm. 1960. *Mambu: A Melanesian Millennium.* Princeton: Princeton University Press.

Charsley, Simon. 1992. "Dreams in African Churches." In *Dreaming, Religion and Society in Africa.* M. C. Jedrej and R. Shaw, eds. Pp. 153–176. Leiden: E. J. Brill.

Craig, Barry, and David Hyndman, eds. 1990. *Children of Afek: Tradition and Change Among the Mountain-Ok of Central New Guinea.* Sydney: Oceania Publications.

D'Andrade, Roy G. 1961. Anthropological Studies of Dreams. In *Psychological Anthropology: Approaches to Culture and Personality.* F. L. K. Hsu, ed. Pp. 296–332. Homewood, IL: The Dorsey Press, Inc.

Eliade, Mircea. 1964. *Shamanism: Archaic Techniques of Ecstasy.* Princeton: Princeton University Press.

Gardner, Donald S. 1981. "Cult Ritual and Social Organisation among the Mianmin." Ph.D. diss., Australian National University.

Geertz, Clifford. 1973. *The Interpretation of Cultures.* New York: Basic Books.

Grunebaum, G. E. von. 1966. "Introduction: The Cultural Function of the Dream as Illustrated by Classical Islam." In *The Dream and Human Societies.* G. E. von Grunebaum and R. Caillois, eds. Pp. 3–22. Berkeley: University of California Press.

Healey, Alan. 1964. "The Ok Language Family of New Guinea." Ph.D. diss., Australian National University.

Hollan, Douglas. 1989. "The Personal Use of Dream Beliefs in the Toraja Highlands." *Ethos* 17(2): 166–186.

Hyndman, David. 1994. *Ancestral Rain Forests and the Mountain of Gold: Indigenous Peoples and Mining in New Guinea.* Boulder: Westview.

Jorgensen, Dan W. 1981. "Life on the Fringe: History and Society in Telefolmin." *In The Plight of Peripheral People in Papua New Guinea, vol. 1: The Inland Situation.* R. Gordon, ed. Pp. 59–79. Occasional Papers, no. 7. Cambridge, MA: Cultural Survival.

Kilborne, Benjamin. 1981. "Pattern, Structure, and Style in Anthropological Studies of Dreams." *Ethos* 9(2): 165–185.

Landau, Paul. 1994. "Evaluation, Illumination and the Image of Christ in the Kgalagadi. "In *Paths Toward the Past: African Historical Essays in Honor of Jan Vansina.* R. W. Harns, J. C. Miller, D. S. Newbury, and M. D. Wagner, eds. Pp. 211–222. Atlanta, GA: African Studies Association Press.

Lepowsky, Maria. 1993. *Fruit of the Motherland: Gender in an Egalitarian Society.* New York: Columbia University Press.

Levy, Robert I. 1973. *Tahitians: Mind and Experience in the Society Islands.* Chicago: University of Chicago Press.

Lincoln, Jackson Steward. 1970 [1935]. *The Dream in Primitive Cultures.* Baltimore: Williams & Wilkins Company.

Lindstrom, Lamont. 1990. *Knowledge and Power in a South Pacific Society.* Washington, D.C.: Smithsonian Institution.

Luhrmann, T. M. 1989. *Persuasions of the Witch's Craft: Ritual Magic in Contemporary England.* Cambridge, MA: Harvard University Press.

MacKenzie, Maureen. 1991. *Androgenous Objects: String Bags and Gender in Central New Guinea.* Chur, Switzerland: Harwood Academic Publishers.

Marks, Arthur. 1963. *Patrol Report Oksapmin No. 7 - 62/63,* Oksapmin Patrol Post: Territory of Papua and New Guinea.

Merrell, William L. 1988. *Rarámuri Souls: Knowledge and Social Processes in Northern Mexico.* Washington D.C.: Smithsonian Institution.

Morren, George E. B. 1986. *The Miyanmin: Human Ecology of a Papua New Guinea Society.* Ann Arbor: University of Michigan Press.

Robbins, Joel. 1995. "Dispossessing the Spirits: Christian Transformations of Desire and Ecology among the Urapmin of Papua New Guinea." *Ethnology* 34(3): 211–24.

———. 1997a. "Six-hundred sixty six, or Why is the Millennium on the Skin?: Morality, the State and the Epistemology of Apocalypticism among the Urapmin of Papua New Guinea." In *Millennial Markers.* P. J. Stewart and A. Strathern, eds. Pp. 35–58. Townsville: Center for Pacific Studies, James Cook University of North Queensland.

———. 1997b. "'When Do You Think the World Will End?': Globalization, Apocalypticism, and the Moral Perils of Fieldwork in 'Last New Guinea.'" *Anthropology and Humanism* 22(1): 6–30.

———. 1998. "Becoming Sinners: Christian Transformations of Morality and Culture in a Papua New Guinea Society." Ph.D. diss., University of Virginia.

Rosaldo, Renato. 1993. *Culture and Truth: The Remaking of Social Analysis.* Boston: Beacon.

Stephen, Michelle. 1979. "Dreams of Change: The Innovative Role of Altered States of Consciousness in Traditional Melanesian Religion." *Oceania* 50:3–22.

———. 1982. "'Dreaming Is Another Power!': The Social Significance of Dreams among the Mekeo of Papua New Guinea." *Oceania* 53:106–122.

———. 1989. "Self, the Sacred Other, and Autonomous Imagination." In *The Religious Imagination in New Guinea.* G. H. Herdt and M. Stephen, eds. Pp. 41–64. New Brunswick: Rutgers University Press.

———. 1995. *A'aisa's Gifts: A Study of Magic and the Self.* Berkeley: University of California Press.

Stewart, Charles. 1997. "Fields in Dreams: Anxiety, Experience, and the Limits of Social Constructionism in Modern Greek Dream Narratives." *American Ethnologist* 24(4): 877–894.

Tedlock, Barbara. 1994. "The Evidence from Dreams." In *Psychological Anthropology.* P. K. Bock, ed. Pp. 279–295. Westport, CT: Praeger.

Tuzin, Donald. 1975. "The Breath of a Ghost: Dreams and the Fear of the Dead." *Ethos* 3: 555–578.

———. 1989. "Visions, Prophesies, and the Rise of Christian Consciousness." In *The Religious Imagination in New Guinea.* G. H. Herdt and M. Stephen, eds. New Brunswick: Rutgers University Press.

———. 1997. *The Cassowary's Revenge: The Life and Death of Masculinity in a New Guinea Society.* Chicago: University of Chicago Press.

Wagner, Roy. 1972. *Habu: The Innovation of Meaning in Daribi Religion.* Chicago: University of Chicago Press.

Wallace, W. J. 1947. "The Dream in Mohave Life." *Journal of American Folklore* 60: 252–258.

Wapnok, Diyos. 1990. Diyos. In *Daring to Believe: Personal Accounts of Life Changing Events in Papua New Guinea and Irian Jaya.* N. Draper and S. Draper, eds. Pp. 154–160. Hawthorn, Australia: Australian Baptist Missionary Society.

Watson, Lawrence C., and Maria-Barbara Watson-Franke. 1977. "Spirits, Dreams, and the Resolution of Conflict among Urban Guajiro Women." *Ethos* 5(4): 388–408.

Weiner, James F. 1986. "Men, Ghosts and Dreams among the Foi: Literal and Figurative Modes of Interpretation." *Oceania* 57:114–127.

Wurm, Stephan A. 1982. *Papuan Languages of Oceania.* Tübingen: Gunter Narr Verlag.

7

Content Analysis of Mehinaku Dreams

Thomas Gregor

Despite the growth of psychological anthropology, dreams remain relatively neglected in the ethnographic descriptions of non-Western peoples. We have a number of systematic examinations of dreams, including those from Australia (Schneider and Sharp 1969), Africa (LeVine 1966), and India (Gray and Kalsched 1971), but many ethnographic regions are virtually unknown territory in terms of dream research. In no case do we have a database that is as scientifically compiled as that of Hall and his collaborators, who have analyzed more than 10,000 American dreams (Hall 1951; Hall and Van de Castle 1966). The purpose of this chapter is to extend the base of evidence on which cross-cultural dream research rests by providing descriptions of the manifest content of 385 dreams collected among the Mehinaku Indians, an Arawakan-speaking people of Central Brazil. Although a number of researchers have effectively utilized dreams as a method of research among South American Indian cultures (see, e.g., Kracke 1978, 1979, and chapter 9 of this volume), I am aware of few published collections of dreams from the peoples of this area.

The eighty-three Mehinaku Indians live along the headwaters of the Xingu River in Brazil's Xingu National Park. They and their culturally similar but linguistically distinct neighbors participate in a well-developed system of intertribal barter, marriage, and collective ritual. (See Gregor 1977.) Unlike that of many of the other native peoples of Brazil, Mehinaku life remains essentially traditional. The presence of an Indian post and a small air force base has had a psychological impact that is visible in Mehinaku dream life, but thus far the villagers remain protected from wage labor and contact with missionaries, squatters, and others who would exploit them or alter their lives.

According to the Mehinaku, dreams occur when the soul (*iyeweku,* literally, "shadow") leaves its home in the iris of the eye to wander about through a nocturnal world peopled by spirits, monsters, and the souls of other sleeping villagers. In the morning, the villagers are careful to recall the adventures of their souls, since they are a clue to the future. Dreamed occurrences are symbols (*patalapiri,* literally "pictures, images") of events to come. The meaning of the symbols is determined by metaphoric equivalences of color, shape, and action. For the most part, the equations are gloomy predictions of misfortune injury, illness, and early death. A dream of collecting flying ants, for example, suggests the death of kin, since the ants are short-lived, and the clouds of flying insects resemble the rain of tears that accompanies a death. Frequently dream symbols have sexual or scatological associations, as in a dream of a vagina, which is a symbol for a knife wound, or a dream of a dirty rectum, which suggests burned manioc bread. (See Gregor 1981 for a full description of Mehinaku dream theory.)

Each morning the Mehinaku remember their dreams and often recount them to their families and housemates. This penchant for recall and immediate verbalization is ideally suited for research, as it ensures that the night's dreams are not lost in the cloud of amnesia that follows waking for most Westerners. During my research, the villagers made superb informants as I circulated through the houses each morning to harvest the previous night's crop of dreams.

In utilizing these data, however, the reader should be aware that in many respects the dream narratives were collected under less favorable conditions than those enjoyed by Hall and others who have worked with American informants. First, my dream reports vary considerably in length, ranging from a sentence or two to several hundred words. Second, the elaborate Mehinaku system of dream interpretation is a powerful incentive for the dream's "secondary revision," in that culturally meaningful elements may be emphasized in the dream reports. We must always keep in mind that we are dealing with accounts of dream experiences rather than the experiences themselves. Finally, although nearly all of the dreams were related to me in the Mehinaku language, I have only a few tape recordings of dream narratives. The bulk of the dreams were written in a notebook in a mixture of Mehinaku and English as they were narrated. With these caveats in mind, it is clear that the dream summaries that follow are not suitable data for the kind of comparative research that may depend on subtleties of verb form or other grammatical nuances of the dream report. We may have more confidence, however, in the dream themes, settings, characters, and emotional tone.

Description of the Sample and the Dimensions of Analysis

All studies of manifest dream content reflect the research interests of the investigator. My own research on the nature of masculinity has led me to examine dream themes dealing with aggression, sexuality, and anxiety. The sample of informants has been weighted toward men (276 out of a total of 385 dreams); among the men two individuals were selected for intensive study. Their sequentially collected dreams constitute about 25 percent of the entire corpus. In all but a few cases, which are noted in the text, their dreams were sufficiently like the others in the sample so that the reported averages are skewed by less than 5 percent. The entire collection of dreams includes at least some narratives from eighteen men and eighteen women, including almost the entire adult population.

The total sample of 385 dreams is examined in tables 7.1 and 7.2 under the following headings:

Dreamer Profile. A brief biographical sketch accompanies each set of dreams included in the sample.

Dream Summary. The summaries are my condensations of the significant elements of the dream in which I list the main dream characters, settings, and action.

Characters. Dreams including relationships with children, parents, and Brazilians are noted in this dimension of content analysis.

Aggression. A dreamed event is scored under this heading if it involves a deliberate physical effort on the part of one dream character to injure another. Killing, chasing, shooting, choking, and robbing are examples of such acts, as are sexual assaults. Limiting the definition of aggression to physical aggression obviously eliminates many important aggressive events from consideration, but has the advantage of defining aggression in a way that is generally unambiguous.

When a dreamer acts aggressively in reaction to an assault, the dreamer is coded as the victim of aggression rather than the perpetrator.

Anxiety. Each of the dreams is rated on a scale of 0 (no perceived anxiety) to 3 (extreme anxiety) as experienced by the dreamer. Anxiety level was utilized for dreams in which the dreamer was threatened but was not in fact injured. This level of anxiety was also scored for diffuse or nonspecific anxiety; for mild anxiety relating to the experience of guilt or shame; for anxiety connected with fear of abandonment, separation, and loneliness; and for any dream, regardless of content, that the dreamer perceived as somewhat disturbing.

Anxiety level 2 was reserved for dreams in which the narrator reports the dream to be frightening (*kowkapapaí*) or otherwise indicates considerable anxiety. These dreams include dreams of slight injury to the dreamer (an insect bite or a fall in the mud), seeing dangerous spirits, or experiences that evoke substantial guilt, separation anxiety, or shame, such as being caught stealing.

Anxiety level 3 is reserved for death anxiety, attacks by dangerous animals (notably jaguars, dogs, snakes, stingrays, and venomous insects) and assaults by other persons.

All the coding for the anxiety dimension of the content analysis involves a subjective judgment on my part based on my impressions of the dreamer's report and the cultural implications of the dream event. Nonetheless, the ratings involved are intended to be roughly comparable to those utilized in other work (c.f. Breger, Hunter, and Lane 1971).

Castration Anxiety. This dimension of analysis follows that of Hall and Van de Castle (1965, 1966: 126–130). A dream statement is coded positively for castration anxiety if it reports an actual or threatened injury or defect in a specifically mentioned part of the dreamer's body; an infantilization of a part of the dreamer's body; a threatened or actual clawing, biting, or stabbing of the body as a whole; or an injury, loss, or defect occurring to an animal or possession in close association with the dreamer. In addition, a dream receives a positive score for castration anxiety when a male dreamer acquires female characteristics or finds that he has difficulty in using a bow and arrow, a gun, or other device that is symbolically phallic in nature.

Passivity/Activity. Dreams are coded as being primarily passive when the dreamer is simply an observer of events or merely responds to the actions of others. The common dream of being chased by an animal, for example, would be coded as passive. When a dream contains mixed elements of passivity and activity, as is often the case, it is scored as active.

Transformation. One of the more interesting distancing mechanisms utilized by Mehinaku dreamers is the metamorphosis of dream characters in the course of the dream. Frequently animals are transformed into people and people into animals, thereby justifying dreamers' hostility or defusing their anxiety. Dreams displaying this feature are noted.

Sexual-Scatological Dreams. A regular percentage of men's and women's dreams incorporate elements that are overtly sexual and scatological in nature. When the dreamer reports seeing or participating in sexual activity or mentions the genitalia or feces, the dream is coded in the appropriate column.

Analysis of the Dreams

Dreams of Aggression

Aggressive dreams that contain at least one violent act are frequent occurrences in Mehinaku dreams, as may be seen in table 7.3.

Men's dreams show nearly one-third more aggressive encounters than do those of the women, a statistic that is understandable given the men's participation in political conflict and their violent interaction with animals. In comparing the Mehinaku data with that of Hall and Van de Castle's sample, it appears that aggressive encounters figure far more heavily in the manifest content of Mehinaku dreams than in those of American subjects. Interestingly, however, the relative differences between male and female dreams are very close. In evaluating this similarity, it is well to post a note of caution. The Mehinaku sample of dreams includes adults of all ages, while Hall and Van de Castle's norms were derived from studies of college students. Further, here and in other tables Hall and Van de Castle calculate their norms from a sample of 200 dreamers, each of whom contributed five dreams to the overall sample. In the analysis of Mehinaku dreams, however, I report averages from fewer dreamers, each of whom has provided more dreams. Finally, as I have indicated in notes to the tables, Hall and Van de Castle's categories are not always strictly comparable to the ones used in this study. The pairing of Mehinaku and American data is therefore intended to be suggestive rather than to be a definitive cross-cultural comparison.

The Role of the Dreamer in Aggressive Dreams

Table 7.4 demonstrates that both men and women are more likely to be the victim of aggression within dreams than the initiator of aggression. The variance between men and women reflects the realities of Mehinaku life. Women consider themselves more vulnerable to the attack of dangerous animals than men do, and are in fact the occasional victims of the men's sexual assault.

The Dreamer as the Victim of Aggression

As shown in table 7.5, men are one of the major sources of aggression in the dreams of Mehinaku men and women. For both sexes, more than one third of these dreamed assaults are by Brazilian men, reflecting a deep-seated insecurity that the Mehinaku have toward whites.

Animals are another major source of aggression in Mehinaku dreams. Jaguars, dogs, snakes, venomous insects, and other dangerous fauna are a part of the natural environment and are cast in a malevolent role in the villagers' dreams. In contrast with the Mehinaku, animal assaults are relatively unusual (although far from absent) in the dreams of Hall and Van de Castle's subjects.

Table 7.1 The Content of Mehinaku Men's Dreams

	Characters			Aggression		Anxiety				
Dream Summary	*Son/Daughter*	*Mother/Father*	*Brazilians*	*Aggressor*	*Victim*	*Level*	*Castration*	*Passive/Active*	*Transformation*	*Sexual/Scatalogical*
Dreamer Profile: A young man of 23, married with two children. A low-status individual within the community, he is attracted to, and yet frightened of, Brazilian life. A new father, he frequently expresses concern over health and well being of his infant son.										
1. Went fishing and caught tiny fish. Brought fish home to family.	S,D	-	-	-	-	-	-	A	-	-
2. A woman attempted to have sex with him. The jealous husband assaulted him and struck him repeatedly with a club.	-	-	-	Jealous husband	self	3	x	A	-	x
3. Lost his belt and could not find it.*	-	-	-	-	-	1	x	A	-	-
4. Desired and approached girl, struck by his jealous wife.	-	-	-	Jealous wife	self	3	x	A	-	x
5. Went to garden with a village child.	-	-	-	-	-	-	-	A	-	-
6. Attacked by a jaguar that turned into a village witch.	-	-	-	witch-jaguar	self	2	x	-	x	-
7. Shot stingray with arrow while he fished.	-	-	-	self	ray	-	-	A	-	-
8. Was frightened of lunar eclipse.	-	-	-	-	-	2	-	P	-	-
9. Fell from tree and injured head and neck.	-	-	-	-	-	3	x	P	-	-
10. Cut down tree and captured two parrots.*	S	-	-	-	-	-	-	A	-	-
11. Turned into a bird and flew above forest.	-	-	-	-	-	-	-	A	x	-
12. Shot a jaguar that turned into a woman.	-	-	-	self	jaguar-woman	1	x	A	x	-
13. Stung by wasps while in woods.	-	-	-	wasps	self	3	x	A	-	-
14. A plane crashed. The bodies were taken from the wreckage.	-	-	x	-	-	1	-	P	-	-
15. A large piece of manioc bread broke as he held it.*	-	-	-	-	-	1	x	P	-	-
16. Shot a pirarucu (a large, 6-foot fish). -		-	-	self	fish-villager	2	-	A	x	-
17. Stung by ant.	-	-	-	ant	self	2	x	P	-	-
18. Caught bird and nurtured it; regarded it like child. (see no. 10.)	S	-	-	-	-	-	-	A	-	-
19. Chased by snake, he turns and kills it with machete.	-	-	-	-	-	2	x	A	-	-
20. Cut self with knife-a deep wound. Sees vagina in dream.	-	-	-	knife-woman	self	3	x	A	-	x

(continues)

Table 7.1 ***(continued)***

	Characters			Aggression		Anxiety				
Dream Summary	*Son/Daughter*	*Mother/Father*	*Brazilians*	*Aggressor*	*Victim*	*Level*	*Castration*	*Passive/Active*	*Transformation*	*Sexual/Scatalogical*
21. Digs for worms, uses them as bait, catches fish which are given to women singers.	-	-	-	-	-	-	-	A	-	-
22. Watched a villager executed as a witch.	-	-	-	village men	distant male kin	2	-	P	-	-
23. Bathed in very cold water in morning.	-	-	-	-	-	-	-	A	-	-
24. Watched as the sun rose.	-	-	-	-	-	-	-	P	-	-
25. Painted self with red urucu body paint.	-	-	-	-	-	-	-	A	-	-
26. Slipped in mud and fell.	-	-	-	-	-	1	-	P	-	-
27. After climbing tree, caught bird and nurtured it. (see no. 10.)	-	-	-	-	-	-	-	A	-	-
28. Too close to the fire, became very hot.	-	-	-	-	-	-	-	P	-	-
29. Struck a spirit-woman with a club for trying to kill his child.	S	-	-	spirit-woman	child	2	-	A	x	-
30. Pursued by ghost of dead mother; cannot escape.	-	M	-	mother	self	2	-	P	-	-
31. Played ceremonial flutes on plaza while women danced behind him.	-	-	-	-	-	-	-	A	-	-
32. After shooting a fish, called to friend from canoe, but friend could not hear or be found.	-	-	-	-	-	1	-	A	-	-
33. Stole and then lost potatoes. Caught by farmer and humiliated.	-	-	-	self	farmer	1	x	A	-	-
34. Went out to the field to get manioc and brought it home.	-	-	-	-	-	-	-	A	-	-
35. Went out to the field to get corn. Harvested it and returned home.	-	-	-	-	-	-	-	-	A	-
36. Shot vulture in the head and captured it. Gave it to parallel cousin who made it his pet.	-	-	-	self	bird	-	1	-	P	-
37. Given tripod by Brazilian. Becomes sick in dream.*	-	-	-	Brazilian	self	-	1	-	P	-
38. After swim in very cold water, huddled near fire to warm up.	-	-	-	-	-	-	-	-	A	-

(continues)

Table 7.1 *(continued)*

Dream Summary	*Characters*			*Aggression*		*Anxiety*				
	Son/Daughter	*Mother/Father*	*Brazilians*	*Aggressor*	*Victim*	*Level*	*Castration*	*Passive/Active*	*Transformation*	*Sexual/Scatalogical*
39. Went fishing and killed many fish with bow and arrow, but missed some, lost arrow.	-	-	-	self	fish	-	1	x	A	-
40. Canoe turned over while fishing. He lost hooks, line, and knife.	-	-	-	-	-	-	2	x	P	-
41. Father was angry at him and set fire to his hair.	-	F	-	father	self	-	3	x	P	-
42. After eating fish, his stomach began to hurt and he vomited.	-	-	-	-	-	-	2	x	A	-
43. Had sex with Brazilian woman and got sore on penis. Removed penis, washed it, put it back on.	-	-	x	woman	self	-	3	x	A	x
44. His infant cries for milk, but mother is with a Brazilian woman and cannot attend to the child.	S	-	x	-	-	-	2	-	P	-
45. Shot fish with arrows. Gave some away and lost others. Became lost in woods.	-	-	-	-	-	-	2	x	A	-
46. Went to traditional village. Ignored by all present.	-	-	-	-	-	-	1	x	P	-
47. Broke an ear of corn and was afraid to wrestle. (see no. 15.)	-	-	-	-	-	-	1	x	A	-
48. Slipped on mud and injured arm.	-	-	-	-	-	-	1	-	P	-
49. Traded his urucu pigments for arrow.	-	-	-	-	-	-	-	-	A	-
50. A small boy started a fire in relatives' house.	-	-	-	-	-	-	1	-	P	-
51. Bathed in very cold water.	-	-	-	-	-	-	-	-	P	-
52. Shot and killed a small bird.*	S	-	-	self	bird-son	-	1	-	A	-
53. Stomach sickened by food he should not have eaten because of taboo, his child is thereby endangered.	S	-	-	self	son	-	1	x	A	-
54. Parallel cousin dies. He cries and mourns for him.	-	-	-	-	-	-	2	x	A	-
55. Woman in the course of a ritual attack him, pull his hair, cover him with their body paint.	-	-	-	women	self	-	3	x	P	-
56. His brother drowns despite his efforts to save him.	S	F	-	-	-	-	2	x	A	-

(continues)

Table 7.1 *(continued)*

	Characters			*Aggression*		*Anxiety*				
Dream Summary	*Son/Daughter*	*Mother/Father*	*Brazilians*	*Aggressor*	*Victim*	*Level*	*Castration*	*Passive/Active*	*Transformation*	*Sexual/Scatalogical*
57. Unable to kill oriole, misses with arrows.	-	-	-	self	oriole	-	1	x	A	-
58. Saw man beating his wife and her lover.	-	-	-	man	wife,lover	-	1	-	P	-
59. Had sex with woman, her husband discovered him and struck him with a club and a machete.	-	-	-	jealous husband	self	-	3	x	A	x
60. Went to the garden.	S	M,F	-	-	-	-	-	-	A	-
61. Captured little bird and nurtured it. It bit him on the finger. (see no. 10.)	S	-	-	bird-son	self	-	1	x	A	-
62. Gave medicine to dying baby.	S?	-	-	-	-	-	2	-	A	-
63. Visited a dangerous neighboring tribe.	-	-	-	-	-	-	1	-	A	-
64. Fell into water while getting his fish trap.	-	-	-	-	-	-	1	x	A	-
65. A house pole carried by many men fell on his finger.	-	-	-	-	-	-	2	x	P	-
66. Forced out of his house by a woman.	-	-	-	woman	self	-	1	-	P	-

Dreamer Profile: A man of 22, married with two children, one an infant. Part of a large kin group, well regarded within the community. An active participant in village rituals and community activities. The considerable anxieties about Brazilians evident in dream material are also consciously expressed.

67. Went with his mother to the Waura tribe to participate in women's ritual, akajatapa.	-	M	-	-	-	-	-	-	A	-
68. Went to Auiti village and stole sugar cane.	-	-	-	self	other tribe	-	1	-	A	-
69. Went to rive with father to fish, but got caught in the rain.	-	F	-	-	-	-	-	-	P	-
70. Played the men's sacred flutes in men's house.	-	-	-	-	-	-	-	-	A	-
71. A plane landed, everyone was afraid of disease. (see no. 37.)	-	-	x	Brazilians	Mehinaku	-	2	-	P	-
72. A child was left out alone in the dark and spirits took her away.	-	-	-	spirits	child	-	1	-	A	-
73. Chased by a black jaguar*	-	-	-	jaguar	self	-	2	x	P	-

(continues)

Table 7.1 (continued)

Dream Summary	*Characters*			*Aggression*		*Anxiety*				
	Son/Daughter	*Mother/Father*	*Brazilians*	*Aggressor*	*Victim*	*Level*	*Castration*	*Passive/Active*	*Transformation*	*Sexual/Scatalogical*
74. Kept pet bird which flew away. (see no. 10.)	S	-	-	-	-	-	1	x	P	-
75. While fishing, shot at stingray, but missed and almost lost arrow.	-	-	-	self	stingray	-	1	x	A	-
76. Almost ate fish in violation of taboo that would have killed son.	S	-	-	self	son	-	1	x	A	-
77. Shot with arrow at Jawari spear –throwing contest-ritual.	-	-	-	man from another tribe	self	-	2	x	P	-
Brought food from house to father to be distributed in the name of sacred flute spirit.	-	F	-	-	-	-	-	-	A	-
79. A poisonous snake bit his parallel cousin.	-	-	-	snake	cousin	-	1	-	P	-
80. Participated in killing of a village witch with a club and a machete.	-	-	-	self	cousin witch-distant	-	2	-	A	-
81. Observed the shamans of the village as they treated a sick kinsman.	-	-	-	-	-	-	1	-	P	-
82. Watched as parallel cousin killed animals with club.	-	-	-	cousin	animals	-	-	-	A	-
83. Brazilians shot and killed his brothers.	-	-	x	Brazilians	brothers	-	3	-	P	-
84. Went to air force base. Soldiers tried to have sex with his wife. They shot at him and the Mehinaku.	-	-	x	Brazilians	self, wife	-	3	x	P	x
85. Killed Brazilians who had threatened them with guns.	-	-	x	Brazilians	self	-	3	-	A	-
86. Frightened by spirit.	-	-	-	spirit	self	-	2	-	P	-
87. Frightened by the ghost of his deceased MoBr.	-	-	-	ghost	self	-	1	-	P	-
88. Frightened by and then kills jaguar.	-	-	-	jaguar	self	-	1	x	A	-
89. Saw an anaconda from his canoe and urged a young man in seclusion to get it for strength magic.	-	-	-	-	-	-	-	-	A	-
90. Caught in a cold wind, he blew on the fire.	-	-	-	-	-	-	-	-	A	-
91. At salt-making village with family; does not participate.	S	M,F	-	-	-	-	-	-	P	-

(continues)

Table 7.1 *(continued)*

	Characters			*Aggression*		*Anxiety*				
Dream Summary	*Son/Daughter*	*Mother/Father*	*Brazilians*	*Aggressor*	*Victim*	*Level*	*Castration*	*Passive/Active*	*Transformation*	*Sexual/Scatalogical*
92. Plane crashes. Mother catches on fire.	-	M	x	Brazilians	self,mother	-	2	-	A	-
93. Brazilian doctor rapes wife and shoots at him.	-	-	x	Brazilians	self,wife	-	3	x	A	x
94. Poisonous snake threatened to bite him.	-	-	-	snake	self	-	2	x	A	-
95. Observed a man rejecting his daughter's suitor as a potential son-in-law.	-	-	-	-	-	-	1	-	P	-
96. Ran from a frightening spirit.	-	-	-	spirit	self	-	1	-	P	-
97. Killed threatening jaguar.	-	-	-	jaguar	self	-	1	x	A	-
98. A jaguar ate a tapir' kills it as it eats.	-	-	-	self	jaguar	-	1	-	A	-
99. Watched with concern as a cousin's husband publicly criticized a man from another tribe.	-	-	x	-	-	-	1	-	P	-
100. A large bat ate his pet parrot.	-	-	-	bat	pet	-	1	x	P	-
101. Young girl saw forbidden sacred flutes. He did not tell other men, thereby allowing her to escape.*	-	M	-	-	-	-	2	-	P	x
102. Drives witch from village, but all still fear the witch.	-	-	-	witch	villagers,self	-	2	-	A	-
103. A Brazilian brought him gifts, but they spread a disease. (see no. 37.)	-	-	x	Brazilian	self	-	1	-	P	-
104. Raced home from fishing to escape stinging mosquitoes.	S	M	-	mosquitoes	self	-	2	x	P	-
105. Killed tapir and gave it to the head of Indian post.	-	-	x	self	tapir	-	-	-	A	-
106. Had frightening dream of jaguar eating turtle.	-	-	-	-	-	-	2	x	P	-
107. With deceased relatives, mourning.	-	-	-	-	-	-	1	-	A	-
108. Refused food and therefore stung by stingray*	-	-	-	stingray	self	-	2	x	A	-
109. Saw growth-medicine spirit and shamans.	-	-	-	-	-	-	1	-	A	-
110. Wrestled with Waura on visit to that tribe.	-	-	-	-	-	-	-	-	A	-
111. Saw fisherman. Ate turtle eggs and meat that father caught and brought home.	-	F	-	-	-	-	-	-	A	-

(continues)

Table 7.1 (continued)

Dream Summary	*Characters*			*Aggression*		*Anxiety*				
	Son/Daughter	*Mother/Father*	*Brazilians*	*Aggressor*	*Victim*	*Level*	*Castration*	*Passive/Active*	*Transformation*	*Sexual/Scatalogical*
112. Bit by a locust while in the garden looking at peppers.	-	-	-	locust	self	-	2	x	P	-
113. Gave up spear gun in trade for tape recorder.	-	-	-	-	-	-	-	x	A	-
114. Shot a bird but missed.	-	-	-	self	bird	-	-	x	A	-
115. Saw spirit and heard its voice, lectured by father to avoid spirits.	-	F	-	-	-	-	1	-	P	-
116. Burned on the body by a spirit fire.	S	F	-	spirit	self	-	3	x	P	-
Dreamer Profile: A man of 21, unmarried, older sister and three younger brothers. A member of one of the village's larger kin groups and likely to become an influential chief. Fascinated yet confused by Brazilians and their civilization. Deep-seated sexual conflicts suggested by dreams have correlates in his ambivalent relationships with woman.										
117. Attacked by women during Yamurikuma role-reversal ritual.	-	-	-	women	self	-	2	x	A	-
118. Had sex with a woman who took his shirt to clean herself off.	-	-	-	-	-	-	-	x	A	x
119. Flies pestered and bit him.	-	-	-	flies	self	-	1	x	A	-
120. Had sexual relations with a woman whose flesh was rotten and breaks open during intercourse.	-	-	-	-	-	-	2	-	A	x
121. Pushed away hands of girl who grasped him because she wanted to dance.	-	-	-	girl	self	-	1	x	P	-
122. Ant bit his finger.	-	-	-	ant	self	-	1	x	P	-
123. Caught playing with Brazilian's camera equipment and was ashamed.	-	-	x	-	-	-	1	-	A	-
124. Placed in jail by Brazilian soldiers. Told he would be released at one o'clock, but could not read watch.	-	-	x	Brazilians	self	-	2	-	P	-
125. A woman gave him her hammock.	-	-	-	-	-	-	-	-	A	-
126. Fell into the mouth of a giant fish.	-	-	-	fish-spirit	self	-	2	x	P	-

(continues)

Table 7.1 *(continued)*

	Characters			*Aggression*		*Anxiety*				
Dream Summary	*Son/Daughter*	*Mother/Father*	*Brazilians*	*Aggressor*	*Victim*	*Level*	*Castration*	*Passive/Active*	*Transformation*	*Sexual/Scatalogical*
127. Offered bad food by a female kin.	-	-	-	woman	self	-	-	-	P	-
128. Pursued by a killer.	-	-	-	man	self	-	2	x	P	-
129. Clubbed a fish which turned into his FaBr.	-	-	-	self	fish-FaBr	-	2	-	A	x
130. Saw kinsman-spirit. The sight weakened his legs.	-	-	-	kinsman-spirit	self	-	2	x	P	-
131. Watched as a woman had sex with a man's foot.	-	-	-	-	-	-	-	-	P	x
132. Carried water from river; injured.	-	-	-	-	-	-	1	x	P	-
133. Watched as a woman wrestled a man and ripped open his cheek with her hand.	-	-	-	woman		man	-	1	-	P
134. Watched as a man washed another's dirty penis with a brush.	-	-	-	-	-	-	1	-	P	x
135. A man died among the Brazilians; they returned only his head.	-	-	x	Brazilians	Mehinaku	-	1	-	P	-
136. A woman lay on top of him; it hurt.	-	-	-	woman	self	-	2	x	P	x
137. Friends jumped from a tree and injured themselves.	-	-	-	-	-	-	1	-	P	-
138. Washed his feet and legs in stream.	-	-	-	-	-	-	-	-	A	-
139. Hauled in fish;jerked free, lost it.	-	-	-	-	-	-	-	x	A	-
140. Wrestled two men from another tribe.	-	-	-	-	-	-	-	-	A	-

Dreamer Profile: A man of 21, recently married, father of infant. Oldest child in family of six children. Well adjusted and highly regarded, takes evident pleasure in his relationship with wife, child, parents.

141. Many passengers get off a plane. Frightening, threatens disease.	-	-	x	Brazilians	self, Mehinaku	-	2	-	P	-
142. Could not get a bird he and brother sought as a pet.	-	-	-	-	-	-	-	-	A	-
143. Showed a wild pig to a child.	D	-	-	wild pig	self	-	1	x	A	-
144. Looked for a baby bird, a pet, with his family.	-	M,F	-	-	-	-	-	-	A	-

(continues)

Table 7.1 ***(continued)***

Dream Summary	*Characters*			*Aggression*		*Anxiety*				
	Son/Daughter	*Mother/Father*	*Brazilians*	*Aggressor*	*Victim*	*Level*	*Castration*	*Passive/Active*	*Transformation*	*Sexual/Scatalogical*
145. Saw a woman have sexual relations.	-	-	-	-	-	-	-	-	P	x
146. Daughter almost drowned. Rescued her.	D	-	-	-	-	-	2	-	A	-
147. Stung by bees.	-	-	-	bees	self	-	1	x	P	-
148. Put out fire he set in thatch grass.	-	-	-	-	-	-	1	-	A	-
149. Had sexual relations with girl friend. Wife saw them and became angry.	-	-	-	wife	self	-	1	-	P	x
150. Rescued drowning brother.	-	-	-	-	-	-	-	-	A	-
151. Shot five fish with bow and arrow from canoe.	-	-	-	self	fish	-	-	-	-	-
152. Shot bird in forest.	-	-	-	self	bird	-	-	-	A	-
153. Attacked by herd of wild pigs.	-	-	-	pigs	self	-	1	x	A	-
154. Shot at threatening jaguar and missed.	-	-	-	jaguar	self	-	2	x	A	-
155. Shot three fish with bow and arrow. Brought them home to his mother.	-	M	-	-	-	-	-	-	A	-
156. Killed a threatening snake in dream. Saw frightening spirit. Reassured by mother.	-	M	-	snake, spirit	self	-	1	x	A	-
157. Glided through flooded forest in canoe.	-	-	-	-	-	-	-	-	A	-
Dreamer Profile: A man in late 20s married with three children. Somewhat marginal to village life in residence arrangements and participation in ceremonial life of the community. More deeply concerned about witchcraft and spirit-induced disease than most villagers.										
158. Eaten by devouring spirits.	-	-	-	spirits	self	-	3	x	P	-
159. Learns in dream that son of distant kin will be eaten by spirits.	-	-	-	spirits	son	-	1	-	P	-
160. Legs were weak. Walked slowly as if old.	-	-	-	-	-	-	1	x	A	-
161. Watched as giant pequi fruit fell from tree.	-	-	-	-	-	-	-	-	P	-

(continues)

Table 7.1 *(continued)*

	Characters			Aggression		Anxiety				
Dream Summary	*Son/Daughter*	*Mother/Father*	*Brazilians*	*Aggressor*	*Victim*	*Level*	*Castration*	*Passive/Active*	*Transformation*	*Sexual/Scatalogical*
162. Had sexual relations with a spirit-woman.	-	-	-	-	-	-	-	-	A	x
163. Gathered flying ants.*	-	-	-	-	-	-	1	-	A	-
164. Flew up in the air, but was shot down by a crowd of armed villagers. Multiple injuries.	-	-	-	crowd of Mehinaku	self	-	3	x	A	-
165. Living at the Waura tribe.	-	-	-	-	-	-	-	-	P	-
166. Eaten by a giant spirit-fish.	-	-	-	spirit	self	-	2	x	P	-
167. Heard a jaguar growling: frightened.	-	-	-	jaguar	self	-	1	x	P	-
168. Chased by pigs. Killed them with knife.	-	-	-	pigs	self	-	2	x	A	-
169. Went to the house of the snake-spirit.	-	-	-	-	-	-	-	-	P	-
170. Bad manioc bread made his stomach hurt.	-	-	-	-	-	-	1	x	P	-
171. An airplane flew low overhead and set fire to the villagers' houses.	-	-	x	Brazilians	self, Mehinaku	-	3	-	P	-
172. Saw ghost and frightening snake.	-	-	-	ghost, snake	self	-	1	x	P	-
173. Man wanted to kill him. A woman protected him.	-	-	-	man	self	-	2	-	P	-
174. Found and nurtured baby turtle.	-	S	-	-	-	-	1	-	A	-
175. Saw the ghost of dead sister.	-	-	-	-	-	-	-	-	P	-
176. Stabbed a troublesome child with knife.	-	-	-	self	child	-	1	-	A	-
177. Saw many male spirit-people building a house.	-	-	-	-	-	-	-	-	P	-
178. Saw distant male kin dressed as a Brazilian. Warned him against Brazilians' diseases.	-	-	x	-	-	-	1	-	A	-
179. Dived under the water.	-	-	-	-	-	-	-	-	A	-
180. Saw the ghost of a man killed as a witch.	-	-	-	-	-	-	1	-	P	-
181. Diseased; covered with sores.	-	-	-	-	-	-	2	-	P	-
182. Had sexual relations with a spirit-woman who looked like a kinsman's wife.	-	-	-	-	-	-	1	-	A	x

(continues)

Table 7.1 (continued)

Dream Summary	*Characters*			*Aggression*		*Anxiety*				
	Son/Daughter	*Mother/Father*	*Brazilians*	*Aggressor*	*Victim*	*Level*	*Castration*	*Passive/Active*	*Transformation*	*Sexual/Scatalogical*
183. Stepped on thorn and injured self.	-	-	-	-	-	-	2	x	A	-
184. Drank manioc beverage which gave him a stomach ache.	-	-	-	-	-	-	1	x	A	-
185. Shot and killed a spirit-fish.	-	-	-	self	spirit-fish	-	-	-	A	-
186. Frightened by the sight of a woman's vagina.	-	-	-	-	-	-	1	-	P	x
187. Rain fell into his house and on the silo of manioc flour.	-	-	-	-	-	-	1	-	A	-
Dreamer Profile: One of the oldest men in the village, in the late 60s. Head of large kin group and household of wife, five children, in-laws and grandchildren. A singer and shaman, well respected in the village.										
188. Visited his sister in another tribe.	-	-	-	-	-	-	-	-	P	-
189. Visited the Auiti village. Saw their underwater silos of pequi mash.	-	-	-	-	-	-	-	-	A	-
190. Shot at fish and lost an arrow.	-	-	-	self	fish	-	1	x	A	-
191. A woman pulled his hair. She wanted to marry him and have sex.	-	-	-	woman	self	-	2	x	P	x
192. Shot at a monkey.	-	-	-	self	monkey	-	2	-	A	-
193. Went fishing and monkey hunting; killed monkey.	-	-	-	self	monkey	-	-	-	A	-
194. Bailed out canoe.	-	-	-	-	-	-	-	-	A	-
195. Working on fish poisoning expedition.	-	-	-	-	-	-	-	-	A	-
196. Threatened with knife by rival within village.	-	-	-	male rival	self	-	3	x	P	-
197. In canoe with wife. She says she is dying.	-	-	-	-	-	-	1	-	P	-
198. Tried to shoot monkey, but missed.	-	-	-	-	-	-	1	x	A	-
199. Bitten by tocandira ant.	-	-	-	ant	self	-	2	x	A	-
200. Went to ancient Mehinaku village.	-	-	-	-	-	-	-	-	A	-

(continues)

Table 7.1 ***(continued)***

Dream Summary	Characters			Aggression		Anxiety				
	Son/Daughter	*Mother/Father*	*Brazilians*	*Aggressor*	*Victim*	*Level*	*Castration*	*Passive/Active*	*Transformation*	*Sexual/Scatalogical*
Dreamer Profile: An outgoing, friendly man of 18; unmarried. As a child persecuted by other villagers on grounds that father was a witch.										
201. Chased by vicious dog.	-	-	-	dog	self	-	2	x	P	-
202. Had sexual relations with an Auiti woman.	-	-	-	-	-	-	-	-	A	x
203. Tried to visit Indian Post, but could not find canoe.	-	-	-	-	-	-	-	-	A	-
204. Wrestled; broke collar bone, back; died.	-	-	-	wrestler	self	-	3	x	A	-
205. Line caught around legs while fishing; tripped and fell.	-	-	-	-	-	-	2	-	A	-
206. Killed monkey with bow and arrow while hunting with cross-cousin.	-	-	-	self	monkey	-	-	-	A	-
207. After eating fermented pequi mash, everyone, including the anthropologist, became sick.	-	-	x	-	-	-	2	x	P	-
208. Sexually aroused by attractive woman on way to river.	-	-	-	-	-	-	-	-	A	x
209. While wearing rituals masks, he and other men teased village women.	-	-	-	self,men	women	-	-	-	A	-
210. Arranged a marriage for cousin and girl friend.	-	-	-	-	-	-	-	-	A	-
211. Returned from fishing trip with big catch. All villagers rejoice on his return.	-	-	-	-	-	-	-	-	A	-
212. Cousin and cousin's wife had sexual relations.	-	-	-	-	-	-	-	-	P	x
213. Got pequi and ate it.	-	-	-	-	-	-	-	-	A	-
214. Went swimming.	-	-	-	-	-	-	-	-	A	-
215. Had sexual relations with little girl and injured her. Sense of guilt within dream.	-	-	-	self	little girl	-	2	-	A	x

(continues)

Table 7.1 *(continued)*

Dream Summary	*Characters*			*Aggression*		*Anxiety*				
	Son/Daughter	*Mother/Father*	*Brazilians*	*Aggressor*	*Victim*	*Level*	*Castration*	*Passive/Active*	*Transformation*	*Sexual/Scatalogical*
Dreamer Profile: A man of 40 married with three children. Somewhat marginal to ritual and social activities, he is ridiculed as a fool by many villagers.										
216. On fish-poisoning trip with deceased brothers. Killed many small fish together.	-	-	M,F	-	-	-	-	-	A	-
217. Stung by ant.	-	-	-	ant	self	-	2	x	P	-
218. Stung on foot by stingray.	-	-	-	stingray	self	-	2	x	P	-
219. Looked for underwater pequi silo.*	-	-	-	-	-	-	1	-	A	-
220. Anthropologist's infant son died.	-	-	x	-	-	-	1	-	P	-
221. Magic witch-killing method split open rotted body of witch.	-	-	-	unstated	witch	-	2	-	P	x
222. Saw dead man's ghost.	-	-	-	-	-	-	2	-	P	-
223. Made sick to stomach by deceased mother's "ghost food."	-	-	-	mother	self	-	1	x	P	-
224. Shot with tiny arrow by spirit.	-	-	-	spirit	self	-	2	x	P	-
225. Found knife in water. An old woman tried to have sex with him and marry him.	-	-	-	-	-	-	-	-	A	x
226. Brought spirit's food to men's house.	-	-	-	-	-	-	-	-	A	-
227. Watched as a Mechinaku woman opened an egg in which she finds her pet chicken.	-	-	-	-	-	-	-	-	A	-
228. Harvested potatoes.	-	-	-	-	-	-	-	-	A	-
229. Washed his necklace.	-	-	-	-	-	-	-	-	A	-
Dreamer Profile: A man of 35, father of three. Affable, outgoing, but somewhat marginal to village life; rejected as a gossip. Long periods of more successful residence in other tribes.										
230. Saw couple having sexual relations.	-	-	-	-	-	-	-	-	P	x
231. Had sexual relations with girl.	-	-	-	-	-	-	-	-	A	x

(continues)

Table 7.1 *(continued)*

	Characters			*Aggression*		*Anxiety*				
Dream Summary	*Son/Daughter*	*Mother/Father*	*Brazilians*	*Aggressor*	*Victim*	*Level*	*Castration*	*Passive/Active*	*Transformation*	*Sexual/Scatalogical*
232. His cheek is torn open by man who had been killed by a witch.	-	-	-	man	self	-	3	x	P	-
233. Attacked by a jaguar.	-	-	-	jaguar	self	-	2	x	P	-
234. Lost his gun.	-	-	-	-	-	-	1	x	P	-
235. Almost eaten by otter monster.	-	-	-	otter-spirit	self	-	2	x	P	-
236. Plane landed on village plaza threatened with disease.(see no. 37.)	-	-	x	-	-	-	1	-	P	-
237. Had sexual relations with village girl.	-	-	-	-	-	-	-	-	A	x
Dreamer Profile: A 13-year-old, well adjusted and sociable. Somewhat marginal to the community in that parents have spent many years in another tribe.										
238. Searched for pequi fruit with comrade.	-	-	-	-	-	-	-	-	A	-
239. Heard sister singing and participating in role-reversal ritual.	-	-	-	-	-	-	-	-	P	-
240. Ran, frightened, from snake-spirit.	-	-	-	snake-spirit	self	-	1	x	A	-
241. Took off in Brazilians' plane.	-	-	x	-	-	-	-	-	A	-
242. Searched for fish underwater, wearing diving mask.	-	-	-	-	-	-	-	-	A	-
Dreamer Profile: A man of 28, married with three children. A powerful shaman.										
243. Had sexual relations with a woman.	-	-	-	-	-	-	-	-	A	x
244. Frightened by spirit seen at air force base.	-	-	x	-	-	-	1	-	P	-
245. Dreamed of sexual relations.	-	-	-	-	-	-	-	-	A	x
246. Frightening spirit appeared as a shaman.	-	-	-	-	-	-	1	-	A	-
247. Dreamed of oral sex with a woman.	-	-	-	-	-	-	-	-	A	x

(continues)

Table 7.1 (continued)

Dream Summary	*Characters*			*Aggression*		*Anxiety*				
	Son/Daughter	*Mother/Father*	*Brazilians*	*Aggressor*	*Victim*	*Level*	*Castration*	*Passive/Active*	*Transformation*	*Sexual/Scatalogical*
Dreamer Profile: A man of 45, married, no children.										
248. Ghosts of dead parents asked him to build a fence.	-	M,F	-	-	-	-	-	-	P	-
249. Wanted to have sex with a girl, but he had no eyes to see her.	-	-	-	-	-	-	3	x	P	x
250. Feeling guilty after having refused to give his wife food, he makes her a present of pequi.	-	-	-	-	-	-	1	-	A	-
251. Angry, he lectures wife's lover, who is hidden.	-	-	-	-	-	-	1	-	A	-
252. Attacked by man who choked him.	-	-	-	man	self	-	3	x	P	-
253. Rejected offer of food from wife.	-	-	-	-	-	-	-	-	P	-
254. Frightened by jaguar.	-	-	-	jaguar	self	-	2	x	P	-
Dreamer Profile: Accomplished well-respected man of 45. Married, six children. Deep-seated insecurities regarding aggression.										
255. Shot a jaguar that turned into a man after death.	-	-	-	self	man-jaguar	-	2	-	A	x
256. Angry at wife because she intended to marry another man.	-	-	-	self	wife	-	1	-	A	-
257. Swam in hot water.	-	-	-	-	-	-	-	-	A	-
258. Frightened by jaguar. Struck it with club and its head fell off.	-	-	-	jaguar	self	-	2	x	A	-
259. Frightening big plane crashed.	-	-	-	-	-	-	2	-	P	-
260. Tried to have sexual relations, but saw woman's genitals and therefor became impotent.	-	-	-	-	-	-	1	x	A	x
261. Smoking like a shaman, fell into trance.	-	-	-	-	-	-	1	-	A	-
262. Pigs attacked him; he rescued child.	S	-	-	pigs	self,son	-	2	x	A	-

(continues)

Table 7.1 *(continued)*

	Characters			*Aggression*		*Anxiety*				
Dream Summary	*Son/Daughter*	*Mother/Father*	*Brazilians*	*Aggressor*	*Victim*	*Level*	*Castration*	*Passive/Active*	*Transformation*	*Sexual/Scatalogical*
Dreamer Profile: Well-adjusted and highly sociable man of 30. Married, two children.										
263. Dug a hole in the ground to escape a bomb.	-	-	x	Brazilians	self	-	2	-	A	-
264. Shot fish and struck them on head with club.	-	-	-	self	fish	-	-	-	A	-
265. Struck wife as she went to have sex with lover.	-	-	-	self	wife	-	1	-	A	x
Dreamer Profile: A man, 40 years; married to two woman; two children.										
266. Could not get his gun from his father.	-	F	-	father	self	-	1	x	A	-
267. Armbands burned in fire. (see no. 3.)	-	-	-	-	-	-	2	x	A	-
268. Killed his pet parrot. (see no.10)	-	-	-	self	parrot	-	1	x	A	-
269. Worked in the forest.	-	-	-	-	-	-	-	-	A	-
270. In canoe. Called by others on bank, but could not come.	-	-	-	-	-	-	1	-	P	-
Dreamer Profile: A boy, age 11.										
271. Chased by jaguar.	-	-	-	jaguar	self	-	2	x	P	-
272. Shot pigs in forest.	-	-	-	self	pigs	-	-	-	A	-
Dreamer Profile: A boy , age 11.										
273. Shot alligator. Transformed itself into fearsome witch.	-	-	-	self	alligator-witch	-	1	-	-	x
274. Caught three fish with friends in river.	-	-	-	self	fish	-	-	-	A	-
275. Went to river and saw birds.	-	-	-	-	-	-	-	-	A	-

(continues)

Table 7.1 ***(continued)***

	Characters			*Aggression*		*Anxiety*				
Dream Summary	*Son/Daughter*	*Mother/Father*	*Brazilians*	*Aggressor*	*Victim*	*Level*	*Castration*	*Passive/Active*	*Transformation*	*Sexual/Scatalogical*
Dreamer Profile: A man, age 40.										
276. Heard jaguar as he sat in canoe.	-	-	-	jaguar	self -		1	x	P	-

Table 7.2 The Content of Mehinaku Women's Dreams

	Characters			*Aggression*		*Anxiety*				
Dream Summary	*Son/Daughter*	*Mother/Father*	*Brazilians*	*Aggressor*	*Victim*	*Level*	*Castration*	*Passive/Active*	*Transformation*	*Sexual/Scatalogical*
Dreamer Profile: A woman of 23, married with three children. Outgoing, enthusiastic, participant in village activities.										
1. Dog attacked and bit her.	-	-	-	dog	self	-	2	x	P	-
2. Collected ants.	-	-	-	-	-	-	1	-	A	-
3. Saw Brazilians and frightened by them.	-	-	x	-	-	-	1	-	P	-
4. Frightened by sight of pregnant woman with enlarged genitalia.	-	-	-	-	-	-	1	-	P	x
5. Village man clubbed her when she refused to have sex.	-	-	-	man	self	-	3	x	P	x
6. Saw cousin eating fish.	-	-	-	-	-	-	-	-	P	-
7. Was bathing.	-	-	-	-	-	-	-	-	A	-
8. Saw villagers eating pequi.	-	-	-	-	-	-	-	-	P	-
9. Participated in woman's ritual of role reversal.	-	-	-	-	-	-	-	-	A	-
10. Processed and skinned manioc tubers.	-	-	-	-	-	-	-	-	A	-
11. Saw and was frightened by feces on path.	-	-	-	-	-	-	1	-	P	x
12. Ate food prepared for spirit festival.	-	-	-	-	-	-	-	-	A	-
13. Saw a man killed as a witch.	-	-	-	man	man	-	1	-	P	-
14. Saw two men on plaza awaiting a jaguar.	-	-	-	-	-	-	-	-	A	-
15. Two men called to her. She held her baby.	D	-	-	-	-	-	-	-	P	-
16. Frightened of men raping her.	-	-	-	men	self	-	1	-	P	x
17. Dreamed of MoBrDa's ghost.	-	-	-	-	-	-	-	-	P	-
18. Saved child from drowning.	-	-	-	-	-	-	1	-	A	-
19. Sank deep in mud as she tried to walk.	-	-	-	-	-	-	2	-	P	-
20. Spilled manioc porridge.	-	-	-	-	-	-	1	-	P	-
21. Pursued by Brazilian motorboat filled with "savage" Indians.	-	-	x	Brazilians, other Indians	self	-	2	-	P	-
22. Married to another man.	-	-	-	-	-	-	-	-	P	-

(continues)

Table 7.2 (continued)

	Characters			Aggression		Anxiety				
Dream Summary	*Son/Daughter*	*Mother/Father*	*Brazilians*	*Aggressor*	*Victim*	*Level*	*Castration*	*Passive/Active*	*Transformation*	*Sexual/Scatalogical*
23. Bitten by dog.	-	-	-	dog	self	-	2	x	P	-
24. Made manioc bread.	-	-	-	-	-	-	-	-	A	-
25. Went bathing, carrying infant.	D	-	-	-	-	-	-	-	A	-
26. Cooked fish for ghost of MoBr.	-	-	-	-	-	-	-	-	A	-
27. Watched as star rose.	-	-	-	-	-	-	-	-	P	-
28. Went to garden to work.	D	M	-	-	-	-	-	-	A	-
29. Ate MoBr's ghost-fish.	-	-	-	-	-	-	-	-	A	-
30. Dreamed of wrestling with another woman.*	-	-	-	-	-	-	1	-	A	-
31. Chased by snake.	-	-	-	snake	self	-	1	x	P	-
32. Defecated in brush outside of the village.	-	-	-	-	-	-	-	-	A	x
Dreamer Profile: A young girl in puberty seclusion, age 14. Intelligent, sociable.										
33. Stole potatoes and ate them. Caught by farmer.	-	-	-	farmer	self	-	1	-	A	-
34. Broke ceramic pot.	-	-	-	-	-	-	-	-	P	-
35. Saw dancing women.	-	-	-	-	-	-	-	-	P	-
36. Saw women wrestling and went bathing.	-	-	-	-	-	-	-	-	A	-
37. Frightened by Brazilians speaking on radio.	-	-	x	-	-	-	1	-	P	-
38. Frightened by deer.	-	-	-	deer	self	-	1	-	P	-
39. Stole sugarcane from garden.	-	-	-	-	-	-	-	-	A	-
40. Frightened by eclipse while bathing with other women.	-	-	-	-	-	-	1	-	P	-
41. Fearful of plane. Mother struck and killed sister. Her corpse turned into an arrow.	-	M	x	Brazilians, mother	self, sister	-	3	-	A	x
42. Saw friend processing manioc.	-	-	-	-	-	-	-	-	P	-
43. Chased and bitten by anaconda.	-	-	-	snake	self	-	3	x	A	-

(continues)

Table 7.2 *(continued)*

	Characters			*Aggression*		*Anxiety*				
Dream Summary	*Son/Daughter*	*Mother/Father*	*Brazilians*	*Aggressor*	*Victim*	*Level*	*Castration*	*Passive/Active*	*Transformation*	*Sexual/Scatalogical*
44. Found and ate foul-smelling pequi.	-	-	-	-	-	-	-	-	A	-
45. Saw woman stirring manioc beverage.	-	-	-	-	-	-	-	-	P	-
Dreamer Profile: A fifty-year-old woman, married with four children. Well adjusted, sociable, outgoing.										
46. Saw woman with ceramic pot.	-	-	-	-	-	-	-	-	P	-
47. Visited another Xingu village.	-	-	-	-	-	-	-	-	A	-
48. Bathed with other women.	-	-	-	-	-	-	-	-	A	-
49. Daughter bitten by rattlesnake.	D	-	-	snake	daughter	-	3	-	P	-
50. Jaguar bit her hand.	-	-	-	jaguar	self	-	3	x	P	-
51. Went to defecate and was transformed into a wolf.	-	-	-	-	-	-	1	-	P	x
52. Went bathing.	-	-	-	-	-	-	-	-	A	-
53. Frightened by dog. Threatened it with stick.	-	-	-	dog	self	-	2	x	A	-
54. Went to "village in sky" (paradise). Saw parents.	-	M,F	-	-	-	-	-	-	A	-
55. Almost drowned.	-	-	-	-	-	-	2	-	P	-
56. Went to distant field. Processed manioc.	-	-	-	-	-	-	-	-	A	-
57. Saw a ghost of a girl in seclusion.	-	-	-	-	-	-	-	-	P	-
58. Saw men bringing fish into village.	-	-	-	-	-	-	-	-	P	-
59. Drifted in canoe to bathing area by river.	-	-	-	-	-	-	-	-	P	-
Dreamer Profile: A woman of 20, married with two young children including newborn infant. Articulate, concerned about and fascinated with Brazilian civilization.										
60. Frightened by sight of rectum of a spirit.	-	-	-	spirit	self	-	1	-	P	x
61. A crying child missed its mother.	S	-	-	-	-	-	-	-	P	-
62. Saw plane landing.	S, D	M, F	x	-	-	-	-	-	P	-

(continues)

Table 7.2 ***(continued)***

	Characters			Aggression		Anxiety				
Dream Summary	*Son/Daughter*	*Mother/Father*	*Brazilians*	*Aggressor*	*Victim*	*Level*	*Castration*	*Passive/Active*	*Transformation*	*Sexual/Scatological*
63. Saw and collected ants with husband.	-	-	-	-	-	-	-	-	P	-
64. Beat her husband and his lover as they had sex.	-	-	-	self	husband,lover	-	1	-	A	x
65. An agouti ate her feces. She killed it with a stick.	-	-	-	self	agouti	-	-	-	A	x
66. A "savage" Indian with a two-headed knife-like penis chased her.	-	-	-	"savage Indian	self	-	2	-	P	x
67. On way to get firewood. Refused to assist grandmother who called her.	-	-	-	-	-	-	1	-	A	-
68. Took an agouti as a pet.*	S,D	M,F	-	-	-	-	-	-	P	-
69. Lost in swamp with family in a canoe.	S,D	M,F	-	-	-	-	1	-	P	-
70. Went to bathe. Path to river ascended toward sky. Frightened.	-	-	-	-	-	-	2	-	A	-
71. Saw spirit woman drinking manioc beverage.	-	-	-	-	-	-	-	-	P	-
Dreamer Profile: A 17-year-old girl, married with two children.										
72. Wrestled on plaza with girl in seclusion. (see no. 30.)	-	-	-	-	-	-	-	-	A	-
73. Visited another person's house.	-	-	-	-	-	-	-	-	P	-
74. Dreamed of pregnancy.	-	-	-	-	-	-	-	-	P	-
75. Attacked by dogs.	-	-	-	dogs	self	-	2	x	P	-
76. Dug potatoes.	-	-	-	-	-	-	-	-	A	-
77. Cleared weeds.	-	-	-	-	-	-	-	-	A	-
Dreamer Profile: A 24-year-old woman, mother of three.										
78. Masturbated daughter; laughed at. Ashamed.	D	-	-	-	-	-	1	-	A	x
79. Singing with other women on plaza.	-	-	-	-	-	-	-	-	A	-

(continues)

Table 7.2 (continued)

	Characters			Aggression		Anxiety				
Dream Summary	*Son/Daughter*	*Mother/Father*	*Brazilians*	*Aggressor*	*Victim*	*Level*	*Castration*	*Passive/Active*	*Transformation*	*Sexual/Scatalogical*
80. Stole pequi mash from deceased man. Caught, lectured.	-	-	-	man	self	-	1	-	A	-
81. Teased a village man about his penis.	-	-	-	self	man	-	-	-	A	x
Dreamer Profile: A 30-year-old women with five children.										
82. Jaguar chased her.	-	-	-	jaguar	self	-	1	x	P	-
83. Kinsman killed monkey.	-	-	-	man	monkey	-	-	-	P	-
84. Brazilian stole her children. Heard them crying to her from far off.	-	-	x	Brazilians	self, children	-	3	-	P	-
Dreamer Profile: A 65-year-old woman.										
85. Jaguar chased and ate her.	-	-	-	jaguar	self	-	3	x	P	-
Dreamer Profile: A 27-year-old woman.										
86. Dreamed of marriage to another man.	-	-	-	-	-	-	-	-	A	-
87. Wrestled with and thrown by woman from other tribe. (see no.30.)	-	-	-	woman self	-	1	-	A	-	
Dreamer Profile: A 20-year-old girl, married with newborn infant.										
88. A flaming plane fell on her.	-	-	x	Brazilians	self	-	3	-	P	-
89. Bitten by ant. Grandparents died.	-	-	-	ant	self	-	2	x	P	-
90. Struck and killed her crying baby.	S	-	-	self	son	-	2	-	A	-

(continues)

Table 7.2 ***(continued)***

	Characters			*Aggression*		*Anxiety*				
Dream Summary	*Son/Daughter*	*Mother/Father*	*Brazilians*	*Aggressor*	*Victim*	*Level*	*Castration*	*Passive/Active*	*Transformation*	*Sexual/Scatalogical*
91. Went to another tribe; missed father.	-	F	-	-	-	-	1	-	P	-
Dreamer Profile: A 12-year-old girl in seclusion.										
92. Bites the penis of sexually aggressive spirit.	-	-	-	spirit	self	-	1	-	A	x
93. Woman with overlarge genitals came to have sex with her.	-	-	-	woman	self	-	2	-	P	x
94. Watched as village man had sex with his wife.	-	-	-	-	-	-	-	-	P	x
Dreamer Profile: A 40-year-old woman.										
95. Brazilian had sex with her, made her sick.	-	-	x	Brazilian	self	-	2	-	A	x
Dreamer Profile: A 40-year-old woman with three children.										
96. Frightened of waterfall.	D	-	-	-	-	-	1	P	-	
97. Husband leaves to have sex with another woman.	-	-	-	-	-	-	1	-	P	x
98. Watched baby agouti nursing.	-	-	-	-	-	-	-	-	P	-
Dreamer Profile: A 65-year-old woman.										
99. Singing ritual on plaza.	-	-	-	-	-	-	-	-	A	-
100. While collecting pequi, man attempts to force her to have sexual relations.	-	-	-	man	self	-	1	-	P	x

(continues)

Table 7.2 *(continued)*

	Characters			*Aggression*		*Anxiety*				
Dream Summary	*Son/Daughter*	*Mother/Father*	*Brazilians*	*Aggressor*	*Victim*	*Level*	*Castration*	*Passive/Active*	*Transformation*	*Sexual/Scatalogical*
Dreamer Profile: A girl of 13 in seclusion.										
101. Bitten and chased by monkey-spirit.	-	-	-	monkey-spirit	self	-	3	x	P	-
102. Found younger brother broken in pieces.	-	-	-	-	-	-	2	-	P	-
103. Told short suitor she wanted a tall lover.	-	-	-	-	-	-	-	-	A	-
104. Saw a villager's dirty rectum.*	-	-	-	-	-	-	1	-	P	x
Dreamer Profile: A girl, age 12.										
105. Saw mother, whom she missed, in Sao Paulo.	-	-	-	-	-	-	-	-	A	-
Dreamer Profile: A 45-year-old woman.										
106. Stung by wasp.	-	-	-	wasp	self	-	1	x	P	-
107. Saw frightening witch-spirit.	-	-	-	witch-spirit	self	-	1	-	P	-
Dreamer Profile: A 15-year-old girl.										
108. Cradled and nurtured bird.	-	-	-	-	-	-	-	-	A	-
Dreamer Profile: A 40-year-old woman with five children.										
109. Husband clubbed turtle.	-	-	-	husband	turtle	-	1	-	P	-

The Dreamer as Aggressor

Noteworthy in table 7.6 is the frequency that children are the victims of men's dreamed aggression. In daily life, children are seldom physically punished even though they are often the source of frustrating experiences for their parents. (See Gregor 1977: 274–275.) The dreamed stabbing of a child (table 7.2, dream 176) and the sexual assault on a little girl (table 7.2, dream 215) are admittedly unusual, but suggest the intensity of the emotions that children may arouse.

The predominance of animals as victims of aggression is understandable, given that the Mehinaku are fishermen and hunters of birds and monkey. It should also be mentioned, however, that animals are often killed for very casual motives, such as getting a closer look at them or making them the butt of children's semisadistic games. It is quite likely, therefore, that within the psychic economy of Mehinaku dreams, the killing of animals is properly understood as "aggression" rather than simply "subsistence."

There is no table corresponding to table 7.6 for women, since the very few women's dreams of aggression (N = 4) do not justify tabular presentation.

Causes of Dream Anxiety

Fifty-five percent of men's dreams and 42 percent of women's dreams reveal at least one level of anxiety. Men's anxiety dreams are not only more frequent but are more fearful than the women's, having an average anxiety level of 1.66 against the women's average of 1.47.

The single major source of anxiety dreams for both Mehinaku men and women is animal dreams, accounting for 30 percent of all anxiety dreams. In the case of women, animal dreams have an anxiety level of 1.78, which makes them among the most distressing of women's dreams. For men, on the other hand, anxiety-charged dream encounters with animals are frequent but less disturbing (anxiety level 1.32). On the face of it, this contrast is unexpected, since men are far more likely to experience encounters with dangerous animals than women. Unlike the women, who do not carry weapons, however, the men can protect themselves against such large fauna as wild pigs, jaguars, and dogs. These animals are especially frightening to the women and are the principal aggressors in 69 percent of their animal anxiety dreams but appear in only 42 percent of the men's. The men are more fearful of insects, snakes, fish, and other fauna against which strength and weapons are a poor defense. I am therefore inclined to attribute the relative intensity of the women's anxiety to their relative helplessness in dealing with dangerous animals, as contrasted with the greater mastery of the men.

Castration Anxiety

As shown in table 7.7, Mehinaku men's dreams reveal 75 percent more castration anxiety than is characteristic of Hall and Van de Castle's American subjects. (See also Winget, Kramer, and Whitman 1972 for additional comparable data.) The significance of this contrast depends on whether this dimension of content analysis actually measures a fear whose root meaning is sexual or is merely an index of concern about assault and injury. Several lines of evidence suggest that the more Freudian, sexual interpretation is correct. There is ample cultural data suggesting castration anxiety in

Table 7.3 Dreams of Aggression

	Mehinaku	*Americans*
Men	45 (N = 25)	24*
Women	34 (N = 37)	15*

Source: American data are derived from Hall and Van de Castle (1966: 168–170), subclasses 5–8 only.
Note: Figures are percentage of all dreams in sample with physically aggressive encounters.

Table 7.4 The Role of the Dreamer as Aggressor, Victim, or Observer in Dreams of Violent Encounters

Sex and Culture of Dreamer	*Dreamer as Aggressor*	*Dreamer as Victim*	*Dreamer as Observer*
Mehinaku men	28	62	10
American men*	23	52	25
Mehinaku women	11	78	11
American women*	11	47	29

Source: *Data are from Hall and Van de Castle (1966: 171), table 14-9, categories 5–8, "reciprocal aggression" being counted as "dreamer as victim." The 4 "mutual" and "self-aggression" categories are not counted for the comparisons in table 7.4.
Note: Figures are percentage of all dreams of aggression.

Table 7.5 The Dreamer as the Victim of Aggression

	Identity of the Aggressor within the Dream			
Sex and Culture of Dreamer	*Men*	*Women*	*Animals*	*Spirits, Monsters, and Others*
Mehinaku men	31	17	42	10
American men*	54	3	14	29
Mehinaku women	41	7	45	7
American women*	53	8	15	24

Source: *Data on American subjects are from Hall and Van de Castle (1966: 74) and represent percentages of aggressive episodes within dreams.
Note: Figures are percentage of all dreams of aggression against the dreamer. N = 78 Mechinaku men's dreams, N = 29 Mehinaku women's dreams.

the areas of mythology, theories of disease, and sexual practices. Sexual relations are said to stunt growth, weaken wrestlers, and cause illness. Myths are redolent with sexual themes, including the vagina *dentata* motif and overt stories of castration. We have already alluded to this pattern in dream symbolism, where a dream of female genitalia portends an ax wound.

The content of men's victim dreams (table 7.5) also suggests that castration anxiety is a psychological reality for the Mehinaku. In dreams of assault, we find that the women are regularly the perpetrators of violence (17 percent of all men's victim dreams) despite the fact that women almost never injure men in daily life. By contrast, in Hall and Van de Castle's sample, women initiated aggression in only 3 percent of

Table 7.6 The Dreamer as Aggressor

	Target of Dreamed Aggression					
Identity of Dreamer	*Child*	*Man*	*Woman*	*Animal*	*Spirit*	*Other*
Mehinaku	15	20	12	50	3	0
American men*	0	58	8	28	0	6

Source: *Data are from Hall and Van de Castle (1966: 74) and represent percentages of aggressive episodes within dreams.
Note: Figures are percentage of aggressor dreams, Mehinaku N = 34.

Table 7.7 Castration Anxiety

Sex and Society of the Dreamer	
Mehinaku men	36
American men*	20
Mehinaku women	12
American women*	9

Source: *American data are derived from Hall and Van de Castle (1966: 94).
Note: Figures are percentage of all dreams in the sample [Men N = 276, Women N = 09] that were scored for castration anxiety.

men's victim dreams. The threatening characterization of women in Mehinaku men's dreams is in accord with a generalized concern about sexual matters and a relatively high level of castration anxiety.

Passive and Active Orientation

61 percent of men's dreams were scored as active and 39 percent as passive. In contrast, only 42 percent of women's dreams were active in character. The substantial differences between men's and women's dreams must be tempered by the fact that long dream narratives are somewhat more likely to be scored as "active" and short ones as "passive." Women, on the average, provided shorter dream narratives than men. Nonetheless, even men's short dreams were more active in orientation than the women's. The relative passivity of women's dreams corresponds to women's position in daily life. Mehinaku society, like many of the small tribal groups of the South American lowlands, is decidedly patriarchal in nature. Men make the political decisions and dominate the religious and public aspects of village life. Even within the domestic arena, the men clearly dominate. Few women buck the system, but those who do seek to control their husbands do so through other men, such as their fathers, rather than by way of their own authority.

Transformation

This relatively rare dream theme appears in only 2 of the 109 women's dreams, and in 9 of the 276 men's dreams. In most of these dreams (table 7.1, dreams 6, 12, 29, 129, 255, 273), the transformation distances the dreamer from a potentially painful aggressive wish.

Thus the dreamer often kills dangerous animals that subsequently turn out to be humans. The heavier use of this mechanism among the men as a way of handling violent encounters may suggest greater male conflict concerning aggression.

Sexual-Scatological Dreams

This dimension of analysis codes dreams with overt sexual and scatological interactions, activities and desires. Among the men's dreams, 35, or 13 percent, were overtly sexual. This figure is virtually identical to Hall and Van de Castle's study of sexual interactions in which 12 percent of the dreams were of this type (1966: 181).

Men's sexual dreams showed great variation from informant to informant in their content and affective tone. One individual's sexual dreams are highly charged with anxiety, having an average level of 2.6 per dream. For others, however, sexual dreams are devoid of anxiety or have a very low anxiety level. Thus the anxiety level of sexual dreams for all the men but two was only 0.74.

Women's sexual dreams occurred with nearly the same frequency (12%) as the men's but with a somewhat higher level of anxiety. The women's dreams often reflected a fear of rape and other violent encounters with sexually aggressive men (table 7.2, dreams 5, 16, 66, 92, 100). In contrast, the men's anxiety-charged sexual dreams show a fear of assault by jealous husbands and paramours. This comparison is understandable in the light of everyday Mehinaku life, since gang rape is institutionalized as a punishment for seeing the men's sacred flutes. (See Gregor 1979: 254.)

An additional interesting characteristic of men's sexual dreams is that they subsume most of the dream plots that can be considered highly bizarre by our own standards, such as dreams 43, 120, 134,and 249 in table 7.1. Among the total sample of 385 dreams we find only 5 scatological dreams, all of which are narrated by women.

Conclusion

Each night Mehinaku men and women enter different dream worlds. The sources and intensity of their anxieties, and their roles as aggressors or the targets of hostility, show substantial variation. For the most part, we were able to point out Mehinaku institutions that reflect and explain the differences in men's and women's dreams. To a large extent, waking life and dream experiences run in tandem.

The special value of dream research, however, is that it takes us beyond the impact of waking experiences on personality to reach conclusions we could only guess at from a knowledge of everyday life. The social anthropologist, for example, would have little basis for predicting the aggressive role played by Brazilians in the villagers' anxious dreams of assault and sexual exploitation. To be sure, the Mehinaku express concerns about the Brazilians and their intentions, but for the most part their history of contact with outsiders has been peaceful. Even today, the villagers' lands are intact and their traditional autonomy is respected by reservation authorities. The impact of the outsider on the Mehinaku is therefore easy to underestimate without the advantage of psychological data.

In a similar way, the prevalence of animals in anxiety dreams leads us to redirect our attention to the villagers' relationship to the natural world. And without the direct evidence of the villagers' dreams, the psychological meaning of the castration themes found in myths and theories of disease would be merely conjectural. Attention to dreams thereby systematically enriches the account of Mehinaku culture provided by descriptive social anthropology.

Beyond the ethnographic value of dream collection, the villagers' manifest dreams provide tantalizing hints of differences in men's and women's dreams that go well beyond the frontiers of Mehinaku culture. The similar percentage of sexual dreams for Mehinaku and American men is especially compelling in this respect. Some of the tables (notably tables 7.4 and 7.5) also display suggestive parallels between the manifest content of American and Mehinaku dreams. With additional cross-cultural data, it may be possible to show that the dream experience is less variant than other aspects of culture. This suggestion is not a new one, for the literature already includes cross-cultural parallels, such as those established by Griffith, Miyagi, and Tago (1958), Hall (1962), and Leman (1966), among such diverse cultures as American, Japanese, Mexican, Yir Yoront, and Hopi. It is my hope that the present study will usefully extend the range of cross-cultural research, so that ultimately it will be possible to make accurate and systematic generalizations about human dream life.

Notes

The field research on which this chapter is based was made possible by grants from the Small Grant Program of the Public Health Service and the Vanderbilt University Research Council. I also gratefully acknowledge the valuable criticism and suggestions offered by Waud H. Kracke, who read a draft of the chapter.

Notes to Table 7.1 [Numbers refer to table items.]

3. A belt and certain other garments are closely associated with the dreamer (see Gregor 1977: 154, 156) and therefore their loss is coded as an example of castration anxiety.
10. All dreams of pets are believed to refer to the dreamer's children, hence the notation under characters of "S" for son.

    Dry bread and other brittle objects are equated with the dreamer's bones. The informant remarked that he feared he would break a bone in the dream.
37. All Brazilian-made objects are symbols of disease, since the Brazilian is said to be responsible for introducing epidemic illnesses to the region.
52. Most small animals are symbolically equated with children.
73. A jaguar is equated with a village witch who intends to assault the dreamer.
101. Women who see the sacred flutes are gang-raped.
108. A frustrated desire or rejected request can lead to illness or injury.
163. Symbolic of death of a kinsman.
219. A *pequi* silo is a symbol of a corpse, hence the indicated level of anxiety.

Notes to Table 7.2 [Numbers refer to table items.]

30. At the time this dream was narrated, the villagers were preparing the role-reversal ritual of Yamurikuma in which the women actually wrestle visiting women from other communities.
68. Within the dream, the narrator regards the pet as a symbol of her children.
104. Informant in recounting the dream interprets the rectum as a symbol of burned manioc, and concludes that she is therefore likely to burn manioc bread later in the day.

References

Breger, L. Hunter, and R. W. Lane. 1971. "The Effect of Stress on Dreams." *Psychological Issues Monographs* 27. New York: International Universities Press.

Gray, A. and D. Kalsched. 1971. "Oedipus East and West, and Exploration of Manifest Dream Content." *Journal of Cross-Cultural Psychology* 2: 337–352.

Gregor, Thomas A. 1977. *Mehinaku: The Drama of Everyday Life in A Brazilian Indian Community.* Chicago: University of Chicago Press.

———. 1979. "Secrets, Exclusion, and the Dramatization of Men's Roles," in *Brazil Anthropological Perspectives,* ed. M. L. Margolies and W. E. Carter (New York: Columbia University Press), pp. 250–269.

———. 1981. "'Far, Far Away My Shadow Wandered . . . ': The Dream Theories of the Mehinaku Indians of Brazil." *American Ethnologist* 8(4): 709–720.

Griffith, R. M., O. Miyagi, and A. Tago. 1958. "The Universality of Typical Dreams Japanese vs. Americans." *American Anthropologist* 60:1173–1179.

Hall, Calvin S. 1951. "What People Dream About." *Scientific American* 184: 60–63.

———. 1962. "Ethnic Similarities in the Manifest Dream Content A Modest Confirmation of the Theory of Universal Man." Unpublished. Santa Cruz: University of California.

Hall, Calvin S. and Robert L. Van de Castle. 1965. "An Empirical Investigation of the Castration Complex in Dreams." *Journal of Personality* 33: 20–29.

———. 1966. *The Content Analysis of Dreams.* New York: Appleton-Century-Crofts.

Kracke, Waud H. 1978. *Force and Persuasion Leadership in an Amazonian Society.* Chicago: University of Chicago Press.

———. 1979. "Dreaming in Kagwahiv Dream Beliefs and Their Psychic Uses in an Amazonian Indian Culture." *Psychoanalytic Study of Society* 8:119–171. New Haven: Yale University Press.

Leman, J. E., Jr. 1966. "Aggression in Mexican-American and Anglo-American Delinquent and Non-Delinquent Males as Revealed in Dreams and Thematic Apperception Test Responses." Ph.D. diss., University of Arizona. Dissertation Abstracts, 1967: 3675–3676.

Levine, Robert A. 1966. *Dreams and Deeds.* Chicago: University of Chicago Press.

Schneider, David, and Lauriston Sharp. 1969. *The Dream Life of a Primitive People.* Ann Arbor: University Microfilms.

Winget, Carolyn, M. Kramer, and R. Whitman. 1972. "Dreams and Demography." *Journal of the Canadian Psychiatric Association* 17: 203–208.

8

Making Dreams into Music

Contemporary Songwriters Carry On an Age-Old Dreaming Tradition

Nancy Grace

If I'm ever asked if I'm religious, I always reply, "Yes, I'm a devout musician." Music puts me in touch with something beyond intellect, something otherworldly, something sacred.

—Sting, Commencement Address at Berklee College of Music, 1994

I was driving home one night several years ago, flipping through radio stations, when I landed on a station just in time to hear a voice say "I think any artist who ignores their dreams is ignoring half of their creative potential." I listened eagerly to hear who was speaking. It turned out to be the tremendously successful pop musician Sting, talking about the creative process.

It was a wonderful stroke of synchronicity—as well as a surprise—to happen upon this admission of the importance of dreams to the creative life of such a mainstream, commercially successful pop icon as Sting. Yet some months prior to this, while listening to Billy Joel speak at Berklee College of Music in Boston, I'd heard something equally striking: Responding to a question about where he gets his ideas for songs, Joel replied that all his songs come from dreams.[1]

Many years earlier, Paul McCartney also was wise to pay attention to his dreams, when he woke one morning with the melody to what became the song "Yesterday." McCartney says, "I liked the melody a lot but because I'd dreamed it I couldn't believe I'd written it. I thought, 'No, I've never written like this before.' But I had the tune, which was the most magic thing. And you have to ask yourself, where did it come from? But you don't ask yourself too much or it might go away."[2] So certain was he that he couldn't possibly have dreamed up a melody so perfect and lovely, he had to play it for many people before he was convinced that it was really his, and not a song of someone else's he had heard but forgotten. When he finally recorded it with the Beatles, it went on to become not only the most successful of all the Beatles' songs but also the most often played song of all time.[3]

Given that the society we live in does not regard dreams as having much value, if any at all, it is surprising that three such well-known stars have dreams to thank for their inspiration.[4] Yet down through history, the importance of dreams to the creative life of a large number of cultures has been well documented.[5] With regard specifically to musical creativity, there exist numerous age-old traditions of seeking spirit songs in dreams and of bringing back sacred melodies and lyrics from the dream world to waking life—for power, for healing, for use in ritual, for community guidance, or for confirmation of a person's calling as shaman, priest, or teacher. Among the many treasures that have been found in the land of dreaming, music most certainly is one of them.

We would likely all agree that modern Western social and religious structures bear little resemblance to the traditional, indigenous, and shamanic cultures that down through time have looked to dreams to bring forth creations of artistic, musical, and spiritual value. Yet despite the radical differences in cultural context, I am suggesting that contemporary musicians who find inspiration in their dreams are the modern-day spiritual descendants of these traditional, indigenous peoples and that it is completely appropriate to place them within the context of this spiritual lineage. In fact, more than appropriate, it is important to do so, in order to properly understand and value the psychological, spiritual, and social dimensions of meaning that are created when dreams are made into songs.

The argument can be made, of course, that not all creating of songs from dreams is equal, and that, despite similarities in result, the differences in cultural context between contemporary songwriters and their traditional counterparts are so substantial as to render the similarities superficial and ultimately meaningless. But my hope is that the examples I share below will demonstrate that this is not the case and will illustrate the enduring potential of dreams to inspire musical creativity that has meaning both for the songwriters themselves and for the community in which these dream-songs are heard.

The words of Sting that open this chapter make a strong argument for the abiding presence of the spiritual dimension of musical experience. In most traditional cultures, this would not be in question, but in the secular and material world of extremely rich and famous pop stars, Sting's words stand out as an unexpected surprise. Given this spiritual orientation to music, it is perhaps not so surprising that Sting finds in his dream life rich inspiration for songwriting.

One very compelling song that came directly from a dream is "The Lazarus Heart," from the 1987 album *Nothing Like the Sun*. In the liner notes to the album, Sting writes, "*Lazarus Heart* was a vivid nightmare that I wrote down and then fashioned into a song. A learned friend of mine informs me that it is the archetypical dream of the fisher king."[6] The song tells the story of a son who finds a sword wound in his chest, which turns out to have been inflicted by his mother. His mother then tells him that the wound will give him pain, but also courage, and that from the pain would come the power to create his life anew. In beautiful metaphors, the song tells a story of transformation, of turning pain into strength and beauty. That the album itself is dedicated to the memory of Sting's mother, who had recently passed away, gives the song special poignancy.

In addition to the psychological and spiritual dimensions of meaning in this song, there is a social dimension of importance, too. *Nothing Like the Sun* sold over 2 million copies, which means that at least that many people have heard "The Lazarus Heart" and likely also read the lyrics, as well as Sting's recounting of how the song was written from a dream. Even if only a modest percentage of people who listen to this song hear its message—that pain can be transformed into strength and beauty—a teaching of both psychological and spiritual value will have been carried, from a dream and through a song, into the culture.

Columbia recording artist Shawn Colvin is another contemporary songwriter who speaks about the inspiration she finds in dreams. On her first major-label album, *Steady On* (1989), there is a song called "The Story," which Colvin says got started in a dream. "I actually dreamed part of the song," she says, "which is something that I've done before. In other words, there have been songs in dreams that I have wanted to remember when I've woken up, but haven't. It's kind of hard to do. And I've tried, I've tried at times, but it hasn't worked out."[7] But this time it did, and the song which resulted from the dream is one of Colvin's most personal and powerful songs. Told in poetry and metaphor, it is the story of her childhood and of the difficult family dynamics that continue to impact her as an adult. In addition to the obvious personal significance of "The Story," Colvin explains that this song has also proven meaningful to many women who have heard it, giving them insight into their own experiences as women living with limited options in the conservative social climate of the 1950s.[8] Here again, a message of value has come from a dream, through a song, into the culture.

Another example of dream-inspired songwriting can be found in the song "Polaroids," from Colvin's 1992 album *Fat City*. In "Polaroids," Colvin writes about the ending of a romantic relationship, of broken promises, and of the desperation that comes from losing love. In this case, most of the song had been written, but Colvin was having trouble finishing it. Then she had a dream, and she knew it was the perfect ending for the song. She explains:

> I had this dream where this couple wasn't walking a plank off of a ship, but they were walking a plank over a huge excavated hole in the ground. And they were totally in love, it was the sweetest damn feeling, you know. And he walked out first and she took a Polaroid, then she walked out and he took a Polaroid as she held up this flash card type of thing that said "Valentine." The good will between these people must have been something that I was striving for because I had had relationships with a lot of ill-will [laughs] which just seems so wrong, but it was in my life.[9]

Set against the emotional upheaval of the previous verses in the song, the final verse that relates this dream scene changes the story from one of disillusionment to one of hope. Obviously, this dream was personally important for Colvin, giving her an experience of the possibility of a more warm and loving relationship than many she had known. But when the dream gets put into a song—a work of art with a life of its own out in the world—it becomes more than one person's particular story. It becomes a statement of possibility with a capital "P," saying to anyone hearing it "this possibility for transformation exists, it can happen to you." From a dream, into a song, a message of hope goes out into the world.

Rory Block is a traditional acoustic blues guitar player who, according to The Blues Foundation, is "widely regarded as the top female interpreter and authority on traditional country blues worldwide."[10] *The New York Times* has said that "her playing is perfect, her singing otherworldly as she wrestles with ghosts, shadows and legends."[11] In addition to interpreting traditional blues, she also writes her own songs. Early in her career, by her own description her songwriting style was somewhat formulaic, relying on catchy lines and clichés. But this was not satisfying, and as she searched for a more personal style of songwriting, using dreams turned out to be one of the keys. Block says that "it was at this point that I really found my voice as a songwriter and began writing songs that had deeper meaning to me and almost without fail, deeper meaning to other people as well."[12]

The song "Silver Wings," from the 1992 album, *Ain't I a Woman,* combines images and stories from four different recurring dreams into a powerful song celebrating the life of a friend who died from cancer, and acknowledging the abiding power of faith to lift us up from despair. In the liner notes to the album, Block tells the story of writing the song and of the dreams that inspired it.[13] The first recurring dream is of flying, a dream Block says she has almost every night. The second is of having a new baby; the third, a recurring dream of the friend who died, whom Block describes as "an endless source of wisdom"; and the fourth, a dream of visiting a cherished house from her past, a dream that gives her great comfort. All four of these dreams contain strong positive images—of new life, of liberation, of wisdom, and of stability—and Block has combined them into a song full of energy and hope, the kind of song that makes you feel good just listening to it, with an infectious refrain that declares in a strong voice, "my faith can pull me up on silver wings." Similar to the previous examples, this song, too, takes inspiration from dreams to create a narrative that is rich in personal meaning for its creator and also brings a message of hope and healing into the community.

In addition to providing inspiration for individual songs, dreams can provide a broader sense of inspiration and focus to a musician's work. Rory Block tells the following story about the making of her 1998 album, *Confessions of a Blues Singer:*

> One night I had a dream and woke with the slide riff from Charley Patton's *Bo Weavil Blues* soaring through my brain with great clarity and volume. This was extremely odd as I had never focused on that particular song nor had I heard it for 30 years. I couldn't even remember the title and had to listen to the entire CD collection to find it. I realized I was meant to record it, and that focused this album. I decided I was going to go for "feel" over "perfection." I wanted to move in the spirit of the early recordings where spontaneity and musical freedom were at the core of everything, all soul and raw power and no technological advantages save the on/off button on the tape recorder. I suddenly felt free to leave the buzzing notes, the imperfect intonation, the unfinished endings, because it's not about a cleanly edited crisp song, it's about joy and dedication to the beauty of music that was the original basis for everything. I asked the engineer to record the vocals a little bit harder and thinner than today's audiophiles would perhaps appreciate, but I wanted to be closer to the old sound. I wanted it to be just a little bit disturbing.[14]

Confessions of a Blues Singer went on to win the WC Handy award for Acoustic Blues Album of the Year in 1999. Clearly, the spontaneous, free, and soulful approach that the dream brought Block was quite effective!

Sting tells a similar story about the making of *The Dream of the Blue Turtles,* his first solo album after a long and successful career with the band The Police. It turns out he really *did* dream of blue turtles, as he explains to Timothy White in the book *Rock Lives:*

> I had a dream that I was back home in Hampshire, looking out the window into this big walled-in garden I have out back with its very neat flowerbed and foliage. Suddenly, out of a hole in the wall came these large, macho, aggressive, and quite drunk blue turtles. They started doing backflips and other acrobatics, in the process utterly destroying my garden. . . . I'm enjoying this curious spectacle, and the dream is so strong I remembered it perfectly when I woke up, to the point where it became part of my juggernaut to complete this record. . . . For me, the turtles are symbols of the subconscious, living under the sea, full of unrealized potential, very Jungian in their meaning. . . . So with the album I wanted to destroy a lot of preconceptions and expectations, and do something unsettlingly different. These blue turtles, these musicians, were gonna help me. And they did.[15]

Similar to the album that resulted from Rory Block's dream, *The Dream of the Blue Turtles* represented a striking departure from the style of music Sting's fans were used to hearing from his days with the Police. It is often challenging for an established musician to go in a new musical direction, given the expectations of fans and record labels, but this album was very successful, selling over 3 million copies and containing several hit singles.

That the dreams of both Sting and Rory Block brought innovative energies to their creative work is a testament to what Jeremy Taylor calls "the archetypal creative impulse woven into the fabric of every dream."[16] Taylor says that dreams always break new ground, and this is certainly the case here (even literally, since the turtles in Sting's dream were destroying his garden!). In light of the dream of the blue turtles, the dream of the "bo weavil blues," and so many other dreams that have led to artistic creations, scientific inventions and discoveries, there is likely something in the very nature of dreaming which inspires this kind of creative upheaval and innovation.

It is worth noting that in addition to recording albums, Sting, Shawn Colvin, and Rory Block all spend plenty of time playing their songs to live audiences, where the power that lies within the music is most accessible to the listener. I believe that live performances play a key role in this process of enabling the energies in dreams to travel through songs and into the community at large.

A more specific reason that live performances bring the energy of dreams into the community is that during many live musical performances, dreams are being told. Given that the oral tradition of community dream-sharing, so common in many traditional cultures, is virtually nonexistent in the modern Western world, the concert hall may be one of the few established social venues where dreams are still spoken about freely, regularly, and with enthusiasm. Because songwriters often find inspiration in their dreams, because songwriters in concert like to talk to the audience, and probably because dreams make for a good story, musicians are often heard introducing songs with a declaration that the entire song, or maybe just a verse or the general inspiration for the song, came from a dream. There seems to be something mysterious, powerful, authoritative, and even romantic about making such a declaration—and sometimes, even something humorous. I heard acoustic guitarist Billy McLaughlin in concert a few years ago, and he introduced a song by saying that he awoke from a dream in the middle of the night with a tune in his head, and he knew he had to capture it right away, before it faded away. Despite concerns that his guitar playing would awaken his wife, he played the tune until he had learned it, and when done, he gave it the title "While She Sleeps."[17]

As I wrote in the beginning of this chapter, many indigenous cultures have traditions of looking to dreams for special songs to bestow power, for healing, for use in ritual, for community guidance, or for confirmation of a person's calling within the community. Although these concepts may be defined differently in modern culture, I believe the examples I have provided of contemporary songwriters' dream songs demonstrate that these traditions are being carried on today. Dreams continue to speak to the creative imaginations and spiritual concerns of present-day songwriters, as they heed the age-old call to bring back from the realm of dreams something of value for themselves and for the world.

In the introduction to this book, Kelly Bulkeley points out that "dreams offer a unique insight into the creative imaginal space where religion, culture, and psyche join together in dynamic interplay." Certainly, the dream-inspired songs of contemporary musicians are one of the most fruitful places to investigate this dynamic interplay. In this barely-researched area, it is impossible to know the full extent to which contemporary songwriters and musicians have been mining the fields of their dreams for music, lyrics, and thematic ideas. But if the truth were known, we would probably be surprised at how many tunes that we've been humming for years have their origins in the fertile land of dreams.

Notes

1. Master Class with Billy Joel, Berklee College of Music (Boston, MA, fall 1992). Also mentioned in Deirdre Barrett, *The Committee of Sleep: How Artists, Scientists, and Athletes Use Their Dreams for Creative Problem Solving—and How You Can Too* (New York: Crown Publishers, 2001).
2. In Barry Miles, *Paul McCartney: Many Years From Now* (New York: Henry Holt, 1997), p. 202.
3. Ibid.
4. For more examples of musicians writing from dreams, see Barrett, *The Committee of Sleep.*
5. Two excellent sources are Kelly Bulkeley, *Spiritual Dreaming* (Mahwah, NJ: Paulist Press, 1995), and Barbara Tedlock (ed.), *Dreaming: Anthropological and Psychological Interpretations* (Santa Fe, NM: School of American Research Press, 1992).
6. From the liner notes to *Nothing Like the Sun,* 1987, A&M Records.
7. Shawn Colvin, from the WUMB Members Concert (October 2, 1989) in Boston, Massachusetts.
8. Shawn Colvin, in an interview in *The Performing Songwriter* (October 1993), reprinted at www.shawncolvin.com.
9. Ibid.
10. Found at www.roryblock.com/reviews.htm.
11. Ibid.
12. Found at www.roryblock.com/interview.htm.
13. Liner notes to *Ain't I a Woman* by Rory Block, 1992, Rounder Records.
14. From the liner notes to *Confessions of a Blues Singer,* 1998, Rounder Records.
15. From Timothy White, *Rock Lives: Profiles and Interviews* (New York: Henry Holt, 1990, pp. 692–709), cited at http://users.sisna.com/clio95/blueturtles.html—"Sting 101."
16. From Jeremy Taylor, *Where People Fly and Water Runs Uphill: Using Dreams to Tap the Wisdom of the Unconscious* (New York: Warner Books, 1992).
17. This song can be found on Billy McLaughlin's 1996 Proton Discs album *Fingerdance.*

Section II

Individuals

9

Kagwahiv Mourning
Dreams of a Bereaved Father

Waud H. Kracke

It is sometimes averred that empathic understanding cannot be gained of the inner experience of a person of a culture very different from one's own, at least not deep enough to make possible depth-interviewing of a psychoanalytic sort, either because the terms in which people in some other cultures conceive and talk about their inner life are so different from ours or because empathy and mutual understanding are too difficult across the barrier of radical cultural difference. Rodney Needham, in one recent phase of his thought, has perhaps espoused this point of view most strongly of recent anthropological writers, arguing that "If individual ideation is in part contingent on changeable cultural convention—there can be no prior guarantees that it will be comprehensible to men whose representations are framed by other cultural traditions" (1972:158).

But the question is at least implicit in many discussions of mental life in non-Western cultures (e.g., Geertz 10973:398–404; Rosaldo [1980]), and positions not too different from Needham's seem implied at times in discussions of human nature with a relativistic emphasis (Geertz 1965)[1].

Such questions, as Needham points out, raise fundamental issues for anthropological investigation (cf. Hanson 1975, chap. 3); but they go especially to the heart of the enterprise of cross-cultural psychoanalytic investigation, which depends sensitively on empathic understanding. Robert LeVine has gone so far as to suggest (1973: 220–224) that, to bridge the gap in understanding, every cross-cultural psychoanalytic investigation might best be carried out in collaboration with a psychoanalytically trained interviewer from the culture in question; but this in part merely shifts the locus of the problem, for the psychoanalytic training of the indigenous interviewer would itself require a cross-cultural psychoanalysis.

When this issue has been raised, it has generally been discussed primarily in abstract, philosophical terms[2] (although the anthropologists who discuss it, of course, draw on their own intercultural experiences) or in terms of methodological prescriptions for evading the barriers perceived. Yet as Needham (1972: 58) justly observed, the question "falls within the scope of empirical determination," and it may be useful to present here the results of an attempt at achieving empathic understanding in an intercultural situation in interviews that I carried out with Kagwahiv Indians in Brazil. I found no such difficulty in establishing empathic rapport with at least some of my Kagwahiv informants. By establishing an atmosphere of relaxed, intimate communication in an interview situation predominantly *a deux,* it was possible to gain many glimpses of the inner life and experience of several Kagwahiv and, to varying degrees, to understand their psychological processes. The main obstacle I had to overcome in order to begin these interviews, I found, was my own reluctance to abandon the relatively protected, semidetached role of anthropologist and to enter the deeper emotional involvement entailed in depth interviewing.

The depth interviews I conducted often tended to focus around dreams, for I found that asking people about their dreams and childhood memories was a way to communicate an interest in their own personal experience (as opposed to the ethnographer's interest in more "official" beliefs of their culture), and led people, in association with their dreams, to open up fantasies and memories of a sensitive kind that were especially helpful in understanding how they felt about themselves and their current lives. I will select one informant with whom I developed a particularly successful working relationship of this kind to show the kind of mutual understanding that is possible.[3] The aspect of this man's psychic processes that was a central focus of my interviews with him was mourning.

The interviews I will describe were carried out from July through September 1968. I did not begin such interviews at the beginning of my fieldwork, but delayed until I had accumulated some six months of contact with Kagwahiv, much of the time spent in the settlement where the interviews described here were conducted (cf. Langness 1965: 35). I was able in that time to acquire some familiarity with Kagwahiv patterns of emotional expression, and a rudimentary knowledge of the Kagwahiv language (although I had to begin the interviews largely in Portuguese, shifting increasingly into Kagwahiv as I mastered it). When I altered my role from that of ethnographic investigator interested in "Kagwahiv life and customs" to the psychological interviewer expressing an interest in individuals and their dreams and fantasies I experienced a dramatic shift in the aspects of themselves that my informants presented to me, opening up a range of personal fantasies of which I had not previously been aware.

It may be that my interviewing was facilitated by some aspects of the culture I was working in—the Kagwahiv Indians, who live on the east bank of the Madeira River, a southern tributary of the Amazon. The fact that dreams are a focus of Kagwahiv cultural interest certainly helped to make it seem less strange to informants to be asked to relate them and discuss them, and the traditional interest of their shamanic curers (*ipaji*) in dreams makes the telling of dreams potentially part of a succorant relationship, although I have no indication that they were used by the *ipaji* of the past (none of whom survive) in anything like the way they are used in our therapy. The Kagwahiv are accustomed to tell their dreams to one another, individually or to the settlement in general, generally first thing in the morning and to discuss their dreams' meanings. The dreams would be interpreted in terms of predictions about game or health, mediated by traditional dream symbols (to dream about a broken-down house means someone will die, for example, or a party means white-lipped peccary will be bagged in hunting), or in terms of other beliefs about dreams, which I have described more fully elsewhere (Kracke 1979). Dreams are in general thought to be a continuation in sleep of the train of thought one was following while falling asleep.

Another helpful factor was the nature of Kagwahiv living arrangements. In their small local groups, of no more than six members each, anthropologists are much more direct participants in the daily life of the people than in an African village, perhaps, where they may live in a separate compound. Under such close conditions, intimacy is much easier to achieve.

The cultural stress on dreams and the Kagwahiv settlement pattern facilitated my establishing such intimate interview relationships; but for informants to open their private thoughts and feelings to an anthropologist in depth-interviews, they must have both a motivation to do so and a basis for trusting in the anthropologist's personal concern. The nature of an informant's motive and basis for trust in the ethnographer will of course shape considerably the aspect of the self that will be revealed in the depth interviews. In this chapter I will examine one informant's motives—what emotional satisfaction or relief he sought from the interviews—and some of the situational factors that I think contributed to his feeling free to confide in me. Then I will consider some of the implications of these observations for anthropologist informant relationships in general. I will limit my discussion to one informant, a young headman whose interviews were perhaps the richest in the insights he gave into his emotional life—partly due to his own self-insight and natural psychological acumen and communicativeness, but partly also due to the strength of his motivation for talking about his feelings. Jovenil was a father who had lost two children three months before the interviews.

As background, I should say a bit about how Kagwahiv deal with death.[4] It is not usual to talk much about such a loss; the accepted thing is to avoid talking about it, because of the painful feelings it arouses. Crying is anathema, leaving one exposed to supernatural dangers. The way to deal with loss is to forget the deceased person as rapidly as possible: You give away all the person's belongings or any utensils the person has used that remind you of him or her. You dismantle the house you have lived in with the person and even move your house, or the whole settlement, to a new spot, in order not to be reminded. The rationale for this in Kagwahiv belief is that, since the person's ghost (*anang*) might return to familiar spots and seek familiar objects, then everything associated with the deceased person is *poky,* supernaturally dangerous. But informants also say, as if it were synonymous with this, "We move so as not to remember, because it makes us sad." New kin terms are used for deceased primary relatives: *ji rava,* "my father, " becomes *ji poria,* "my late father"; *hy,* "mother," becomes *ymbora;* and so on. Everything is done to push away the memory of the deceased and the immediacy of the death. Under these conditions, mourning is all the more a problematic period.

In retrospect, the illness of Jovenil's two children was an important transition point in my relationship with him and the others of his group. For a few weeks, my research activities practically came to a halt as I spent most of my time giving what rudimentary medical attention I was able to give to the two children and others in the settlement suffering from complications to a measles epidemic. Beforehand I was a stranger with a rather peculiar interest in Kagwahiv lifeways and a periodic source of relatively cheap trade goods. After the episode of illness I became more a part of the group, or at least someone who cared, who valued Kagwahiv lives and had shown I shared some of their concerns and feelings. I also took on a more medical kind of role in the group from then on I had been giving injections to one or two members of the group as part of a series of treatments for tuberculosis, but now this role became more a part of my identity in the group and of my contribution to it. This, I think, made possible the kind of interviewing I was to carry on in my last three months of fieldwork during that field trip.

The first time I arrived at Jovenil's settlement, I was welcomed quite hospitably as a visitor (in some contrast to a rather cooler reception on my initial contacts some months earlier with a neighboring group that a pair of missionaries had made their center of operations when "in the tribe"); but I was strictly (and somewhat ambivalently) regarded as a transient guest. In a conversation the second evening I was there, Jovenil compared me with other American visitors who had come and enlivened things, showing their generosity by distributing fish they caught, but passed on. He forecasted that, like them, I would get married and never come back.

This visit grew into a period of mutual testing. For a time, I became the visitor who overstayed his welcome, with the distribution of my last food supplies at a time of sparse hunting and fishing becoming a rather focal issue toward the end of this initial one-month visit. My return a few months later (albeit still unmarried) impressed Jovenil with my commitment, and at the beginning of this second, longer visit, Jovenil negotiated with me the construction of a house for me in the settlement. It was only later in this visit, however, that the episode of illness occurred that was to more substantially alter my relationship with Jovenil and his group.

Several of Jovenil's children were sick when I arrived in November 1967 for a three-month stretch of fieldwork, in the aftermath of a measles epidemic. But the climax came around Christmas when his one-year-old daughter became extremely ill. He was at first reluctant to have me give her injections, fearing that in her weak state the strong medicine would be too much for her. At one point she reached the unresponsive state the Kagwahiv call death, and her mother had started wailing. Antibiotics did pull her through that crisis, however, and with continued treatment she gradually improved. I also treated Jovenil's cherished five-year-old son, Alonzo, who had also gotten seriously ill, although not quite to the same extremity. Unfortunately, I had to leave to replenish my supplies at the end of February, before they had fully recovered; but both were definitely on the mend when I left, and seemed well on the way to recovery. A month or two later, however, both had relapses (or in their weakened state contracted new illnesses) and, one right after the other, they died.

It was in my next three-month stint of fieldwork, after a break of several months, that I began the intensive, psychologically oriented interviews. It was the last of four stints of fieldwork in 1967 to 1968, the first three of which were devoted to more general ethnography participant observation primarily in Jovenil's settlement and a neighboring one and shorter visits to several others. The psychological interviews were saved for the last one, when I had some feel for Kagwahiv culture and modes of emotional expression and a little grounding in their language.

I learned of the children's deaths as I was returning from the break in June 1968. I went in with some trepidation, with vivid images of what their reaction to the deaths might be. My worst fantasies were not realized. But on arriving, I realized later, I did commit something of a faux pas in asking Jovenil's wife, Aluza, about the deaths, expressing sympathy—thus reminding her of the painful event she was trying to forget.

Jovenil was the first informant with whom I began the intensive interviews when I got up to his settlement. I established a pattern of daily interviews with him, varying in length from under an hour to more than two—"fifty minutes" would of course have no significance whatever to a Kagwahiv—asking him to tell me whatever he felt like talking about, including dreams, childhood memories, or whatever thoughts he had. We sat either on a bench in the clearing in the middle of the settlement or on the open platform of the house in which I was staying—an uncompleted house without walls, affording much greater privacy than would any more secluded, walled spot at which the children would indubitably gather to listen.

Jovenil did not mention the deaths of his children for the first week and a half of the interviews, with the exception of one indirect allusion. This allusion arose in telling me for the first time, in his fourth interview, about an incestuous affair he had had in adolescence with a parallel cousin, a woman of his own (Kwandu) patrimoiety. He observed that the consequence of such behavior is that "your child dies, or else your father." Except for that, he made no explicit reference to it until the ninth interview.

In the latent content of his dream, however, allusions to his children's death begin to appear much earlier. In the sixth interview, Jovenil told me a dream that was rather startling in its frankness. At first sight, it seems to have little to do with his loss, but closer examination reveals strong allusions implicit in it.

> José Bahut [an older man, of the opposite moiety] was having intercourse with his wife [Camelia]. Everyone saw it. Suddenly his dick was very big. Patricio [Camelia's younger half-brother] grabbed his dick and pulled it, and it snapped. "Why did you break my dick?" "Because you were screwing my sister." Patricio was fixing José's dick with a vine thong, and it got real thin.—It's funny, my dream. Ai, they said, "Did your dick snap?" Ai, a lot of blood came out, his dick got rotten. Patricio fixed his dick, it got real thin. Homero [Patricio and Camelia's father] scolded Patricio, "Why did you snap his dick? He'll die." "No, he won't die," he said.

He followed the dream with a series of associations that underscored the danger to the dreamer of such a dream—"If you dream of a woman's genital, it's a wound you are going to get, you cut yourself"—suggesting that the wound represented in the dream may be his own.

I pointed out that this was the second time in two days he had mentioned to me a dream of José Bahut's big penis. In the previous interview, he had told me of a dream he had upriver that "José Bahut had a dick this long." Could it be, I asked him, that he had sometime seen a grown man's big penis when he was little? Yes, he replied, he had. At five years of age, he saw José Bahut's penis, when he went swimming in the river as José was there bathing. He had asked José how he got such a big penis, and José responded, "I make my wife a lot, that's why it gets so big." Excitedly, Jovenil ran back to report his observation and new knowledge to his mother, only to receive a severe scolding. "When you see someone else's dick like that," his mother told him, "when you get older, you will go blind." "She scolded with a stick, a belt," Jovenil recalled, "for me not to ask him any more."[5]

Further memories led him to recollections of a childhood phobia of pigs and cows. "It seemed as if they wanted to eat me." Sometimes he couldn't sleep at night for fear of ghosts, so he would go to sleep in his father's hammock.

All of this shows a remarkable access to memories of his own childhood phobias and conflicts; but so far we see little connection with his mourning of his children. A hint of some dream thoughts related to this mourning appears, however, when we note that the woman José Bahut was making love with in the dream—José's current young wife at the time of the dream, not his wife of the time of Jovenil's five year-old memory—was the very same parallel cousin of Jovenil's with whom Jovenil had had an incestuous affair in adolescence. In Kagwahiv terminology, she was his "sister." If we put Jovenil himself, the dreamer, in the place of José Bahut in his dream, then some of the comments in the dream take on new significance. "Because you were screwing my sister" may be an echo of Jovenil's own self-accusatory guilty conscience; and Homero's exclamation "Why did you do that? Now he'll die" may refer to the punishment for such incestuous activity, the death of a close relative—perhaps that of his child. The dream, then, is a self-accusation, saying that he himself was responsible for his five year-old son's death, represented in the dream as a castration. In the imagery of the dream, it was his own incestuous desires that brought about his "castration."

This guess is confirmed by the somewhat more open expression of the idea in a dream he reported in his interview the next day. Daniel Aguarajuv (a neighbor and close friend of Jovenil's) and his older Brazilian wife had a pet monkey that, since they were childless, was like a child to them. In the dream, Daniel went out hunting and shot what he thought was a wild monkey—but it turned out to be his own pet monkey, which had run away. Daniel's wife was furious when she found out and chased him out of the house. Jovenil, this dream seems vicariously to aver, had inadvertently killed his own child. Jovenil's associations, just to confirm this, went back to earlier losses and finally to that of his first child, who had many years earlier died young, with his wife almost dying at the same time; they then focused on the various prohibitions that surround the birth of a child: "When he is born, you don't go working . . . If you do, the child won't grow up—he'll die."

He listed the animals one should not hunt—including monkey—to avoid bringing harm to one's infant, and recalled how another of his children was seriously ill in infancy because he was negligent in observing the taboos. The mood of the interview was sad, and it was clear that his thoughts were returning to his lost children, with allusions to his own sense of responsibility for their death.

The next day, Jovenil elaborated much more on his teenage affair with Camelia, who was then single, vividly describing the incident that terminated his relationship with her. The dog barked as he and his companion snuck into her settlement, and they were almost caught. In that interview, he also described a recent fight in which José Bahut almost killed a man who had slept with his wife Camelia. And, toward the end of the interview, he commented on a dream he had reported in it:. "When you dream that your clothes are all torn, you dream your own death. You're afraid in the morning, because sometimes something can happen to you. Sometimes you can get sick. You get sad when you dream like that. If you dream of a house, it's a bad dream like that, a house full of holes, it's a child of yours that's going to die." (The literal prediction of this dream element, a falling-down house, is that a close relative will die.)

It was the following day, in his ninth interview, that Jovenil finally brought up his son's death explicitly—through a dream. "I had a dream," he said right off. "A bad dream . . . My son died. Alonzo. They drowned him in the deep—in the water. 'Why did you guys kill my son?' 'No, he died.' 'Where did you bury him?' 'In the bank.' They buried him in the bank."

Jovenil elaborated that it was three Brazilians who had drowned him, then revised it they hadn't drowned him; Alonzo went out in a canoe with them and the canoe turned over.

The drowning in the "deep water" is a punning reference to the sin Jovenil felt he was being punished for. When he first told me of his incestuous relationship with Camelia, he had used a Kagwahiv word for "incest"—*typyowy*—whose literal meaning is "deep green/blue water." But what of the three Brazilians in the dream? They could refer to the thought that came out toward the end of the interview, his suspicion that a woman jealous of his healthy family had hired a Brazilian sorcerer. But they may also be an allusion to my treatment of the children, holding me responsible (in the end) for not saving them. ("Three" may include the two missionaries, who had a part in the treatment.)

In the rest of this interview, Jovenil went on to describe the children's deaths in detail, with deep affect. It was the first time, with me at least, that he had fully experienced and expressed his grief—an important step in his mourning. It would seem that he had to deal with his conflicts over it, his sense of guilt and remorse over having, as he felt, caused his own children's death—and, in this last dream, his anger at me for not saving them—before he could go on with the mourning.

In the rest of the interviews, he went on to mourn further and deal with other facets of these conflicts. In the tenth interview, in association with a dream with a theme of being lost in the jungle, he acknowledged another contribution to his guilt over Alonzo's death was some ambivalence toward the child. I suggested that some planks he was carrying in the dream might be for a coffin, which he agreed was a conventional interpretation of that dream image; and I suggested that they might refer to Alonzo's death, to which he replied "I dreamed of Alonzo too."

> He went to the Festa with me. "Ah, Alonzo, there you are, after so much time!" Alonzo said, "I died at first, now I came alive again."
>
> The Brazilians [Jovenil went on] say it is God who gives the orders. If you scold your child too much, He kills him. If you scold your child too much, God is watching and says, "He doesn't like his son. I'm going to kill him, to see if he will be sad." [Did you feel you scolded him too much?] I scolded him a lot. Afterward, Papa said to me, "One doesn't scold one's son."
>
> First I thought one's children didn't die. That's why I married, to have children. A single woman doesn't have children. It happens a lot when you are married. If your wife doesn't die, your child dies.

Here he remarked on a plane passing over "*Puxa!* One after another, the airplanes!" and a moment later, returning to this theme, he observed "From Porto Velho, you took a plane to Rio." This referred to my movements after I left his settlement in February; so his train of thought went from Alonzo's death to my departure a couple of months prior to it. If I had not left, he may have been thinking, I might have been able to save his children's lives with my medicines. By leaving, I let them die. In addition, a week hence I was to go to a neighboring settlement where I was doing other interviews—the first interruption since I had started these interviews with Jovenil—and there awaited a small float plane that would take me out for a two-week sojourn in Porto Velho. It would be just a three-week interruption (after three intense weeks of interviews), but it no doubt reminded him of my permanent departure planned for two months later as well as of my previous absence that had been so disastrous for him. He felt he was about to be deserted.

In casual conversation later that morning he mentioned that Maria, a Kagwahiv girl who had flirted with me in earlier field trips and was jokingly regarded as my amour and bride-to-be, had gotten married. *Opohi he nde-hugui,* he said. "She discarded you." But this husband of hers was very jealous, and she left him to go to Porto Velho, at which he cried piteously. "He was old and crippled, that's why she didn't like him." These spontaneous remarks, although not in the interview itself, may be taken as further free associations. They again express the theme of abandonment and anger—perhaps a fear that his anger, like the husband's jealousy, might drive me away, as it had led to Alonzo's being taken away.

Jovenil had to work through all these feelings as part of the emotional process of mourning the loss of his children. The sense that one might in some way have caused the death of someone with whom one is close, even in our culture, which does not have concepts of supernatural retribution to rationalize such ideas, is a normal part of the reaction to bereavement (Pollock 1961). So is anger at others for not preventing it. We tend to rationalize these ideas in medical terms—one should have called the doctor sooner, or recognized the symptoms earlier, or the doctor was not competent; Jovenil rationalized them in terms of breach of taboo.

These interviews, a situation decidedly out of the ordinary in Kagwahiv society (as it would be in ours), seem to have given Jovenil significant help in carrying through the mourning process. (Although that was not their intent, nor was I fully aware to what degree Jovenil was using the interviews in this way until I reviewed the interviews in the perspective of later psychoanalytic training.) That his uncompleted mourning had been affecting his life was suggested by a remark he had made to me early in July, before we started the interviews. "I don't want any more children," he said. For Jovenil, usually immensely proud of his prolific family, this was a very unusual remark. I asked him why, but he only said, "It seems I already have enough." The source of these feelings in discouragement and anger over the loss of a favorite son comes out clearly in the remark just quoted: "If your wife doesn't die, your child does." His depression over the death thus interfered with his full emotional involvement with his children and his pleasant anticipation of having more. By the end of the summer, he had recovered some of his good spirits and enjoyment of life. After I left, Aluza became pregnant again and has since had three more children.

But it was not only the conflicts immediately pertaining to the loss of his child that Jovenil had to work through before he came to directly experiencing the loss in his interviews. The first dream alluding to the loss—the castration dream—was one directly modeled on a childhood memory of seeing José Bahut's big penis and learning that its size (erectness, presumably) had something to do with "making his wife." The conflicts he needs to work out over his current loss are related, then, to interests and feelings he had had when he was five years old. His guilt feelings about his incestuous experimentation in adolescence may be derivatives of guilt over childhood curiosity in the same area, perhaps related to the blindness his mother threatened in punishment for his curiosity. The loss of his child in punishment for incest is represented in his dream as castration—the loss of that about which he was so curious at five. Perhaps the threat of loss of eyesight for his visual curiosity may have suggested the loss of another member in punishment for illicit pleasures involving it. Perhaps, too, this representation suggests why he felt with special intensity the loss of his male child.

The exact nature of Jovenil's conflicts as a five-year-old need not concern us here—just what response he wished from his mother when he approached her with his new discovery, and why in the dream the young boy, Camelia's brother, literally pulls off José's erect penis. The details of this did come out in a later dream,[6] but the point here is that he had to work through these conflicting feelings from childhood that were stirred up by the loss of his child as well as the adult guilt feelings about having caused his child's death that were closer to consciousness before he could really begin to experience the grief he felt over his children's deaths. It was only after recalling these conflict-laden childhood experiences that he had the first dream directly expressing his sense of being to blame for his children's death, the dream of shooting the monkey. It would seem, then, that his childhood conflicts interfered with his mourning process; articulating them helped him to sort them out, separating past fantasy from current reality, and freed him to face the present mourning task. It was his needs in mourning, then, that prompted his relating to me these deep childhood conflicts; this is why his interviews are so rich in childhood memories.

I have presented in great detail what was going on in the interviews with one informant, down to the infantile conflicts that were engaged in the interviews, in order to suggest the depth and complexity of the motives an informant may have for participating in interviews. The interviews were of course not carried out for therapeutic purposes. Yet every informant who engaged in them—not just Jovenil—used them to express and sort out conflicting feelings and to work out (and seek some help with) personal problems.

I should make it clear that I was not aware of all of these themes and conflicts during the interviews. Some of the connections became clear to me only as I went over the materials after coming back from the field (as is of course the case with other more straightforward anthropological data), and some of the important themes became evident to me only during my subsequent training in psychoanalysis. In particular, it was not until much later that I realized how much Jovenil was dealing with the mourning of his son throughout these interviews, although in retrospect it seems obvious that he was skirting the issue through several interviews before he finally explicitly brought it up.

Various circumstances make Jovenil's case a special one, as any single case is. Mourning a loss, particularly the loss of one's own child (Pollock 1961) is an emotional task that calls for much support from others. While Kagwahiv beliefs facilitate the articulation of certain frequent emotional conflicts surrounding mourning—such as blaming oneself or someone else for the death—Kagwahiv norms do not give much opportunity or communal support for recalling and working through grief and the attendant conflicts, although they do provide support for separation and forgetting. For these reasons, the interviews came at an especially opportune time for Jovenil's needs.[7] Yet all the other informants I interviewed had some personal crisis they were facing or had recently undergone and were working through, or some adaptation they had to make, which provided a motive for talking to someone willing to listen. For Jovenil and for all informants, a strong motive to participate in interviews is the opportunity to talk to a sympathetic listener about things that are disturbing them.

The nature of the crisis or adaptation facing each informant as they came to the interviews must have made some difference in regard to what aspects of their personality came to the fore, which childhood memories surfaced, or generally what they talked about and how they saw it. Awareness of an informant's personal motives for participating must help anthropologists evaluate the information they get from the informant, not only when the information is of such a personal nature as what I was looking for, but even when it is more abstract social and cultural data.

There are other preconditions for such interviews as these, however, besides motivation. The interviewees must have confidence in the trustworthiness of the interviewer not to abuse their confidences. My involvement in the treatment of Jovenil's children I think played an important part not only in my relationship with Jovenil, but in preparing the way for these interviews with *all* the informants, in demonstrating that I was a person who could be trusted to be concerned personally. Such a point of transition, where one becomes a person who can be trusted with confidences and to respect personal feelings, must be a significant one in the field experience of any anthropologist with a group that he or she gets to know reasonably well. Doubtless there is not one but many such points in any field sojourn, at different levels or in different domains.

The issues of mourning his children were intertwined for Jovenil, especially in the later interviews with the issue of impending separation from me. Owing to the transitory nature of fieldwork and, at the same time, to the intensity of relationships that are built up during it, the issue of separation from anthropologists and mourning them after their departure[8] (as well as anthropologists' mourning their informants)[9] must be, as Edgardo Rolla suggested to me in personal communication, a general one in ethnographer-informant relations.

The anthropologist's involvement with an informant includes not only the anthropologist's personal needs and professional goals (not discussed here) but also the personal needs of the informant that are fulfilled (or frustrated) in the interviews and the personal gratifications the informant seeks. Understanding these processes that go on in the relationship with one's informants should be of help not only in conducting the interviews but also in evaluating the nature of the information communicated in them—and in tuning in to levels of information that are present in all interviews (or conversations) but that are not usually made use of in anthropological interviewing. It enables us to see more clearly some of the gratifications and aids that we are, knowingly or unknowingly, offering informants—for better or for worse—in exchange for being our collaborators in research. Being aware of what we may be offering an informant and what the informant may be seeking from us may help make the exchange more rewarding for both parties.

But the more fundamental point demonstrated here is that cultural difference is not an insuperable obstacle to communication and to the understanding of psychological states in another person. Jovenil, at least, was able to verbalize his feelings and fantasies to me clearly enough that I could achieve a psychoanalytic understanding of the mourning process that he was engaged in and the conflicts that blocked it, and even help him surmount that blockage. This is not to say that I could communicate as easily with every Kagwahiv I interviewed as I did with Jovenil; some were far less communicative than he, others were less able to put their thoughts and feelings into words, and still others were beset with conflicts far more severe and crippling than his, which would have required a longer and more difficult series of interviews to unravel. Such variations and difficulties of course exist just as much in our own culture. But all of the individuals I interviewed worked on some inner problems in the interviews and in doing so revealed some of the psychological processes involved in grappling with their problems (Kracke 1978, 1979). If the investigator is willing to make the additional effort of understanding the cultural world of the person being interviewed and to be receptive to the subtle, implicit, and not always culture-syntonic messages that the person conveys about his or her emotional state, psychological understanding can be both possible and beneficial.

Notes

An earlier version of this chapter was presented in a symposium on psychological sensitivity in anthropological field work at the 76th annual meeting of the American Anthropological Associabon in Houston, Texas, on December 1, 1977. It grew out of an earlier presentation to the Interdisciplinary Colloquium on Psychoanalytic Questions and Methods in Anthropological Field Work, then chaired by L. Bryce Boyer, at the annual fall meeting of the American Psychoanalytic Association, December 8–9, 1976.

1. When discussing the issue most specifically, Geertz takes the middle position—but one still rendering cross-cultural psychoanalysis a highly tenuous enterprise—that "the ethnographer does not, and in my opinion, largely cannot, perceive what his informants perceive. What he perceives—and that uncertainly enough—is what they perceive 'with' or 'by means' of or 'through' or whatever word one may choose" (1975: 48).
2. Two notable exceptions are Kenneth Read's account of his poignant communication with Makis in the High Valley (1965: 84–88) and Paul Riesman's perceptive thoughts on empathic intuition in his fieldwork with the Fulani (1974: 151–153). Intercultural communication has been a central theme of some noted works of fiction (Bowen 1954; Forster 1949), but only in Devereux's classic *From Anxiety to Method* (1967) did it become the subject of a systematic theoretical discussion in anthropology.
3. Interviews with this and other individuals I interviewed are presented and discussed more fully in Kracke (1978 and 1979).
4. Although much has been written about mortuary ritual in anthropology, to my knowledge there has been rather little research on the mourning experience in non-Western societies. In a later publication that will focus more specifically on Kagwahiv mourning I discuss the literature on this topic more fully, but some brief comments are apposite here. Of special relevance here is Lewis's (1975) interesting reports of a "Culturally Patterned Depression in a Mother after Loss of a Child" among the Trio of Surinam. A particularly important contribution is Pollock's (1972) article discussing mourning ritual as a culturally constituted defense mechanism that articulates the psychological process of mourning. I am somewhat skeptical of Goldschmidt's (1973: 98) contention that the Sebei do not experience a loss deeply enough to mourn, but clearly, as among the Kagwahiv, their grief is vigorously suppressed. This and other important contributions (Matchett 1974; Woodward 1968) will be discussed more fully elsewhere.
5. Kagwahiv modesty forbids a man to be seen without his penis sheath, so Jovenil's mother may have been simply giving him a lesson in modesty.
6. In interview 11, Jovenil reluctantly recounted to me a frightening dream: he was watching a family of forest spirits (*anang*) from behind a tree, while the father-*anang* was making love to the mother-*anang,* teaching his five-year-old son how it was done. Terrified at the sight, Jovenil ran back to the settlement and told about it. Another man in the settlement was all for going out to hunt the *anang* family and kill the father; Jovenil tried to dissuade him, but he went ahead and did it.

   This dream is a blatant portrayal of a childhood fantasy which, to judge by the age of the onlooking child—Jovenil must have had at the age of five—the same age as the earlier reported childhood memory, which also involved watching and learning about sex. The fantasy was a little too openly expressed for Jovenil's comfort; even the last-ditch distancing mechanism of presenting the action, as it were, "on the stage," (Jovenil was watching the scene take place before him), was not enough to allay his anxiety. Not only was he afraid in the dream, but he did not at first want to tell it to me.

   If we regard this as a second edition of the first dream that referred to memories at the same age, the child's intent in pulling off Jose Bahut's penis becomes clearer. If the two dreams are parallel, then Jovenil's fantasy was of borrowing Jose's penis (or his father's) for his own use, just as in the second dream he learned from his father how to use it.

The theme of learning in the *anang* dream also has a reference to me, for I had, just two days earlier, suggested in casual conversation that he learn to give injections (note possible analogies) so that he could continue the tuberculosis treatment I was giving to his wife.

7. It is an interesting but perhaps unanswerable question whether Jovenil would have resolved his conflicts in the same way without having these interviews with me, or whether my interviews offered him a support for his mourning process that would have been unavailable in his own culture. This raises further questions about the part that anthropologists play in the lives of the people they study and how anthropologists' contributions to their lives affect the data and the image of their culture. It also raises the question of to what degree any culture provides satisfactorily for all the needs of its people. In any case, though, Jovenil was quite ready to use the interviews with me to his own benefit in working out his conflicts over mourning. It seems likely that he might have worked out some, although perhaps not all, of these problems in conversations with some other person.
8. Dorothy Eggan's informant, Don Talayesva, expressed this issue very neatly in the dream image of his "white wife" who was eager to watch Hopi rituals, but who "gets homesick" and wants to leave (Eggan 1949: 182–183).
9. The idealization that one often sees in an anthropologist's memories of his or her principal informants (cf. Casagrande 1960) may be a consequence of mourning them, for the mourning process often results in some idealization. I am indebted for this observation to Laura Kracke.

References

Bowen, Elenore Smith. 1954. *Return to Laughter.* New York: Natural History Press.

Casagrande, Joseph B., ed. 1960. *In the Company of Man.* New York: Harper.

Devereux, George. 1967. *From Anxiety to Method in the Behavioral Sciences.* The Hague: Mouton.

Eggan, Dorothy. 1949. "The Significance of Dreams for Anthropological Research." *American Anthropologist* 51: 177–198.

Forster, E. M. 1949. *A Passage to India.* New York: Harcourt Brace.

Geertz, Clifford. 1965. "The Impact of the Concept of Culture on the Concept of Man." In *New Views of the Nature of Man* (J. Platt, ed.), pp. 93–118. Chicago: University of Chicago Press. Reprinted in *The Interpretation of Cultures* (New York: Basic Books).

———. 1973. "Person, Time and Conduct in Bali." In *The Interpretation of Cultures* (New York: Basic Books).

———. 1975. "On the Nature of Anthropological Understanding." *American Scientist* 63: 47–53.

Goldschmidt, Walter. 1973. "Guilt and Pollution in Sebei Mortuary Ritual." *Ethos* 75–105.

Hanson, F. Allan. 1975. *Meaning in Culture.* London: Routledge & Kegan Paul.

Kracke, Waud H. 1978. *Force and Persuasion: Leadership in an Amazonian Society.* Chicago: University of Chicago Press.

———. 1979. "Dreaming in Kagwahiv: Dream Beliefs and Their Psychic Uses in an Amazonian Indian Culture." *Psychoanalytic Study of Society* 8: 119–171.

Langness, Lewis L. 1965. *The Life History in Anthropological Science.* New York: Holt, Rinehart and Winston.

Levine, Robert. 1973. *Culture, Behavior and Personality.* Chicago: Aldine.

Lewis, Thomas N. 1975. "Culturally Patterned Depression in a Mother after Loss of a Child." *Psychiatry* 38: 92–95.

Matchett, William Foster. 1974. "Repeated Hallucinatory Experiences as a Part of the Mourning Process among Hopi Women." In *Culture and Personality* (Robert LeVine, ed.), pp. 222–231. Chicago: Aldine.

Needham, Rodney. 1972. *Belief, Language and Experience.* Chicago: University of Chicago Press.

Pollack, George H. 1961. Mourning and Adaptation. *International Journal of Psychoanalysis* 42: 341–361. Reprinted in *Culture and Personality* (Robert LeVine, ed.), pp. 65–94. Chicago: Aldine, 1974.

———. 1972. "On Mourning and Anniversaries: The Relationship of Culturally Constituted Defensive Systems to Intrapsychic Adaptive Processes." *Israel Annals of Psychiatry* 10: 9–41.

Read, Kenneth. 1965. *The High Valley.* New York: Scribners.

Reisman, Paul. 1974. *Freedom in Fulani Social Life.* Chicago: University of Chicago Press.

Rosaldo, Michelle. 1980. *Knowledge and Passion: Ilongot Notions of Self and Social Life.* Cambridge, England: Cambridge University Press.

Woodward, James A. 1968. "The Anniversary: A Contemporary Diegueno Complex." Ethnology 7: 86–94.

10

Reflecting on a Dream in Jungian Analytic Practice

Jane White-Lewis

"Last night I had a dream—well, a fragment of a dream," a patient tells me as she is settling into her chair. "I dreamed of a woman with a bunch of balloons," she adds.

Closing my eyes for a few seconds, I imagine the dream. I see the dream, my version, in my mind's eye. In my dream of the dreamer's dream, I am in a smallish room and am looking at a stocky older woman to my left sitting quietly, holding a bunch of balloons. The image feels familiar.

And at this moment, I am barely aware that my heart jumps a bit—a mix of excitement, inadequacy, and fear. This feeling, so familiar now, still takes me by surprise. I used to think the odd flash of terror was certain evidence of my inexperience and limitations. How could I ever understand this dream? How could I possibly come up with a helpful, insightful response?

Early in my training I read Jung's comment that "for a long time I have made it a rule, when someone tells me a dream and asks for my opinion, to say first of all to myself: 'I have no idea what this dream means.'"[1] At the time I thought, "How could Jung, after working with and analyzing thousands of dreams, feel so insecure and inadequate? Surely this passage was just false modesty, posturing." But from time to time I would hear others—experienced analysts, training analysts, colleagues—saying the same thing.

Now I think that this twinge is not just a matter of lack of training or knowledge but evidence of a magic moment when the unconscious enters in and when we are confronted with the unknown, the unexpected. With this modal shift to the symbolic, imaginal realm, we move beyond the puny ego and touch and are touched by the spiritual dimension of the psyche, which is both awesome and mysterious.

In former/ancient times, dreams were thought to come from God or the gods. Now we say dreams come from the Unconscious or the Self—as if we were saying something. Are not these constructions synonyms for a mystery we do not fully understand? Maybe the ancients were correct, and the "twinge" we feel in hearing another's dream is awe in the face of this mystery.

Certainly it is possible to do solid therapeutic work without considering dreams, but dreams do make a difference and are generally central in a Jungian analysis. But what is that difference and how do dreams contribute to the analytic process? How do my Jungian training and sympathies color the work I do, and how do dreams inform my work? Perhaps my reflecting on a dream and on my own process may provide some answers.

With a not-unexpected prompt from me ("Do you have any thoughts about the dream?"), the dreamer continues. I say little at this point. The dreamer is familiar with dream work in the context of a Jungian analysis. Before our first meeting three years ago, she had worked with another Jungian analyst for a relatively brief period. She knows that personal associations are a key to appreciating a dream, are central to understanding a dream, and are a natural place for her/us to start when "working" on a dream. (Accessing the feelings in the dream, dream "reentry" does not come easily.) So, slowly and thoughtfully, she offers her associations. "I think of parties. . . . and bubbles in comic strips (you know, what the character is thinking or saying) . . . and a balloon payment and . . . hmm, pollution" A longer pause follows; another association surfaces. *The Red Balloon,* which was a movie . . . and, I think, a book as well." She appears thoughtful and sad as she tries to recall the story. "I don't remember the ending," she eventually says. She then returns to the dream image and adds more descriptive detail. "In the dream I am in a small room. The balloons are filled with helium, standing straight up, touching the ceiling. I am interested, but detached. The balloons are of various colors—blue, purple, green."

At that moment I am startled by the "coincidence" of the colors of the balloons and the colors of the skirt she has chosen to wear today. It is a skirt she has never worn to a session before—a bold, floral print of blue, purple, and green. I comment—perhaps too cheerfully, too quickly, "Just like the splendid colors in your skirt!" Clearly uncomfortable, she quickly and sharply replies, "This is an old skirt."

My spontaneous remark was perhaps ill-timed, ill-considered. The dreamer is suspicious of compliments. Any comment about her appearance is problematic and suspect, given her history of a scanning, judging, nonaccepting mother. My possibly clumsy comment popped out, I think, from my delight at seeing the connection between the dream and reality coupled with my unconscious (at that moment) desire to connect with the dreamer (a major issue in the analysis).

While the dreamer was offering her associations, I was listening attentively as well as registering (to myself) my own associations to her dream. I imagined seeing a dog walker in the city with a bunch of lively charges on the way to the park—an event that always reminds me, for some reason, of balloons. I thought too of balloons, an image that resonates, for me, with both happy and sad memories, of birthday parties, of hospitals. And even before the dreamer mentioned it, I thought of *The Red Balloon*—both the extraordinary and beautifully filmed French short film and the book based on clips from the film, a book I read many, many times to my children. Also a murky image emerged of a painting of a woman with balloons that I had seen years ago, a childhood memory. Where had I seen it? My grandparents' house? The dream, I realize, delights me, and I wonder for a narcissistic moment if this image of balloons is possibly a belated birthday present. This thought is, perhaps, not too far-fetched. As the dreamer was leaving her last session, a delivery man arrived, wished me a "Happy Birthday," and handed me a bunch of flowers!

Meanwhile, of course, I was also taking mental notes on the dreamer's associations. Her first association, "parties," was not surprising, not unexpected. Given what I know of her history from the time we have been meeting, I do have a strong sense of what "parties" might lead to—painful memories of longing, being excluded, and perhaps of special moments (birthday parties?) as well. We can explore those associations later. The dreamer had already elaborated a bit on her second association, "bubbles in comic strips," in adding "like what the character is saying or thinking about." I can imagine that her image might be useful at a later date with this dream (or with any dream, for that matter)—for example, "If there were a 'balloon' next to the Balloon Woman's head, what might she be thinking?." The third association, "balloon payment," is unusual and needs clarification; the fourth, "pollution," seems definitely off the chart. Bizarre responses, however, are often therapeutic "gold." (It is worth noting, I think, that Jungian analysis grew out of Jung's "Word Association" studies early in his career, when he learned to explore with his patients their unusual responses to the mention of certain words.)

Not certain myself, I ask her what a "balloon payment" is. "I'm not exactly sure," she replies, "but I think it may be a large payment, perhaps at the end of a certain kind of mortgage, perhaps it's called a 'balloon mortgage.'" "Hmm, a curious metaphor! What is the meaning?" I think to myself. The thought crosses my mind that the "mortgage" agreement and payments may well relate to the analytic process and the analytic relationship. Surely there are connections between images of money and inner resources, psychic energy and personal power—all something to keep in mind.

"What is the connection between balloons and pollution?" I ask. She tells me that environmentalists are very concerned with the impact of latex balloons on the environment. Each year thousands and thousands of helium balloons end up in trees and in the sea and are a definite hazard to wildlife. Fish, dolphins, a variety of sea creatures lose their lives.

Clearly, letting go of balloons is hazardous and not good for the environment; it is dangerous, toxic, and possibly fatal to live creatures. In the dream, the balloons are contained (touching the ceiling), but there is an inherent danger of popping, of being let go. What do "balloons" represent and how can we understand the "environment"? When I think of balloons being filled with air, being filled with "pneuma" (breath, spirit), I feel certain that this dream relates, in some way, to the dreamer's current spiritual concerns and distress. Although not overtly a spiritual dream in content, I strongly suspect a spiritual dimension.

So how will we work with this dream fragment? The dream would not be considered a "big," "intensified," "highly significant dream"; there is no feeling of numinosity or transformative power. Some (including the dreamer) might well consider the dream "little," "trivial," "forgettable," or "only a fragment." The dream, however, feels like a precious gift as I sense boundless possibilities of working (and playing) with it, this bit of poetry.

We have already started to "unpack" this "gift" by considering some of the dreamer's associations. As Jung would say, we will continue to "circumambulate" the images, that is, "walk" around them, come back to them as the complexities of their meanings are revealed and as the dream space is known and felt. First we will consider an "objective" understanding of the dream, but probably we will move quickly to a more subjective, symbolic and feeling level given that the dream setting and dream figure are unknown to the dreamer and have no evident connection to her external world. We will explore the feeling tone of the images and associations as we reenter the dream landscape.

Assuming, as Jung did, that the dream is a compensation for conscious attitudes, we will repeatedly consider what the dream is trying to tell us. How does the dream shed some light and stretch our understanding of the dreamer's current professional, relational, and spiritual concerns? Can we identify the polarities in the dream to better understand the unresolved psychological issues that fed it? How does this dream relate to the present and the future and to the dreamer's own individuation process of becoming who she is meant to be? Especially important will be an examination of the transference and countertransference issues raised by the dream. The dream, this readout from the unconscious, will give us clues as to how to proceed in our analytic endeavor. Throughout this process we will want to "befriend" the dream, as James Hillman would say, "to participate in it, to enter into its imagery and mood, to want to know more about it, to understand, play with, live with, carry, and become familiar with—as one would with a friend."[2]

Outside of the session, I will do my "homework" and "homeplay" with the dream as well. Starting on a personal level, I might call my sister and ask her if she has memories of a balloon painting in my grandparents' house. Always interested in the etymology of a word, I might check out the etymology of "balloon" to get a deeper sense of its family history, its soul sense. I might consider the archetypal level of the dream and the symbols implicit in the dream, such as balls, spheres, air, the Wise Woman, the Great Mother. In the process, myths, folk tales, and other amplifications will undoubtedly surface. Considering the various levels of interpretation—personal history, present concerns, future possibilities, archetypal underpinnings, transference and countertransference dynamics, the spiritual dimension—will enrich my understanding and appreciation of the dream. The results of my musings and explorations will waft their way into the analytic hour. While some of the information may be interesting and useful, "informing" the patient is generally alienating, problematic. (Jung was a major offender in this realm, I suspect.)

Given that the dreamer and I meet once a week and lead full and complicated lives, it is unrealistic to expect that we will accomplish such extensive dream work. Other dreams and pressing life issues demanding attention will intervene. I sense, however, that this dream will continue to play in our imaginations, to reverberate through our sessions, and will play a part in shaping the unfolding of the analysis. Furthermore, given the content and the timing of this dream, it seems very much like an "initial" dream.

Initial dreams are usually defined as the first dream brought to an analytic session or the first dream experienced after the first phone call or first session. They are often valuable indicators of the major issues of the analysis to come. I believe that comparably revealing dreams can also surface at the beginning of a new phase of therapy. The "balloon dream" is a good example, because it coincides with a recent remarkable shift in my analytic relationship with the woman. Establishing a strong therapeutic alliance has been a major struggle from the beginning of our work together. Although the dreamer seldom missed or canceled a session, she was usually late and often seemed uninvolved. We seemed to be going through the motions; many of the sessions were lukewarm. A real split was evident, and her feeling life was lived elsewhere. Any efforts on my part to discuss the issue failed. Several months ago, however, with some discomfort and trepidation, she reported a conversation with a friend in which she had described her lack of enthusiasm for our work. The friend had suggested that she consider another therapist. She courageously broached the sensitive issue of our lack of connection, and we spoke honestly about our difficulties. It had taken time to develop enough trust to take such a risk. That session was a turning point that was reflected in deepening in our relationship and in the analysis. As a result, both of us are more involved in the analysis. She arrives on time, and I look forward to seeing her.

Three weeks after hearing the balloon dream, I considered asking the dreamer for permission to write about her dream. I am always reluctant to use a patient's material and, as a result, have written little about my clinical work. The thought of "using" a patient's imaginal material has always been troubling to me and feels a bit like a violation of the analytic container. I do not want to jeopardize the analysis; I do not want to take a risk that might negatively impact on our work. I realize, however, that either risking or not risking to speak to the dreamer will have an impact on the work. That is, my asking to write about the dream could be positive or negative; my *not* asking could be positive or negative. Can I not trust that the analytic relationship is strong enough to weather this challenge?

I remember the dreamer's courage in speaking to me about her dissatisfaction with therapy and her risking my possible displeasure, hurt, and retaliation. She was able to trust the relationship, to speak honestly and to work with me on resolving the issues. Can I not do as much at this stage in our work together? If my request does, in fact, lead to some intense, negative response, can I not trust that this "grist for the mill" can be worked thorough analytically and our work deepened?

Obviously, I decided to ask her if I could write about her dream. When I did, she smiled broadly and said simply, "Of course you can use it. I feel flattered." There may well be complications because of this decision, but I trust the strength of our connection and our courage to work through the issues.

In any case, this story is not over. The images and metaphors of this dream will continue to color our work, and elements of the dream may well appear in her dreams and mine. We will refer to the Balloon Lady; balloons will have a special loaded, layered meaning for us. As other dreams resonate with elements and associations from this dream, a complex imaginative tapestry will emerge in time. Because dreams exist in a continuous present, this particular dream will continue to live in the dreamer's imagination, in my imagination, and perhaps, my reader, in yours.

Notes

1. C. G. Jung, "On the Nature of Dreams," in *Dreams,* trans. R. F. C. Hull (Princeton: Princeton University Press, 1974), p. 69.
2. James Hillman, *Insearch: Psychology and Religion* (Dallas: Spring Publications, 1967), p. 57.

11

Group Work with Dreams

The "Royal Road" to Meaning

Jeremy Taylor

I have dreamed in my life dreams that have stayed with me ever after, and changed my ideas; they have gone through and through me, like wine through water, and altered the colour of my mind.

—*Emily Brontë*[1]

Humankind has ascribed important symbolic meanings to dreams, in all societies around the world, throughout history. The evidence of archaic iconography and remnants of prehistoric oral tradition strongly suggests that our individual and collective preoccupation with dreams and their deeper meanings has persisted from our earliest human beginnings. In the modern era it has become fashionable in some academic circles to say that dreams have no intrinsic meaning, reflecting only the "random firing of neurons in sleep," and are, at best, merely the epiphenomena of disordered metabolism. Even so, there remains a huge, growing, and compelling body of evidence which indicates very clearly that the experiences of the dreaming mind are the source not only of meaningful ideas and feelings but are a primary stimulus for some of the deepest religious intuitions, artistic inspirations, scientific and technological innovations, successful creative problem solving, clarifications of philosophical meaning, and epiphanies of spiritual significance that human beings are capable of experiencing and formulating into words and images.

The Proof Is in the Pudding

The difficulty of "proving" this ancient wisdom that dreams are a primary and intrinsic source of meaning in our lives in anything other than anecdotal ways lies in the fundamental nature of symbolic experience itself. By definition, symbols always carry multiple meanings and layers of significance simultaneously—as distinct from "signs," which are supposed to carry only one single message or valance.[2] These multiple meanings defy objective measurement and analysis and therefore tend to disappear from the scientific/academic discourse that relies on clear definition and objective, reproducible measurement as its primary tool of analysis. The fact that these multiple meanings that all dreams carry cannot be adequately demonstrated or measured by scientific analysis does not mean that they are unreal, or that they do not exist.

Carl Jung puts the problem very succinctly: "Whether a thing is a symbol or not depends chiefly on the attitude of the observing consciousness . . ."[3] Jung goes even further and defines the way in which the existence and importance of symbols can be "verified": "In psychology the exact measurement of quantities is replaced by an approximate determination of intensities, for which purpose, in strict contrast to physics, we enlist the function of *feeling* (valuation). The latter takes the place in psychology of concrete measurement in physics."[4]

I had a conversation with the eminent laboratory dream researcher Dr. Milton Kramer at the Association for the Study of Dreams international conference in New York City a few years ago. At that time he summed up his estimation of the modern laboratory dream research efforts to date in the following way: "The question that twentieth-century dream research set out to answer is 'Do dreams constitute "signal," or are they merely "noise"?' We can now say with certainty as the century comes to close that they are 'signal.'"

Not only do dreams communicate meaningful "signal," because of their fundamentally symbolic nature they communicate many multiple layers of signal simultaneously.

The Universality of Dreaming

The laboratory evidence is in—all human beings, indeed, all complex warm-blooded beings (with the possible exception of the *Echidna,* the spiny ant eater of Australia), dream during sleep on a regular basis. Any person who claims "I don't dream" is simply admitting that he or she fails to pay any conscious attention to this universal aspect of human experience.[5]

When the question of the deeper meanings of dreams is approached in actual practice, by men and women who are willing to undertake the sustained moral and psychospiritual effort required for this kind of self-examination of previously unconscious dramas and motivations, it turns out that all dreams come in the service of health and wholeness and speak a universal language.

I have been working as professional dream worker for more than thirty years. While I was writing this chapter, I recorded the 11,900th of my own dreams in my personal dream journal. At a conservative estimate, I hear and read ten dreams from other people for every dream of my own that I am able to recall and record, so I now have a "sample" of something well in excess of 100,000 dreams upon which to draw in making generalizations about dreams and their deeper meanings. In all that time I have not heard a single dream or had an experience working a dream that has not contributed to my conviction that all dreaming is deeply involved with the health and wholeness, not just of the individual dreamer, but the entire species.[6]

I grant that at first glance, this may not appear to be the case. Anyone interested in dreams has almost certainly experienced at one time or another a dream or two that were so nasty that when the dreamer awakened, these experiences did not seem to have anything even remotely to do with health and wholeness. We usually call these dreams nightmares.

Nightmares and Human Evolution

What I would ask the reader to consider with regard to the nightmare form is our evolutionary history as a species. The fossil record provides compelling evidence to suggest that we human beings have been struggling for the last four and a half million years or so to maximize our ability to survive in a wide range of ecological circumstances. One of the primary strategies we have cultivated to achieve this end (if not *the* primary strategy) is this trick of consciousness that allows us to identify threat at an early enough stage of its development to allow us to make educated guesses about its speed and direction and to *get out of the way*. Simple contemplation will demonstrate that creatures able to pull off this trick of consciousness have a much greater tendency to survive and thrive than creatures that blunder around and can not quite get it together to do that.

Thus, we contemporary humans have been shaped by natural selection (if you prefer that nineteenth-century, scientific-sounding language), or the hand of God, or the hand of the Goddess, (if you prefer that more resonant, post-modern-sounding language), so that we are now all inherently predisposed to pay particularly focused attention to nasty threatening stuff. We know, literally "in our bones" (probably twined into the DNA itself), that paying close attention to nasty threatening stuff is a survival issue. We also know that paying attention to more seemingly benign and supportive experience is interesting and entertaining but that it is not a survival issue in the same way as staying alert to threat is.

One consequence of this evolutionary history is that when the deep unconscious, not-yet-speech-ripe part of ourselves has information of particular importance and potential survival value to impart to the waking mind (particularly if that waking mind is not accustomed to paying attention to dreams), it is very likely to dress up that information in the form of a nightmare, because we are all inherently more disposed to pay attention to information that enters our field of awareness in that form than we are to pay attention to precisely the same information if it were to come into our field of awareness in some more seemingly benign form.

With that thought in mind, I would like to suggest that the generic message of every nightmare you have ever had, of every nightmare that your kids ever crawled into bed and woke you up with, is: "Wake up! Pay attention! There is a *survival* issue at stake in your life right now that you can *do* something about, if you only notice and acknowledge it in time!"[7]

Archetypes in Dreams and Sacred Narratives

If you can at least see why a person with my experience might come to such a conclusion (whether you are convinced yourself or not), you have at least one fairly clear example before you of what Carl Jung is talking about when he talks about archetypes of the collective unconscious. The nightmare is itself an archetypal form—that is, a symbolic form that addresses all human beings in essentially the same form, with essentially the same generic message, regardless of the gender and cultural differences and psychological uniquenesses that appear to separate us from one another.

Archetypes of the collective unconscious comprise the vocabulary and grammar of the universal language of myth and dream. They appear as symbolic motifs and forms that recur in the dreams of individuals and the sacred narratives of world religions in all periods of history.[8] The spontaneous, repeating appearance of archetypal forms demonstrates that the health and wholeness served by the dream is not limited by the envelope of skin of the individual dreamer but plays a role in the health and wholeness of the entire species (and, by implication, in the whole biosphere, without which the species could not survive, and by further implication, in the entire universe, which continues to preserve this little, seemingly anomalous, wet, warm, green place that we call home). The archetypal foundation of every remembered dream implicates the dreamer as a direct participant, even a co-creator, in the largest cosmic/spiritual drama.

Dreams come in the service of individual health and wholeness to be sure—and they also serve successively broader and deeper patterns of complexity and interdependence simultaneously. This breadth of significant resonance means that dreams do not come to serve or flatter the ego. In fact, dreams often come to confront the waking mind with disturbing information about its weaknesses and failings, which makes remembered dreams particularly valuable in the effort to overcome that most insidious human failing—self-deception.

Overcoming Self-Deception

One of the most important self-deceptions that dreams regularly address is the sense that a situation is hopeless and that there is nothing the person can do about this situation in his or her life. In my experience, no dream ever came to anyone to say, "Nyeah, Nyeah—You have these problems and there's nothing you can do about them!" Thus if a person has a dream and understands upon awakening that the dream makes reference to a seemingly unsolvable problem in his or her waking life, it means that, in fact, some creative, potentially effective response *is* possible, and in the service of health and wholeness the dream is directing the dreamer's attention to those as-yet-unperceived possibilities. If this were not the case, the dream would simply not have been remembered. In fact, this is a generic implication of all remembered dreams: If a dream is remembered at all, it suggests that the dreamer's waking consciousness is capable of playing a creative, positive, even a transformative role in the further unfolding of whatever issues and situations are taking symbolic shape in the dream.

Dreams come from an unconscious source that is much deeper than the conscious mind. This dreaming source simply ignores even the most passionate and sincere opinions of the waking mind when they are rooted in self-deception and denial. For instance, you can be an underpaid graduate assistant in a neurophysiology department sleep lab, and you can be absolutely and sincerely convinced that Dr. Allan Hobson is correct and that dreams are simply the meaningless result of random firings of neurons in the cerebral cortex during sleep, *and your nightmares will wake you up with your heart pounding anyway* . . . The depth and sincerity of one's waking convictions and prejudices makes no difference (thank goodness!); the dreams come in the service of health and wholeness, arising from and directing our attention back toward the deepest shared aspects of our common humanity.

All humankind are one folk. This is not just liberal rhetoric or a pious hope about something that may come about "later"; it is a statement of the bald and simple truth of our individual and collective lives. The universality of the archetypal symbolic forms that emerge spontaneously from our dreaming experience demonstrates the reality of deeply shared common humanity on a daily and nightly basis.

Dreams and Nonviolent Social Change

This fact was borne in on me with great force when I undertook the first piece of organized group dream work that I ever did, back in 1969, as part of a church-sponsored community organizing effort devoted to overcoming racism. The work was undertaken as part of a community organizing effort in Emeryville, California. The participants in the volunteer training seminar were of diverse racial and cultural backgrounds, and although each of us was intellectually convinced that racism was a bad idea, we were also subject to unconscious racial stereotypes and prejudices to such an extent that we drove one another crazy. It was only when we began to share our remembered dreams with one another, paying particular attention to those that revealed racial and class sentiment as part of their manifest content, that we actually began to surface and address the deep unconscious sources of our prejudices and to transform them. It was as a result of that amazing, profoundly moving experience that I first devoted myself to group dream work.[9] As we explored our dreams together, cobbling together the " . . . if it were my dream" form to facilitate responsible, candid, adult group discussion, we uncovered our internal repressions and projections, which are always at the root of prejudice and collective oppression and injustice in the world.

The only person who can confirm that these or any other deeper meanings actually reside in any dream, beyond and below the surface of obvious appearance, is the original dreamer. When the dreamer discovers something true about the deeper meaning(s) of his or her dream, this discovery is most often confirmed by an "aha!" of recognition.[10] My experience convinces me that this "aha!" is a function of memory. The dreamer discovers *words* for an understanding and an awareness that were previously unconscious—"not yet speech-ripe," as the ancient Anglo-Saxons would say—and in that moment *remembers* what he or she "knew" the dream meant all along but had no words for until the "aha!" of insight. The only person who can remember what a dream means is the person who first experienced it. However, since the archetypal symbolic language of the dreaming mind is, in fact, universal—since we human beings are inherently predisposed to symbolize the most important events and passages of our lives in essentially the same ways—the chances that the comments, suggestions, and projections of others will awaken the "aha!" of recognition in the dreamer are very high. These "ahas!" are not limited to the original dreamer. In my experience, the benefit of working on a dream in a group is always shared liberally among all those taking part in the work. Everyone in the group is doing his or her own interior work in projected form on the gift of the original narrative.

The "Aha!" of Self-Recognition

When working with dreams in a group, this "aha!" is always the focus of the search. Only the original dreamer can ever say with any certainty what deeper meanings his or her dreams may have, but in solitude, the original dreamer is always uniquely and selectively blind to those deeper meanings. This is the primary reason why dream work undertaken in solitude is generally not as valuable as dream work carried out in company with others. The dreamer is always selectively and uniquely blind to the deeper meanings of his or her dreams. This is not a result of lack of intelligence, or dedication, or failure to bring one's best effort to the task: It is a consequence of the current state of human evolution itself. Conscious human self-awareness rests on a foundation of selective perception that filters out the details of subtle, interior experience, allowing the limited energies of consciousness to be focused outward on the challenging details of waking life. The dreamer exploring his or her dreams in solitude will certainly have any number of exciting and valuable "ahas!" of insight and understanding, but over time, those insights will always fall into the patterns of what that person already knew and believed to begin with.

One of the great truths about our dreams is that they never arrive in waking awareness just to tell us what we already consciously know. Dreams always come to tell us something new, and it is precisely these levels of novel meaning and startling new awareness that solitary dreamers are always uniquely blind to. Whenever dreamers gather cooperatively to explore one another's dreams, they provide each other the uniquely valuable gift of the fresh ears with which they are able to hear and the fresh eyes with which they are able to imagine the dreamer's experience.

The Universal Process of "Projection"

When dream work is undertaken cooperatively with the participation of others in a group setting, each member of the group imagines his or her version of the dream and speculates, that is, "projects" about the deeper meanings of the dream below the surface of obvious appearance. In the technical literature of psychoanalysis, projection is usually called "transference" and "countertransference" and is seen primarily as an annoying source of bias and confusion in analytical work. In fact, it is a natural and inevitable unconscious human process, which, properly understood and consciously acknowledged, can become a way of deepening our appreciation of our shared human predicament, our mutual longing for greater connection with one another, and our common hunger for greater communion with the Divine.

Whenever a person tells a dream to others, the people listening always imagine their own versions of the dream as they listen. As we imagine the dreamer's narrative, we "redream" it for ourselves, automatically imbuing our own imagined version of the dream with all our own unconscious dramas and energies in the process. From that point onward, each person is actually exploring his or her own imagined version of the dream. Thus anything that is said to the dreamer about the possible meanings of his or her dream is always a projection, based on the speaker's own imagined version of the dream. It also means that any "aha!" that anyone has in the course of exploring another person's dream is completely valid for that person, whether it is confirmed by the original dreamer or not, (because, of course, it is actually an "aha!" of insight about the deeper meaning and significance of that person's own imagined version of the original dream).

In order to facilitate responsible and productive group exploration of the deeper meanings of people's dreams, group participants must have as clear and conscious a grasp as possible of the inevitable nature of unconscious psychological projection. We all project, all the time. For this reason, in the groups that I train and facilitate I insist that participants preface any comments they are going to make to one another with some version of the idea "if this were my dream . . ." and keep the ensuing remarks in the first person. Participants might say "When I, as a man, imagine being a woman and having this dream, the following things seem true to me . . ." or "When I imagine this dream for myself in the light of the life experiences you have shared, it seems to me that . . ."

This mode of discourse sometimes seems a little stilted and awkward at first. It goes against the language habits of lifetime. Often people slip back into the "you" form of address, out of excitement and enthusiasm if for no other reason. I have developed the habit of patting my hand on my chest, gorilla fashion, as a quick, wordless reminder to people to stay true to the group's agreement about consciously owning the projections that give birth to our speculations about the deeper meanings of each other's dreams.

If This Were My Dream . . .

Every time a dream group participant says some version of "If this were my dream," he or she is saying to the dreamer (and to everyone else who imagined the dream for themselves), "There is nothing in you, or your dream, or your unconscious—no matter how strange, or bizarre, or confusing, or downright repugnant the imagery of your dream may be to me—that I am not also perfectly prepared to find in myself at this moment." The practice becomes an operational affirmation of the deep, shared common humanity out of which the dream springs and back toward which the dream directs our attention. It is a way of respecting the dreamer, the dream, and everyone else engaged in the effort to explore and "unpack" the dream.

Over the years I have noticed that this mode of discourse, with its attendant increased sensitivity to the universality and inevitability of projection and its affirmation of empathy and the effort to understand rather than judge, tends over time to "jump the fence" and become a useful conversational habit outside of the dream group. Many people have reported that the increasingly comfortable "If it were my dream . . ." habit of speech turns into an "If it were my life . . ." way of speaking, making conversations outside of the group much more intimate, interesting, and productive.

Ensuring Emotional Safety

To undertake the work of exploring the deeper meanings of dreams productively and responsibly, everyone in the group needs to feel safe. To accomplish this in the groups I work with, we stress an initial agreement of anonymity in any conversation about our experiences outside the group. We also emphasize that every group member also has both the right and the responsibility to request strict confidentiality at any point in the process, any time he or she feels drawn to do so. Thus, if no member of the group has exercised his or her responsibility to ask for strict confidentiality, any participant is free to talk about what happens in the group with anyone else, as long as no one in the group is identifiable in the details of what is said. Whenever any group member asks for confidentiality, even retroactively, all other group members are pledged to move into that more restrictive mode until they are released from that obligation by the person who originally made the request.

Over the thirty-plus years that I have been doing this work as a professional, I have become convinced that these simple principles are sufficient for anyone to undertake, responsibly and productively, the work of exploring dreams, looking for their deeper meanings. Over that same period, I also have become reluctantly convinced that if dream work is undertaken with basic assumptions significantly different from the ones just discussed, there is an ironic tendency for dream work itself to become yet another instrument of tyranny in our lives. It is ironic, because the better the "ahas!" the more tyrannous the work tends to become.

Finding the Truth Within

If anyone involved in the work fails to understand that the "aha!" is a function of the dreamer's own previously unconscious, not-yet-speech ripe understanding, and comes from within, then the better and more moving the potentially life-shaping "ahas!" of insight are that flow out of the work, the more likely it is that the dreamer will return to the seemingly external source of wisdom for "more." People who make this mistake indefinitely postpone their arrival at the center of their life experience, with their own creative and decision-making powers intact. In my experience, this is true even when the mistakenly identified external source of wisdom and authority is as abstract as a theory or a book, and it is particularly rampant when the unconscious projection of authority is focused on an actual person—whether therapist, spiritual counselor, trance-channel, or hair-dresser. Whenever the dreamer or the dream worker forgets the ever-present influence of unconscious projection, then the better the "ahas!" are and the more tyrannous the work tends to become. The best way that I know to avoid this ironic pitfall is by following the set of basic hints for projective group dream work outlined above.

Dream Work as a Spiritual Discipline

When dream work is undertaken in this "If it were my dream" fashion, it regularly transcends the limitations of a mere intellectual exercise in analyzing symbols and begins to transform into a spiritual discipline. Any activity, regularly undertaken, that reliably generates greater conscious awareness and understanding of the deepest sources and patterns of meaning and value in my life and the lives of others (in other words, any activity that increases the experience of the ultimate worth of self, of others, and of life itself, generating an increased felt sense of the presence of the Divine in the process) is, by definition, a spiritual discipline. Group dream work, especially when it is done in the "If it were my dream" format, regularly has this effect.

Let me offer an example of experiential group dream work to illustrate these principles.

A woman in the last third of her life, an avowed atheist with a schizophrenic son and a healthy daughter, dreams:

> I am a disembodied observer. I see a man, a "potter," talking with a woman. The woman is a great admirer of the potter's work and asks him to make a piece especially for her. He agrees and makes her a small bowl, about the size of two hands cupped together. When he gives her the bowl, she admires it greatly and says that it's "too beautiful" to actually use. Instead, she wants to display the bowl as an art piece, and so she asks the potter to modify his creation so that "invisible fish line" can be strung through it, and it can be hung up on the wall. She goes on to say the inside of the bowl is as beautiful as the outside, and she wants to be able to display it either side out and shift from one view to the other. The potter takes the bowl and, "against his better aesthetic judgment," drills two holes in the base and two holes in the rim. He has to "reinforce" the thin rim of the bowl to accommodate the unplanned-for holes. He does all this because he is in love with the woman and wants to give her a love gift that is to her liking. She accepts the

> bowl with rapture but does not notice the potter's gentle hints about wanting to court her and have a more intimate and personal relationship with her. Time goes by, and the woman calls the potter up in great distress and tells him that the bowl is broken. He visits her house and she shows him the bowl split in half. The potter takes the two pieces from her and drops them, shattering them into even more fragments on the floor. He departs and creates another, even more special bowl for his love, even though she has not asked him to do so. He changes the design so that there is now a rhythmic pattern of holes all around the rim of the new bowl, fully integrated into the aesthetic conception, as well as regularly spaced holes incorporated into the base. He makes a single loop of invisible fish line that passes through two of the holes in the rim and two of the holes in the base, so that the bowl can be easily displayed on the wall to exhibit either side. He brings the new bowl to the woman and gives it to her as a gift. She is ecstatic to receive the beautiful, new bowl. The potter believes that her joy means that she really does want to have a deeper relationship with him. He proposes marriage to her, but she rebuffs him—she loves his work, but she doesn't love him . . . The disembodied observing dreamer feels "sadness" for the potter and his unrequited love.

The dreamer brought this dream to a seminar focused on "Dreams and Spiritual Development" held at a Catholic college near San Francisco, California, in the summer of 1999. The work exploring the dream was carried out in a classroom setting with seven other students, lifelong learners as well as graduate students in counseling. Each member of the class shared and worked one of her dreams in depth with the full participation of all the other members of the class, using the "If it were my dream" technique.

Working with the Dream in the Group

When the group began to explore this dream of "The Two Bowls & the Potter's Unrequited Love," using these techniques of facilitating group interaction, a number of "ahas!" emerged. The first set of shared "ahas!" occurred during the initial exploration of the dreamer's strongly felt sense of the beauty of the two bowls. An "aesthetic response" to *beauty* in the dream world is very often an archetypal metaphor of the encounter with deeper psychospiritual truth. When Keats says in *Ode to a Grecian Urn,* "Truth is beauty, and beauty truth / That's all we know, and all we need to know," he is giving voice to an ancient archetypal symbolic equation. In the waking world, there are undoubtedly many things that present a deceptively beautiful face to the observer, a face that hides all manner of nastiness, but in the dream world, the experience that something is *beautiful* is a very reliable indication that the beauty in the dream is a living symbol of a higher and deeper order of truth in the dreamer's life, even if that order of truth may also involve sorrow and bitterness.

As we explored the dream further, it came out that the dreamer harbored some bitterness about the "unfairness" of her son's schizophrenia and the tragic limitation of her son's (and her own) life and ability to love and be loved that is the result. It was, in fact, one of the things that turned her toward atheism, since she found it impossible to sustain belief in an "all-good" deity who would randomly visit such a scourge upon the innocent. At this level, the dream depicts in symbolic narrative form the dreamer's quarrel with the Divine. At the same time, the woman's excitement over the second bowl is a symbolic representation of her transpersonal gratitude for her second, beautiful, healthy child. It was a shock to her realize, as demonstrated by her own "aha!," that she "loved the potter's work but not the potter"; that is to say, she loved her children, but not the Divine, which she had once believed was the source of all love.

Unrequited Love as a Symbol of Spiritual Longing

The love of individuals (or the lack of it) in a dream is often a metaphor of even deeper longings and desires, the most compelling of which is the universal, archetypal desire of all human beings to live in a universe that makes sense, the deep desire to inhabit a cosmos that is not simply a meaningless consequence of random events and brutish collisions. All humans have a deep desire to live lives that are animated by a deep and reliable sense of purpose and value beyond their physical and emotional comfort or discomfort at any given moment. The longing to relate to something "beautiful" that is infinitely larger than the waking ego or the individual life remains alive in our unconscious depths, even when conscious experience has led to the abandonment of active psychospiritual searching and struggle. The exigencies of alienated, postmodern, industrial life often lead to deep disappointment and disillusionment with flawed religious institutions, and to the sense of frustrated idealism. These feelings often emerge as a consequence of even the most sincere spiritual search. In this dream, that spiritual longing for deeper meaning was given shape by the "potter's" unrequited love as well as by the dream woman's attraction to "his work." It also echoes in the disembodied dreamer's sense of "sadness" upon realizing that the "potter's" desire to love more deeply and intimately is not shared by the woman.

Unprepared for the Final Exam

The problem of disappointment and disillusionment occasioned by apparently failed religious and spiritual search is very common in our postmodern world. It regularly finds symbolic shape in dreams and in the psychospiritual struggles of many dreamers. Any person using dreams as a focus of spiritual counseling and direction is almost certain to meet this issue in the work with clients. It is important to understand that this drama takes many apparently different symbolic forms. In this dream, it is given shape by the potter's unrequited love, and it is also often reflected in the very common dream of "discovering that I have been enrolled in a class that I totally forgot about. I never went to class. I never did any of the reading, and now I suddenly discover that it is time to take the final exam!" Whenever a person abandons his or her deepest spiritual longings and unresolved questions because of the frustrated failure to find adequate answers, that person increases the likelihood that he or she will have a version of this "classic" dream.

The ubiquitous appearance of this dream, at the larger, collective level, is quite an indictment of Western civilization in general and Western higher education in particular. Widened access to higher education and the products of scientific/technological achievement have offered the promise of answering our deepest questions about ourselves and the nature of the universe, and have delivered only larger and more complicated versions of the same unanswered questions and unsolved psychospiritual problems. At first glance, it might seem utterly absurd that two images as diverse as the potter's unrequited love and the anxiety occasioned by final exam in the forgotten course could be related to one another in any meaningful way, but in fact, they are *both* clear symbolic and emotional metaphors of unfulfilled spiritual longings.

We Each Have Our Own "Broken Bowls"

As the group continued to project on this dream, it became clear that at one level, the "beautiful broken bowl" was a metaphor of the dreamer's schizophrenic son and the "beautiful replacement bowl" a symbolic picture of her sane and healthy daughter. At another level, the "bowls" were symbols for injured and uninjured parts of her own psyche. The "broken bowl" is particularly resonant with the child's simplistic faith that was "shattered" by the adolescent's initial encounters with the world's imperfections and later with the adult's experience of "unfair" birth defects. The "second, even more beautiful bowl" symbolizes her slowly dawning intuition that the significance of creation, (the stunning beauty and grandeur of nature and the amazing human capacity to create) is greater than the seemingly individual and separate things created.

At yet another level, the "two bowls" evoke the two halves of the dreamer's adult life: the first half, when she was married and working to serve her family and hold it together, and the second half, after being deserted by her husband who left her with the two children to look after on her own. At that level, the "holes" drilled into the first "bowl" represent the disruptions and unexpected disappointments of her early married life and her efforts to make the best of them. The "beautiful bowl with the holes 'fired' directly into the clay" represent the ironic truth that it was only after being deserted by her husband and facing the "imperfect" world of single motherhood (particularly single motherhood of a child with dramatic special needs) that she began to discover the depth of her own "beautiful" authentic character and deeply creative energies. It was as a result of these "holes" and this trial by fire that she began to have a more conscious appreciation of the true extent of her own strength and potential.

Deus Faber

The "potter" has long been an archetypal metaphor of the divine demiurge, *Deus Faber,* who longs to enter into and love his creation even more fully, if we will only open ourselves to it. Even in this dream of an avowed atheist, the "potter" turned out (as confirmed by the dreamer's own "aha!") to be an image of God longing to love and be loved more fully.

As we explored the dream further, the "potter" also emerged as a metaphor of personal loneliness. At one level, *everything* in a dream is a symbolic representation of aspects of the dreamer's own psyche and character. At this level, the dreamer *is* the "potter." The "potter" in the dream is not only an archetypal figure, "he" also stands for the dreamer's own frustrated desire to love and be loved by more than just the members of her immediate family. This personal loneliness, in turn, also reflects her previously unacknowledged longing to be related to something *more* than the ethical ideals and principles that for her, decades earlier, took the place of her belief in a personal deity. Working with this dream, she realized with a shock that this part of her that longs to love and be loved in a more transcendent fashion, both personally and spiritually, is not just a childish atavism but a robust and valuable part of her mature psyche. The exploration of dreams almost always leads to the revelation of intimate personal details of the dreamer's emotional life. Most often, through sharing these details, as they are revealed and emerge from dreams, the energies for psychospiritual growth, transformation, and healing are awakened and released.

The Shared Benefits of the Work

As the group continued to explore this dream, other people in the seminar began to realize that the ability to imagine and project upon this narrative was affording them an unparalleled opportunity to explore their own particular versions of the universal "frustrated longing to love and be loved MORE . . ." Several participants experienced their own "ahas!" about the ways that their own abandoned or disappointed spiritual searches had caused them to place an undue burden on their interpersonal love relationships. Because their desire for personal, direct experience of the Divine had been abandoned out of frustration, several people realized that they had unconsciously tried to make their human loves carry the weight of the longing for divine love. Of course, this impossible demand had made these inevitably imperfect relationships seem all the more inadequate.

Each person in the group began to see some of the emotional/relational dramas in their own lives more clearly. There was a shared "aha!" that some of them were also "loving the bowl(s)" without realizing that they were also "gifts of love from the potter." Several people commented that one of the things the group work with the dream was making more clear was their competitive desire to put their long-term loves and relationships "on display"—to " drill holes in them and hang them on the wall for others to appreciate," worrying about "how things *look*" and "what other people think" without giving the same attention to how those relationships actually *are.*

Spiritual Search and Alchemy

The exploration of this dream points to the fact that atheism is often just a thinly conscious abreaction, an instinctively outraged response to deep pain, injustice, and incredible life difficulties, and not a true rejection of the possibility of more conscious relationship with the Divine. Atheism is often just an emotionally theatrical stage of a lover's quarrel.

The work with this dream also demonstrated another great spiritual truth: that only when a person's spiritual perspective extends completely into the darkest and most distressing and evil aspects of both personal and collective life—into the most noxious and base of base matter, as the alchemists avow—can the true gold of authentic and reliable spiritual perspective be created.

Throughout our lives, our dreams continually bring us metaphors of the worst that is in us and the worst that is in the world (along with all the other joyous and wonderful things our dreams do!), to provide us with the opportunity of turning our own base matter, whatever it may be, into the gold of authentic and reliable spiritual experience.

Any spiritual perspective that systematically avoids "the worst," either personal or collective, in the final analysis will also reveal itself to be illusory "false gold." When a dreamer who has used piety to shield him or herself from confronting his her worst demons faces death, alone, confronted with the previously repressed and denied worst things (which the false religious and spiritual perspective has been carefully designed to suppress and ignore), there appears to be no hope. In such a situation, spontaneously manifesting grace alone can lift the dreamer up from despair. It has been said that "Luck favors the prepared mind." It could be said equally that "Grace favors the sincere soul," and attention to dreams is a profoundly reliable touchstone of sincerity, even beyond the pitfalls of self-deception. Dreams are the eternal enemy of premature closure and self-deception. Even casual attention to our dreams makes it much more difficult to ignore these worst-case aspects of our lives and psyches. When we confront and embrace our own most problematic and difficult experiences and desires in our dreams, it is much more likely that we will deal with these aspects of ourselves more responsibly and creatively in waking life. In this way, we also open ourselves to the Divine.

Conclusion

Working with dreams in spiritual direction and companioning, particularly with the clear acknowledgment of inevitable projection on and from all parties, can be an invaluable practice for the only alchemy that really matters—transforming even our worst fears and experiences into the dance of deepening encounter with the Divine.

History is filled with examples of profound creative breakthroughs, innovations, and psychospiritual insights that were generated first as experiences in dreams. This ancient and natural source of wisdom, creative inspiration, and more conscious connection to the Divine is as available to us postmoderns as it was to our ancestors. The face of contemporary intellectual fashion may have turned momentarily away from the "magic mirror" of the dream, but anyone who is truly interested in the creative, transformative gifts dreams have to offer will soon discover that making the effort to remember and share dream experience with others, joining with them in the serious play of uncovering their deeper meanings, is one of the most enjoyable and mutually productive activities yet discovered.

Notes

1. Emily Bronte, *Wuthering Heights* (New York: Washington Square Books, 1972), p. 94.

12

Wish, Conflict, and Awareness

Freud and the Problem of the "Dream Book"

Bertram J. Cohler[*]

Freud's study *The Interpretation of Dreams* (1900), often referred to as the "Dream Book," remains a controversial work even a century after its publication. In this work Sigmund Freud (1856–1939) both demonstrates a technique for understanding subjectivity and elaborates a theory for understanding mental life. However, it was founded on perspectives from the neurosciences (Sulloway 1979), and there has been considerable critical discussion regarding Freud's theory of dream formation (Fiss 2000, Hobson 1988, Hartmann 1998; Pribram and Gill 1976). Recognizing the validity of this critique (which Freud himself, as a biologist of the mind [Sulloway, 1979], would likely have endorsed), the "Dream Book" still remains Freud's most systematic and programmatic statement of a theory of mental life, informing his subsequent work across half a century and providing an approach to the study of mental life that has had a major influence on contemporary culture (Freud 1930).

Of central importance to clinical and cultural perspectives alike is Freud's claim made in the book that attention as a mental state is determined by a tabooed wish founded in early childhood but preserved for a lifetime. However, this wish has both force and direction, seeking satisfaction, forcing a compromise in which the wish is partially satisfied through adopting a disguise that is both socially and personally acceptable. So-called "unintended" actions and slips of the tongue (Freud 1901), hysterical and obsessional symptoms (Freud 1896), sublimations reflected in culturally valued artistic expressions (Freud 1910a), and enactments anew in relationships with others across a lifetime (Freud 1914) all are similarly determined by this socially reprehensible wish for intimacy with the parent of the opposite gender arising spontaneously as a consequence of child care within the bourgeois family of the West. Freud's rhetorical problem in writing this book is that he must convince the reader of the existence of another level of awareness, the unconscious (noted by Freud as the system Ucs), which by definition is not knowable and that is founded on desire experienced within the family of early childhood.

Further, recognizing the controversial nature of this approach to the study of awareness, in the effort to convince the reader of the validity of this claim, Freud cannot rely on the accounts of his analysands, for they could be all too easily dismissed as the musing of persons suffering psychological distress. Instead, believing that his own intellectual stature and his reflexive self-awareness provides evidence less likely to be suspect than the accounts of his analysands, Freud relied on his own experiences in order to show the validity of his claim. Freud is both concerned about the impact of self-revelation for his professional reputation and yet too intellectually honest not to make such revelations, as they bear on his effort to convince the reader of the validity of his perspective regarding the foundation of conscious awareness. As a result, Freud employed a rhetorical strategy in which he provided the evidence that he believed would support his claim, but did so in a discrete reference in a footnote to a paper on the role of early memories and memory recall, written during the same time that he was writing the "Dream Book," and published in a scientific journal (Freud 1899).

The "Dream Book" and the Discovery of the Nuclear Neurosis of Childhood

When he began the "Dream Book" early in 1898, Freud had more than a decade of experience working in that genre of psychotherapy that he termed psychoanalysis. In his editorial introduction to the text, translator James Strachey tells us (1953: xiv) that by 1895 Freud had obtained evidence from his psychoanalytic work that his analysands felt it necessary to bring into association with each other any ideas of which they were presently aware. The belief that we continually make meanings of lived experience, connecting our thoughts with each other in the continuing search after a coherent narrative, is essential to the claim that mental life can be understood as motivated. Those thoughts of which we are aware and the connections between these thoughts are founded on wishes first arising in early childhood, seeking satisfaction across the course of life.

It was only following his father's death in October 1896 and his recognition of the complex and mixed feelings that accompanied his mourning that Freud began his period of self-scrutiny leading to recognition of both sadness and also some feeling of joy following his father's death, which he recognized as ambivalence. In turn, this ambivalence reflected rivalry of son with father, inevitable as a part of the family romance of son and daughter seeking the affection of the opposite-gender parent. Well-read in classical texts and long fascinated with Sophocles drama (Rudnytsky 1987), Freud saw in his own case, as more generally, ambivalence based on this early struggle of little boys and girls for affection and rivalry within the family as the basis for all later relationships.[1]

The "Dream Book" was published 1899 but carried a 1900 inscription in order to reflect a modern approach to the study of mental life. It is significant that this book, which is so symbolic of modernity and its discontents, was published on the eve of the new century. As such the book stands on the portal between the old and the new. Ernest Jones (1953) reports that Freud regarded the "Dream Book," together with the volume of three essays on the theory of sexuality, as the most important books of his career of more than a half century and twenty-three volumes of written work. Reflecting the importance that Freud attached to this work, he saw the "dream book" through eight revisions over more than a quarter of a century from 1900 to 1926. It should be noted that the book was written backward: Chapter VII, providing a theory of mental life founded on the study of dreams, was actually a revision of an effort, published only posthumously (Freud 1895), to develop a model of mental functioning fashioned in terms of the neurosciences (then as now a preoccupation of psychoanalytic explanation). The central chapters (II–VI) were written following completion of chapter VII, and then chapter I was written (essentially a review of the literature on dreaming, dispelling notions of dreams either as prophecy or as merely expressions of superficial wishes easily understood in terms of a compendium of such dreams).[2]

Freud had been aware since 1895 of the formulation, stated in chapter III, that dreams are founded on wishes. Reviewing Freud's interest in the psychology of dream life, Jones (1953), in his encyclopedic biography, maintains that Freud had long been interested in the psychology of dream life. However prior to his self-analysis, beginning in July of 1897 and nearly a year after his father's death, while struggling with the complex feelings with which this grief had aroused, Freud had not appreciated two central aspects of dreaming which became the focus of the "Dream Book": Dreams reflect wishes that are socially and personally reprehensible, and these are determined in turn by nuclear wishes founded in the experiences of early childhood. The first hint of this discovery appears in a draft ("N") from May 1897, in which Freud observes that "It seems as though this death wish is directed in sons against their fathers and in daughters against their mothers" (1897/1985: 250). Some five months later (October 1897), Freud reported to his colleague in Berlin, Wilhelm Fliess, that he is preoccupied by his self-analysis and observes that "I have found, in my own case too, [the phenomenon of] being in love with my mother and jealous of my father, and I now consider it to be a universal event of early childhood" (1897/1985: 272).

Freud's "Specimen" Dream of Irma's Injection and the Problem of Revealing the Wish

Freud begins his substantive discussion in chapter II with an example, his so-called specimen dream of Irma's injection, which he describes as the first fully analyzed dream. He concludes that the wish portrayed in the dream was that of the wish to be innocent of a series of possible accusations against him in the recent past. The problem with the chapter is that, having made the claim that the Irma dream is a completely analyzed dream, Freud's discussion falls short of his own goal. In section C of chapter VII, Freud informs the reader that:

> My supposition is that a conscious wish can only become a dream-instigator if it succeeds in awakening an unconscious wish with the same tenor and in obtaining reinforcement from it . . . we bear firmly in mind the part played by the unconscious wish and then seek for information from the psychology of the neuroses. We learn from the latter than an unconscious idea is as such quite incapable of entering the preconscious and that it can only exercise any effect there by establishing a connection with an idea which already belongs to the preconscious by transferring its intensity on to it and by getting itself "covered" by it. Here we have the fact of "transference" which provides an explanation of so many striking phenomena in the mental life of neurotics. (591, 601)

The problem with the discussion of the dream of Irma's injection is that while Freud carefully informs the reader of the day-residue and of the conscious wish—that he not be held responsible for Irma's slow progress in her treatment—he does not reveal the nature of the unconscious wish whose intensity is transferred on to the day residue. Without this aspect of the explanation, the analysis is incomplete. Assuming that Freud is aware of the contradiction in his discussion of the Irma dream, the problem posed by his analysis of the dream in this chapter is in finding out how he resolves the rhetorical dilemma that, while he claims this as the first fully analyzed dream, he does not make reference to those unconscious determinants, which, as he tells us in Section C of Chapter VII, are essential for the complete analysis of a dream. What Freud does is to use a series of dreams throughout the text to provide an answer to the question of the unconscious wish instigating this "specimen" dream.

Freud is well aware that the explanation of the origins of the wish to be held innocent of Irma's failure to make progress in her treatment is but the tip of a psychic iceberg whose origins lie within the system unconscious, constructed in early childhood, and continuing to exercise an influence over mental life. The problem is solved by reordering the presentation of dreams across the text, which moves from surface to depth as the book progresses, in a manner that follows the model of the mental topography portrayed in chapter VII of the "Dream Book": The Irma dream is the surface, or conscious awareness, while the Botanical Monograph represents the unconscious wish. Most significantly, an innocuous footnote in the first discussion of the Botanical Monograph dream (205) to another paper, published separately but written during the period of the writing of the "Dream Book" (Freud 1899), provides the clue to the entire work, since it portrays the nuclear neurosis that determines all else.

The report of the Irma dream is among the most carefully studied in all of Freud's work. As a result, we know far more than Freud had ever intended about the circumstances of this dream, including those supposed "indifferent" events of the time immediately preceding the dream that served as the day residue or the kernel around which the dream is formed. Imagine a sultry summer night in July 1895, in the hills overlooking Vienna. The lights of the city float languidly over the horizon. Sitting on the veranda of an old hotel with a grand foyer, now converted for residential use, Freud and his visitor from the city are relaxing after a satisfying meal with cigars and conversation, the visitor's gift of a bottle of anise liquor on the table before them.

The visitor, Oscar Rie (Otto of the dream), Freud's protégé at the children's neurological hospital and a promising young academic pediatrician, is collaborating with Freud on a monograph on infantile paralysis. Otto and the Freuds are both friends with the Freuds' neighbors whose daughter, Anna Hammerschlag Lichtheim (Irma in the dream), is one of Freud's analysands at that time. Freud's wife has also just informed him that she has invited her good friend Anna Hammerschalg to her forthcoming birthday party. Anna's father, Samuel, was Freud's esteemed Hebrew instructor in Gymnasium, and he is none too comfortable with Freud's daily sessions with Anna, a recent widow after a tragically short one-year marriage to Rudolph, a wealthy merchant, who died of tuberculosis. Rudolph's brother was a neurologist fervently opposed to Freud's theories. Freud cannot resist fishing for a compliment, and asks Oscar how he thinks Anna is recovering from her recent loss. Oscar, feeling a bit awkward at this request for information, which breaches the frame of the analysis, replies cautiously that Anna is doing better, but that she is not yet cured.

The conversation goes on to other subjects, but the momentary rebuff in Freud's search for assurance of the success of his work continues to trouble him as he prepares for bed. That night he dreams that there is a large reception hall; there is a party that they are throwing for numerous guests, including his patient Irma. One of these guests appears to question Irma's progress while Freud seeks to be held innocent for this apparent lack of progress, as well as for three other incidents: the death of an old lady treated by Freud who died while on holiday and under the care of another physician whose dirty syringe led to her death following an attack of phlebitis; the death of his admired teacher Fleischl von Marxow, one of Brucke's laboratory assistants who overdosed on cocaine recommended by Freud for resolving continuous pain caused by a laboratory accident; and the wish to be held innocent of an operation on Emma Eckstein, one of Freud's first analysands, and perhaps the first person after Freud himself to practice psychoanalysis.

Concern regarding the old lady actually treated by another physician is significant, not only because it reflects Freud's distaste for aging, including his own, but also because she is a "stand-in" for his nursemaid of childhood, Resi Wittek, a devout Catholic who spoke to the young Freud in Czech much of the time and took him with her to mass. Resi may have been involved in a seduction of Freud when he was between ages two and four (Krull 1986). Freud (1897/1985) himself recalls being cared for by his nursemaid around the time of the death of his younger brother Julius, who was born when Freud was about eleven months old and died of enteritis at about six months of age, and the death of his young mother's own brother, also named Julius, who died of tuberculosis one month before the infant's death. Freud (October 3, 1897/1985) reports to Fliess that the self-reproach accompanying his wish for the death of this early competitor for his mother's affection had haunted him all of his life. Further, Freud's mother Amalie herself is portrayed by Krull (1986) as a very pretty but cold and volatile woman who adored her son Sigismund.

In the aftermath of these two closely spaced losses in his mother's life, Freud's mother may have withdrawn into her own grief, leaving the nursemaid as the particularly significant person in the young Freud's life. Krull (1986), who has been able to read the unedited Freud letter to Fliess, reports that the letter goes on to narrate that Resi chided Freud for being clumsy and not being able to do anything, that they bathed together in water that her self-care had turned reddish, and that he recalled being chased up the stairs by Resi. Freud comments:

> Now these other dreams were based on a recollection of a nurse in whose charge I had been from some date during my earliest infancy till I was two and a half. I even retain an obscure conscious memory of her. According to what I was told not long ago by my mother, she was old and ugly, but very sharp and efficient. From what I can infer from my own dreams her treatment of me was not always excessive in its amiability and her words could be harsh if I failed to reach the required standard of cleanliness . . . it is reasonable to suppose that the child loved the old woman who taught him these lessons, in spite of her rough treatment of him. (1900: 280–281)

It is clear that Freud at least experienced in thought or in deed some seduction and accompanying erotic stimulation at the hands of his nursemaid.

The third person of whom Freud wished to be absolved was Fleischl, his friend and laboratory instructor who had injured his hand in a laboratory accident some time prior to meeting Freud. It is well known that Freud had a brief cocaine addiction from which he cured himself during his self-analysis. Freud had been using cocaine medically for some time, including as a topical anesthetic during surgery. He had participated with Dr. Konigstein (of the Botanical Monograph dream) in an operation on his father's cataracts; Freud had suggested that the distinguished opthamologist attempt this surgery using cocaine.

The Irma dream refers obliquely to the wish to be absolved of yet another event, surgery performed on Freud's analysand Emma Eckstein. Freud and Fliess had been discussing for several years the place of sexuality in the neuroses. This position was presented systematically in a book Fliess published in 1902 reporting on a presumed causal connection between the nose and the genitals. Fliess had maintained that the seat of the neuroses was in the nose and that an operation on the turbinal bones or bridge of the nose would resolve the neurosis. Hypochondriacal, Freud was anxious to have this operation performed upon himself, and Fliess did perform that operation in February 1895, using Freud's beloved cocaine as a topical anesthetic. During the same time that Fliess was in Vienna, Freud asked him to examine a young woman, Emma Eckstein, with whom he had just begun working, and whose abdominal symptoms he believed to be of nasal origin. Fliess undertook this second operation as well, and with Freud serving as his assistant in the surgery, the two men operated on Freud's hapless patient.

Initially disclosed by Freud's own physician, Max Schur (1966), and later elaborated in some detail by F. Hartman (1983), Grinstein (1968), Masson (1984), Anzieu (1986), and others, this surgery and Freud's response has become something of a scandal in the popular press. Masson (1984) maintained that Anna Freud and Ernest Jones conspired to cover up the embarrassing incident. Emma Eckstein (1865–1924) would have remained a shadowy figure in psychoanalysis were it not for Masson's detailed exposition of her life and contributions to psychoanalysis. Eckstein came from a prominent socialist family in Vienna. Terribly afflicted by her hysterical symptoms, she was unable to walk and spent much of her time as an invalid confined to her bed.

It is still puzzling why Freud should have encouraged Fliess to operate. Fliess had virtually no experience as a surgeon, and the operation had no documented successes. However, both men believed that symptoms could be displaced from one part of the body to another, Freud as a psychological symptom and Fliess as a physical symptom. Fliess also maintained that there was a close connection between menstrual pain and masturbation, and believed that an operation on the nose would cure both problems. Freud worshipped Fliess, indeed, to such an extent that he had permitted Fliess to operate on himself. Further, he sought increased closeness to Fliess and enhanced collaboration.

Masson (1984) maintains that Fliess's treatment would have appeared as unorthodox in 1895 as at the present time; however, Freud appreciated unorthodox approaches, since he regarded his own approach as revolutionary. Archivist for the Freud collection, Masson was in a position to see the complete correspondence and has provided a particularly lurid and dreary account that goes even beyond the more acceptable presentation of Schur, who was Freud's physician during his illness, and Grinstein, whose discussion of Freud's dreams is the most complete to date. Within a month following this operation, Eckstein developed severe swelling and hemorrhaged. After the senior surgery consultant, Gersuny, was called in, it emerged that Fliess had left a quantity of gauze in the wound. Eckstein's condition worsened across the weeks of March and April 1895, and she nearly died on several occasions. Indeed, it was not until the end of May, just two months preceding the fateful dream of July 25, 1895, that Freud was able to write Fliess that their patient was finally recovering from surgery.

Understanding the factors that led Freud to encourage Fliess to undertake this operation is central to showing the infantile unconscious wish and conflict underlying the dream of July 25, 1895 that would fulfill Freud's claim that this was the first complete analysis of a dream. Freud recognized the factors leading to this decision as a consequence of his self-analysis in the intervening two-year period; portrayal of that conflict is necessary in order that he might live up to his own promise that the dream of Irma's injection was the first completely analyzed dream. (The dream analysis cannot be complete unless the latent dream wish is portrayed.) Again, Freud's need to protect his reputation made it difficult for him to explain why he decided to proceed with the reckless surgery on Emma Eckstein that nearly took her life.

The Botanical Monograph Dream and the Secret Revealed

The question is what motivated Freud to undertake this unnecessary surgery, which he, as a prudent and sober physician, knew was not appropriate. The clue to this question and the motivation for this surgery is found in the Botanical Monograph dream of March 10, 1898 (Mautner 1991). It is important to recognize that in the first edition of the "dream book," presentation of the dream of the Botanical Monograph (pp. 202–209) was not as widely separated from the specimen dream as appeared in the seven later editions in which much additional material had been inserted. The Botanical Monograph dream is told in two different places within the text (pp. 202–209, 315–318). The two tellings of the dream differ in one critical respect; the first telling includes the additional information "as though it had been taken from the herbarium." The day residue, an apparently innocuous event of the time immediately preceding the dream, which provides the kernel for the dream, included looking at a new book on the genus Cyclamen in a bookshop window and receipt of a letter from Fliess describing his fantasy of the whole manuscript lying open before him.

In the dream, Freud saw a book before him and was turning over a folded colored plate. There was a preserved copy of a plant, as if taken from a herbarium. The most significant dreams often are those that are highly condensed. The next set of associations take Freud back to boyhood and the dried specimen of plant. Reporting his associations to this dream, Freud recalls that these dried specimens were crucifers which, it turns out, were the only species he later had difficulty identifying on his medical school botany exam. (This exam, together with his other examinations, earned him much-coveted honors.) Crucifers are then associated to a third species of flower, the compositae, of which the vegetable artichoke is a member. Artichokes were his favorite flower; his wife frequently brought them to him (recall the earlier association to forgetting to give flowers); artichokes are eaten by pulling apart the leaves.

Freud recalls his pleasure as a student at seeing another kind of leaf, the colored plates in books. Recollection of this enjoyment at looking at these colored plates then recalls a scene when he was five, in which he and his next youngest sister, three-year old Anna, had been given a book by their father containing colored plates of a journey through Persia, which they were able to destroy. Freud (Page 205) continues: "the picture of the two of us blissfully pulling the book to pieces (leaf by leaf, like an artichoke, I found myself saying), was almost the only plastic memory I retained from that period of life."

Freud then recalls that he had been a bookworm, again referring to the herbarium, his hobby of learning out of books, his enjoyment now of preserving rather than destroying the colored plates, the large bills he later runs up at the bookseller as a result of his interest in owning such books. This hobby of collecting and saving is contrasted with his criticism of his father permitting he and his sister to pull a book with colored plate to pieces.

At this point, Freud introduces a footnote "2," "Cf. my paper on screen memories [Freud, 1899]." This discrete footnote referring to the screen memory paper unlocks the unconscious determinants of the dream of Irma's injection and fulfills Freud's requirement for the analysis of a dream, that it must include infantile determinants. (The use of the footnote and the "secret" it contains may be understood as a compromise between Freud's effort to preserve his professional reputation, disguising a revelatory and somewhat embarrassing incident from his youth, and his intellectual honesty and effort to show the impact of early childhood experiences upon adult mental life).[3] In this paper Freud describes the analysis of a young man with a university education, a man whose age and social position are not unlike himself, who has an annoying travel phobia.[4]

The screen memory, from a time when the subject of the memory (Freud) was three or four, is of playing with his nephew John and sister Pauline in a mountain meadow in which there were large numbers of dandelions. The three of them are picking bouquets of the yellow flowers.[5] Freud then narrates that: "each of us is holding a bunch of flowers we have already picked. The little girl has the best bunch; and, as though by mutual agreement, we—the two boys—fall on her and snatch away her flowers" (1899/1953: 311). Pauline then goes running up the meadow. As consolation, a peasant woman watching the scene gives her a big piece of black bread. The two boys see this offering and run up the meadow for their share, which the peasant woman cuts with a long knife!

The screen memory paper raises a number of issues regarding Freud's struggle to portray the origins of his neurosis. Recall the issue of Emma Eckstein's operation and the question of why Freud joined Fliess in a sadistic operation with little medical justification. Recall next that the footnote is inserted just following Freud's recollection that he and his next younger sister, two years apart in age, were pulling the leaves (plates) out of a travel book with their father's permission. In the screen memory paper Freud places great emphasis on the action of snatching the flowers away from the girl as an allusion to deflowering her, which then connects the artichokes of the Botanical Monograph dream, the pulling of the plates from the travel book, and the actions that Freud and John carried out with Pauline.

The operation on Emma Eckstein was an enactment anew of another deflowering whose origins were out of conscious awareness and that symbolically represented a repetition of Freud and John and their childhood sexual explorations in the meadow with Pauline. In each case, two men were operating on a woman in a sadistic manner. Freud wishes not be to be held responsible in the Irma dream for the actions he and John performed upon Pauline in the meadow that afternoon and that are symbolically represented by the yellow flowers. It is possible to explain the operation being performed on Freud himself as yet another effort to make retribution for the action of that afternoon, turning active into passive and subjecting himself to Fliess's cruel operation.

The question, then, is posed regarding the determinants of the first enactment, the meadow scene reported in the screen memory essay. Again, we are helped by Freud's honesty in his correspondence with Fliess. In the letter of October 3, 1897, Freud lists three factors that would account for his infantile neurosis:

> . . . the old man plays no active role in my case . . . I drew an inference by analogy from myself onto him; that in my case the "prime originator" was an ugly, elderly, but clever woman who told me a great deal about God Almighty and hell and who instilled in me a high opinion of my own capacities; that later [between two and two and a half years] my libido toward matrem was awakened, namely on the occasion of a journey with her from Leipzig to Vienna, during which we must have spent the night together and there must have been an opportunity of seeing her nudam (you inferred from the consequences of this for your son long ago, as a remark revealed to me); that I greeted my one-year-younger brother (who died after a few months) with adverse wishes and genuine childhood jealousy; and that his death left the germ of self-reproaches in me. I have also long known the companions of my misdeeds between the ages of one and two years; it is my nephew, a year older than myself, who is now living in Manchester, and who visited us in Vienna when I was fourteen years old. The two of us seem occasionally to have behaved cruelly to my niece who was a year younger. This nephew and this younger brother have determined, then, what is neurotic but also what is intense, in all my friendships. You yourself have seen my travel anxiety at its height. (October 3, 1897/1985: 268).

Two weeks later, still referring to this ugly, clever, governess, Freud observes: "I asked my mother whether she still remembered the nurse. 'Of course,' she said, 'an elderly person, very clever, she was always carrying you off to some church; when you returned home you preached and told us about God Almighty'" (October 15, 1897/1985: 271). Freud goes on to describe his mother's discovery during her confinement with Anna that this nursemaid had been a thief, stealing from the children and later serving time in prison for this misdeed.

Based on the enactment in the dream of Irma's injection, the screen memory paper of 1899, the Botanical Monograph dream written down a year earlier when the screen memory paper was being written, and Freud's recollections in his correspondence with Fliess, we can arrive at the following formulation: Freud is preoccupied with issues of guilt and self-reproach on account first of the death of his next younger brother, Julius, the subject of the usually jealous and hostile wishes of an older brother accompanying the birth of a younger rival for his mother's affection, the experience with his nephew John and his sister Pauline in the meadow, probably at age four, just before the family moved from Freiborg to Vienna (the move occurred when he was four, and not when he was two and a half), and the thinly disguised repetition of this sexual activity with his sister Anna pulling apart plates from the travel book when he was five and she was three (Mautner 1991).

The terror that Resi Wittick instilled in her young charge may well be responsible for the enormous antipathy Freud later showed toward all of religion as represented in the several significant texts on religion, notably *Totem and Taboo* (1913), *The Future of an Illusion* (1927), and *Civilization and its Discontents* (1930). Resi also may have been responsible for Freud's earliest sexual education. Krull (1986) notes Freud's (1905) observation that: "It is well known that unscrupulous nurses put crying children to sleep by stroking their genitals" (1931: 180; 232). Krull wonders if this veiled remark may have applied to Freud. Regardless of the reality, Freud experienced her care as seductive. Krull further observes that:

> There is little doubt but that his nursemaid's relationship with Sigmund had sexual overtones to which the small boy reacted with sexual feelings, for only in this way do Freud's associations to his dreams about the nursemaid become comprehensible . . . it is equally possible that she thought nothing of playing sexual games with him but that at one point she was caught by Freud's parents, and that it was not until then that the child gathered something was wrong . . . he must have suffered violent conflicts, for the combination of active stimulation by adults with threats of castration for self-stimulation must have utterly confused him. (Krull 1986: 121)

This premature experience of sexual stimulation, difficult for a young child to master, was further enhanced by the experience of traveling in his mother's sleeping compartment on the train from Freiborg to Vienna and seeing his mother naked, as he reports in his letter to Fliess. This was yet one additional experience in which he felt sexually stimulated and was unable to respond (one determinant of Freud's phobia of traveling by train). This passive experience of early childhood was then reenacted in an effort at mastery with his younger sister Anna. Mautner (1991) notes that within two weeks of the Botanical Monograph dream, Freud had written to Fliess (June 20, 1898) of a novel portraying a complex triangle involving a mother merged with the image of a maid and a sister, all important figures in Freud's own life. This shows again Freud's guilty preoccupation with the experienced destructive sexual play of his childhood, which was enacted anew in the operation with Fliess on Emma Eckstein as a further effort to master the feelings of being overwhelmed with excitement, perhaps by turning passively endured stimulation into active stimulation.

The sexual play first with Pauline and then with Anna enacted anew in adulthood in the operation on Emma Eckstein shows that Freud was turning passive into active, doing what had been done to him. In his self-analysis, he became aware of the reason for these researches and operations. Having gained this awareness, he then felt particular self-reproach for what he had done but was too honest not to present both the infantile and adult aspects of this collaboration with Fliess, who represented in the operation his nephew John, just as Emma Eckstein stood for both Pauline and his sister Anna.

Conclusion

The secret of the interpretation of dreams is the progressive elaboration of the principle that Freud so clearly states in section C of chapter VII: A dream represents a wish formed in infantile life and formed on the basis of a nuclear wish unacceptable in everyday life, which is partially satisfied through fresh transference of energy across the repression barrier into the system Preconscious where it is potentially accessible to conscious awareness, albeit in an appropriately disguised manner. This wish is disguised through the dream work which consists of the fusing together of several images, condensation, or displacement, placing a situation of greater personal intensity into one of lesser intensity.

The conflict between wish and anti-wish is then disguised or subjected to secondary revision and then is represented by socially constructed understandings of what is reprehensible within a particular culture. It is then told in a story in which images represent the conflict. In Freud's case, the nuclear conflict is determined less by the so-called oedipal configuration related to the family romance than to possibly sexual experiences in Freud's early childhood that fostered both excitement which could not be mastered by the young boy and/or fantasies occasioned by stimulating experiences for this child, both with his nursemaid Resi and also his mother, which were then enacted anew in a disguised manner both in the incident with John and Pauline (two men performing an "operation" on a woman) and, later, in a parallel manner, through the unnecessary operation on Emma Eckstein. Freud's associations to the Botanical Monograph dream provide the evidence necessary for understanding the meaning, out of conscious awareness, for the self-reproaches reflected in the dream of Irma's injection, and fulfill Freud's claim that the Irma dream is indeed the first fully analyzed dream. Indeed, the "Dream Book" is less a theory of dreams than a theory of the origins of mental life and, particularly, a demonstration that the things we think and say are meaningfully connected. These meanings can be explicated through the study of the connections that we report through the study of these associations.

Notes

* Revision of paper presented at St. John's College, Annapolis, Maryland, and Santa Fe, New Mexico, and at the University of Chicago. Discussion of issues presented here with students and staff of the general education course entitled "Self, Culture and Society" at the University of Chicago has been particularly helpful in understanding Freud's "Dream Book." I am particularly indebted to Yaokov Jackson's careful reading and important suggestions for revision of the chapter. For the sake of consistency with the corpus of secondary literature, references in the present text are to the James Strachey translation (one-volume paperback edition), a part of the so-called Standard Edition, a twenty-three volume English translation of all of Freud's psychoanalytic writings, complete with detailed bibliographic notes, and based on the often-revised text through the eighth printing of the book in 1930. However, the Joyce Crick translation, based on the first edition, including important historical notes by Ritchie Robertson that clarify many textual allusions that would have been familiar to the reader in Vienna at the time the book was published, and taking into account critiques of the Strachey translation (Bettelheim 1983; Ornston 1992), is in many ways more readable than the Strachey translation. Unencumbered by Freud's later efforts to clarify and amend his earlier claims, the Crick translation is useful in understanding Freud's initial claims regarding his theory of dreams.

1. The "Dream Book" is itself such a compromise, perhaps making reparation for such ambivalent feelings. Freud makes clear in his 1908 introduction to the second edition of the "Dream Book" that writing the book was an important part of his own work of mourning. The idea of a dream book emerged in discussion and correspondence with Fliess sometime during the autumn of 1897, and several months after beginning his self-analysis. The sequence of events beginning with his father's death, his discovery through his self-analysis of inherent ambivalence regarding feelings toward the same-gender parent, and his effort to write his theory were all of a piece. Indeed, the book may be regarded as the vehicle Freud used to work through his grief following his father's death. Freud belatedly (1900/1908) came to realize this significance for the volume when he concludes the preface to the second edition of the book with the following observation: "this book has a further subjective significance for me personally—a significance which I only grasped after I had completed it. It was, I found, a portion of my own self-analysis, my reaction to my father's death—that is to say, to the most important event, the most poignant loss, of a man's life" (xxvi).
2. We know much about Freud's life and work during the period (1897–1899) when he was working on the "Dream Book" and formulating the concepts on which it is based through his collaboration with Wilhelm Fliess (1858–1928), a physician in

Berlin specializing in disorders of the nose and throat. Initially recommended by Josef Breuer (1842–1925), a senior medical school faculty member who was Freud's early mentor and then collaborator (Breuer and Freud, 1893–95), Fliess sought to learn neurology from Freud. Discovering that they shared a worldview, the two became fast friends, and Freud worked out many of his ideas in occasional meetings and frequent correspondence across the years 1887 to 1904 (Freud 1887–1904/1985). For the sake of convenience, these letters are referred to in the present text by date in the volume edited by Masson (1985). Fliess's widow saved correspondence by Freud, but there is little report of Fliess's responses to Freud's often complex musings regarding the progress of his own self-analysis and his effort to understand the place of wish, fantasy, and memory in mental life.

3. Freud frequently uses footnotes to present ideas that are controversial or not fully worked out. The footnote as a rhetorical device serves the function of being accessory to a text and, presumably, not central to the argument made in the text (Grafton 1997). It is a kind of disguise, permitting insertion of ideas whose very importance is actually highlighted by their absence from the text. The discrete footnote to the screen memory paper (and who actually follows up on such references?) reflects both Freud's effort at discretion and also his concern that he maintain personal and intellectual integrity.
4. Bernfeld (1946) provides considerable detail connecting the phobic man of the screen memory paper with Freud, while Jones (1953) provides additional detail regarding the facial scar that both Freud received in an accident at the age of two and the analysand of the written account shared in common.
5. Freud reports a temporary memory lapse or temporary inhibition in identifying crucifers, yellow flowers including the dandelion in his final medical school examination (1900/1953:204). Bernfeld (1946) reports that on his eightieth birthday, Freud was given a gift of a bunch of *yellow* alpine flowers by his students at the Vienna Institute for Psychoanalysis. Freud very much appreciated receiving them!

References

Anzieu, D. 1986. *Freud's Self-Analysis,* trans. P. Graham. London: Hogarth Press and the Institute of Psychoanalysis.

Bernfeld, S. 1946. "An Unknown Autobiographical Fragment By Freud." *American Imago* 14: 3–19.

Bettelheim, B. 1983. *Freud and Man's Soul.* New York: Knopf.

Fiss, H. 2000. "A 21st Century Look at Freud's Dream Theory." *Journal of the American Academy of Psychoanalysis* 28: 321–340.

Freud, S. 1871–1881/1991. *The Letters of Sigmund Freud to Eduard Silberstein,* ed. W. Boehlich, trans. A. Pomerans. Cambridge, MA: Harvard University Press.

———. 1887–1904/1985. *The Complete Letters of Sigmund Freud to Wilhelm Fliess,* ed. J. Masson. Cambridge, MA: Harvard University Press.

———. 1895/1966. "Project For A Scientific Psychology." In *The Standard Edition of the Complete Psychological Works of Sigmund Freud,* ed. and trans. J. Strachey. London: Hogarth Press, 1: 295–398.

———. 1896/1962. "Further Remarks On The Neuro-Psychoses Of Defence." In *The Standard Edition of the Complete Psychological Works of Sigmund Freud,* ed. and trans. J. Strachey. London: Hogarth Press, 3: 162–188.

———. 1899/1953. "Screen Memories." In *The Standard Edition of the Complete Psychological Works of Sigmund Freud,* ed. and trans. J. Strachey. London: Hogarth Press, 3: 303–322.

———. 1900/1953. *The Interpretation of Dreams,* trans. J. Strachey. New York: Avon/Discus Books (*Standard Edition* 4–5).

———. 1900/1999. *The Interpretation of Dreams,* trans. J. Crick with notes by R. Robertson. New York: Oxford University Press.
———. 1901/1953. "The Psychopathology of Everyday Life." In *The Standard Edition of the Complete Psychological Works of Sigmund Freud,* ed. and trans. J. Strachey. London: Hogarth Press, 6.
———. 1095/1953. "Three Essays on the Theory of Sexuality." In *The Standard Edition of the Complete Psychological Works of Sigmund Freud,* ed. and trans. J. Strachey. London: Hogarth Press, 7: 130–243.
———. 1910a/1957. "Leonardo da Vinci and a Memory of his Childhood." In *The Standard Edition of the Complete Psychological Works of Sigmund Freud,* ed. and trans. J. Strachey. London: Hogarth Press, 11: 163–176.
———. 1910b/1957. "A Special Type of Choice of Object Made by Men (Contributions to the Psychology of Life, I)." In *The Standard Edition of the Complete Psychological Works of Sigmund Freud,* ed. and trans. J. Strachey. London: Hogarth Press, 11: 163–176.
———. 1913/1953. *Totem and Taboo.* In *The Standard Edition of the Complete Psychological Works of Sigmund Freud,* ed. and trans. J. Strachey. London: Hogarth Press, 13: 1–161.
———. 1914/1958. "Remembering, Repeating and Working Through: Further Recommendations on the Technique of Psychoanalysis." In *The Standard Edition of the Complete Psychological Works of Sigmund Freud,* ed. and trans. J. Strachey. London: Hogarth Press, 12: 146–156.
———. 1927/1961. "The Future of an Illusion." In *The Standard Edition of the Complete Psychological Works of Sigmund Freud,* ed. and trans. J. Strachey. London: Hogarth Press, 21: 5–58.
———. 1930/1953. *Civilization and Its Discontents.* In *The Standard Edition of the Complete Psychological Works of Sigmund Freud.* London: Hogarth Press, 21: 59–148.
Gay, P. 1988. *Freud: A Life for Our Time.* New York: W. W. Norton.
Grafton, A. 1997. *The Footnote: A Curious History.* Cambridge, MA: Harvard University Press.
Grinstein, A. 1968. *Sigmund Freud's Dreams.* New York: International Universities Press.
Hartman, F. 1983. "A Reappraisal of the Emma Episode and the Specimen Dream." *Journal of the American Psychoanalytic Association,* 31: 555–586.
Hartmann, E. 1998. *Dreams and Nightmares: The New Theory on the Origin and Meaning of Dreams.* New York: Plenum.
Hobson, J. A. 1988. *The Dreaming Brain.* New York: Basic Books.
Jones, E. 1953–1957. *The Life and Work of Sigmund Freud* (3 vols.). New York: Basic Books.
Krull, M. 1986. *Freud and His Father.* New York: W. W. Norton.
Masson, J. M. 1984. *The Assault on Truth: Freud's Suppression of the Seduction Theory.* New York: Farrar, Straus, Giroux.
Mautner, B. 1991. "Freud's Irma Dream: A Psychoanalytic Interpretation." *International Journal of Psychoanalysis,* 72: 275–286.
Miller, A. 1981. *Prisoners of Childhood,* trans. R. Ward. New York: Basic Books.
Ornston, D., ed. 1992. *Translating Freud.* New Haven, CT: Yale University Press.
Ross, J. M. 1982. "Oedipus Revisited: Laius and the 'Laius Complex.'" *Psychoanalytic Study of the Child,* 37: 167–200.
Rudnytsky, P. 1987. *Freud and Oedipus.* New York: Columbia University Press.
Schur, M. 1966. "Some Additional 'Day Residues' of 'The Specimen Dream of Psychoanalysis.'" In *Psychoanalysis—A General Psychology: Essays in Honor of Heinz Hartmann,* ed. R. M. Lowenstein, E. Kris, et al. New York: International Universities Press, 45–85.
Sulloway, F. 1979. *Freud: Biologist of the Mind.* New York: Basic Books.
Solms, M. 1997. *The Neuropsychology of Dreams.* Hillsdale, NJ: Lawrence Erlbaum.
Weiss, S. 1985/1989. "How Culture Influences the Interpretation of the Oedipus Myth." In *The Oedipus Papers,* ed. G. Pollock and J. M. Ross. Madison, CT: International Universities Press, 373–388.

13

Penelope as Dreamer

The Perils of Interpretation

Kelly Bulkeley

No matter where it is practiced, the interpretation of dreams is fraught with difficulties, uncertainties, and ambiguities. In contemporary Western society the most common location for dream interpretation is private psychotherapy: A client suffering some kind of mental distress tells a dream to a professional therapist, whose job it is to discover what the dream might be saying about the client's life situation. The methods used by most psychotherapists are drawn in one way or another from the clinical practices of Sigmund Freud and Carl Jung. These methods include asking for personal associations, identifying puns, metaphors, and wordplay, and seeking homologies between particular dream images and broader cultural symbolism. Although some psychotherapists report great success in the use of dream interpretation to treat their clients,[1] many other healthcare professionals remain wary. One of the major reasons for this wariness is a lack of uniform standards and guidelines to use in the practice of dream interpretation—Freud said one thing, Jung said another, and their followers have gone on to say a thousand other things. With no settled, commonly accepted method for determining how exactly dream image "A" is related to waking life situation "B," dream interpretation appears inherently unstable, unreliable, and therapeutically suspect.

If dream interpretation is a perilous endeavor in psychotherapy, it must be even more so when practiced in cross-cultural contexts. Anthropologists who seek to understand the dreams of informants from other cultures must contend with languages, religions, and community traditions that in many cases are radically different from their own. (These cultural factors are also present in psychotherapeutic contexts, but in most cases therapists and their clients share significantly more common cultural ground than do anthropologists and their informants.) A further difficulty is that many cultures regard dreams as spiritually powerful experiences that must be honored and carefully guarded, a belief with two important consequences: One, it makes informants cautious about what they do and do not report to the inquiring anthropologist; and two, in most cases the informants have their own interpretive ideas about what their dreams mean, ideas that are often very different from those of the anthropologist. Unlike psychotherapists, whose clients usually grant the therapist's greater knowledge about dreaming, anthropologists often work with informants who have developed their own distinct ideas about the meaning of their dreams. If the integrity, intelligence, and sophistication of these "non-Western" approaches to dream interpretation are taken seriously (as many anthropologists argue we should—see chapters 6, 7, 9, and 16 in this volume), grave questions are raised about the adequacy and universal applicability of the hermeneutic methods of Freud, Jung, and their conceptual progeny.

At least anthropologists and psychotherapists are able to speak in person with their informants. Historians interested in dream interpretation have no direct personal access to the subjects of their research, no way of asking for associations, no way of questioning the dreamers about what they think their dreams mean. Added to the formidable difficulties of cross-cultural understanding, historians have this further problem of being confined in their interpretive efforts to the impersonal analysis of textual records. When the temporal distance between historians and their subjects is combined with the inevitable distortions that arise in copying, editing, and transmitting texts over hundreds or in some cases thousands of years, it makes the practice of historical dream interpretation seem a nearly impossible affair.

In each of these arenas—psychotherapy, cross-cultural investigation, historical research—the methodological challenges are daunting for those who seek to interpret dreams. Anyone who continues in the face of these challenges must do so with deep humility and chastened expectations. Critics will always have ample material to use in questioning the validity of a particular interpretation of a dream.

I regret having to say that this is not the worst of it. The greatest difficulty of all facing those who pursue the interpretation of dreams remains to be mentioned. This last difficulty is so serious that it threatens to destroy the very possibility of dream interpretation as a legitimate, worthwhile, knowledge-producing enterprise. Even if all the aforementioned methodological obstacles could somehow be overcome, this one problem would still remain, and it would still pose a potentially fatal challenge.

In what follows I will explore this greatest of all interpretive dangers by telling a story. This story is a very old one, a story you probably have heard many times before. I would like to tell it again because even though it is just a fiction, just a make-believe tale from a faraway place and time, I believe it illustrates as nothing else can the *reality* of the ultimate methodological challenge facing any would-be dream interpreter.

The story I would like to tell is of the meeting of Odysseus and Penelope in Book 19 of *The Odyssey.* In many respects this encounter is the most dramatically intense moment in the entire poem, and at the heart of the scene is a dream—Penelope's dream of the twenty geese that are suddenly slaughtered by a mountain eagle. Odysseus, after leading the Achaean army to victory against the Trojans and after enduring a seemingly endless series of trials and adventures, has returned at last to his island home of Ithaca, where he has found a mob of rude noblemen besieging his palace. The crafty warrior has disguised himself as an old beggar in order to gain entrance into the palace without being recognized, and he is plotting violent revenge against the men who would steal his throne. Penelope, who for many years has desperately clung to the hope that Odysseus would someday return to her, has invited this strange wanderer into her private chambers to ask if he can tell her any news of her husband. The beggar fervently promises the Queen that Odysseus is very close and will return very, very soon.

Penelope replies to the beggar's story by saying she wishes his words would come true, but she doubts they will. She asks her old servant woman, Eurycleia, to bathe the stranger and arrange a comfortable place for him to sleep. The Queen steps away while the old nurse washes the beggar's feet. Then, before parting for the night, Penelope returns to the beggar and they have one final exchange:

> "Friend [she says to the beggar],
> Allow me one brief question more . . .
> Interpret me this dream: From a water's edge
> Twenty fat geese have come to feed on grain
> Beside my house. And I delight to see them.
> But now a mountain eagle with great wings
> And crooked beak storms in to break their necks
> And strew their bodies here. Away he soars
> Into the bright sky; and I cry aloud—
> All this in a dream—I wail and round me gather
> Softly braided Akhaian women mourning
> Because the eagle killed my geese.
>
> Then down
> Out of the sky he drops to a cornice beam
> With mortal voice telling me not to weep.
> 'Be glad,' says he, 'renowned Ikarios' daughter:
> Here is no dream but something real as day,
> Something about to happen. All those geese
> Were suitors, and the bird was I. See now,
> I am no eagle but your lord come back
> To bring inglorious death upon them all!'
> As he said this, my honeyed slumber left me.
> Peering through half-shut eyes, I saw the geese
> In hall, still feeding at the self-same trough."
> The master of subtle ways and straight replied:
> "My dear, how can you choose to read the dream
> Differently? Has not Odysseus himself
> Shown you what is to come? Death to the suitors,
> Sure death, too. Not one escapes his doom."
>
> Penelope shook her head and answered:
> "Friend,
> Many and many a dream is mere confusion,
> A cobweb of no consequence at all.
> Two gates for ghostly dreams there are: one gateway
> Of honest horn, and one of ivory.
> Issuing by the ivory gate are dreams
> Of glimmering illusion, fantasies
> But those that come through solid polished horn
> May be borne out, if mortals only know them.
> I doubt it came by horn, my fearful dream—
> Too good to be true, that, for my son and me."[2]

What has just happened here? What is going on between Odysseus and Penelope, and what is the significance of her dream and their exchange about its meaning? The traditional interpretation of this scene, shared with near unanimity by scholars from antiquity to the present, is this.[3] Odysseus has heroically controlled his desire to rejoin Penelope and hidden his identity from her for two reasons. One is to test his wife's fidelity during his long absence; Odysseus is well aware that when his compatriot Agamemnon returned home from the Trojan war, he was viciously murdered by his wife Clytemnestra and the lover whom she had taken in his absence.[4] The second reason for Odysseus' continued disguise is to pick up information about how to destroy the hated suitors. The traditional view is that Penelope's dream of the twenty geese is a straightforward prophecy, whose true meaning the disguised Odysseus instantly recognizes. But Penelope, who has shown a stubborn skepticism throughout the story, refuses to accept the dream's obvious meaning. Indeed, perhaps she unconsciously enjoys the attention of the suitors and does not really want Odysseus to come back.

My dissatisfaction with this widely held interpretation centers on its strange depreciation of Penelope's intelligence. This is a woman whom several characters have praised for her unrivaled perceptiveness, cunning, and guile; this is the woman who devised the famous ruse of the funeral shroud, by which she successfully deceived the suitors for three years. All of the evidence in the poem makes it clear that Penelope is not a fool: She is extremely perceptive and capable of remarkably subtle deceptions. So why, when we come to Book 19 and her meeting with the "beggar," should we now forget all that and regard Penelope as a pathetically unwitting dupe in the vengeful scheming of Odysseus?

The Iliad and *The Odyssey* together contain, up to the point of Penelope's dream of the 20 geese, four major dream episodes: Agamemnon's "Evil Dream" from Zeus (2.1–83), Achilles' mournful dream of the spirit of dead Patroklos (23.54–107), Penelope's reassuring dream from Athena (4.884–946), and Nausicaa's arousing marriage dream from Athena (6.15–79). Viewed in this context, Penelope's dream is unusual in at least two ways. First, this is the only dream that occurs "offstage," out of direct view of the audience. We do not "see" the dream while it is happening; we only hear the dreamer describe it, after the fact. Second, this is the only "symbolic" dream, with its meaning encoded in stylized imagery. The dream thus poses a riddle, which must be accurately interpreted for the true meaning to emerge.

I believe these two details suggest a very different interpretation of the encounter between Penelope and the disguised Odysseus. Could it be that this is not a "real" dream at all, that in fact Penelope has made it up? Could it be that Penelope is deliberately using the riddle of her dream as a test to find out the intentions of this man, whom she consciously suspects is Odysseus? Could it be that while he thinks he is deceiving her, she is really the one deceiving him? This would not be the first time in Homer's poems that dreams have been used to deceive and manipulate others—in fact, it would be the fourth time: Zeus sending the "Evil Dream" to Agamemnon, Athena sending the "marriage dream" to Nausicaa, and Odysseus (at the end of *The Odyssey,* Book 14) making up a story about the "real" Odysseus making up a dream in order to steal another warrior's cloak on a cold, windy night (14.519–589).

But why would Penelope fabricate such a dream? The answer emerges if we think carefully about what is happening at that crucial moment when the old nurse Eurycleia is washing the beggar's feet.[5] Penelope has removed herself and is standing alone, after a long and intimate conversation with a man who has detailed knowledge about Odysseus, who looks and sounds very much like Odysseus, who insists with passionate certainty that Odysseus will return to the palace the very next day. The question could hardly not arise for this most intelligent and perceptive of women: Is this stranger Odysseus himself? If he is, then why is he not revealing himself? Penelope has just poured her heart out to him, saying how terribly she has suffered over the years—why will he not drop his disguise and reunite with her this very moment?

When Eurycleia finishes washing the beggar's feet, Penelope returns to him and says she has one last question: What is the meaning of her dream of the geese and the mountain eagle? Without a second's hesitation the disguised Odysseus agrees with the words of the mountain eagle: The dream means "death to the suitors, sure death, too."

Penelope, however, disagrees. Her "two gates" speech that follows is a subtle but unmistakable way of saying "I don't think so" to the beggar's interpretation. She cannot agree with him for a simple reason: The mountain eagle and the beggar have both misinterpreted the dream. There are twenty geese in her dream, but more, many more than that number of suitors in the palace. As we learn in Book 16.270–288, where Telemachus tells Odysseus who all the suitors are and where they come from, there are a total of 108 men besieging the palace. Penelope's refusal to accept the interpretation of the mountain eagle and the beggar is not due to stubborn skepticism, pathetic ignorance, or unconscious desire—she rejects the interpretation because it is wrong. The true meaning of the symbol of the twenty geese is surprisingly easy to find if we do not automatically assume that the mountain eagle and the beggar are right (i.e., if we do not automatically privilege the hermeneutic perspective of Odysseus). The twenty geese symbolize the twenty years that Odysseus has been away fighting the war at Troy and journeying through the world. The exact length of Odysseus' absence, twenty years, is mentioned five separate times in the poem.[6] The fifth mention is the most significant as a kind of "day residue" because it involves the beggar/Odysseus, who comments to Penelope just a few lines earlier in the same scene that Odysseus has been gone for twenty years.

Thus, the first part of Penelope's dream symbolically, and very accurately, describes her emotional experience of what has happened between them: Odysseus, by going off to fight in someone else's war, has destroyed the last twenty years for her. What should have been the prime years of their marriage, the wonderful years of raising a family and creating a home, the years that Penelope would have "loved to watch" and care for, have been slaughtered by Odysseus. The second part of the dream expresses Penelope's fearful perception of Odysseus right now, still standing apart from her in the disguise of a beggar. He does not recognize her and what the last twenty years have been like for her; all he can see are the suitors and a galling challenge to his honor. By posing this dream riddle to the beggar, Penelope is in effect asking if her suspicion is true: Is the "real" Odysseus as blind to her feelings and as obsessed with killing the suitors as is the "dream" Odysseus? When the beggar agrees with the mountain eagle's words in the dream, Penelope knows the unfortunate answer.

The mysterious poetry of Penelope's two gates speech becomes all the more powerful when it is understood as a response to Odysseus' failure of the dream interpretation test. To his reprimanding words ("My dear, how can you choose to read the dream differently?") Penelope replies that dreams are always difficult to understand, and they do not always come true. The danger is that we will allow our desire to cloud our perception—taking as divine prophecy what is merely human fantasy. But some dreams, she goes on to say, do have the potential to come true, "if mortals only know them." That is precisely what Odysseus has failed to do. He has failed to see past his own desire for revenge.

I am reluctant to finish with this story, because there is so much more to be told (and so much more to be questioned, if you happen to disagree with my admittedly unorthodox reading of this scene).[7] But let me come back to the opening discussion of the difficulties confronting those who pursue the interpretation of dreams. The encounter between Penelope and Odysseus is, in the context of our discussion, a cautionary tale about the most profound challenge facing any form of dream interpretation. More than the barriers of language and culture, more than the ambiguous symbolic connections between dream imagery and waking life, more than the subtle complexities of social exchange between interpreter and dreamer, the greatest challenge facing the interpretation of dreams is the danger of self-deception. The human propensity for self-deception threatens the legitimacy of dream interpretation in psychotherapy, anthropology, historical research, and every other context in which it is practiced. Put in the simplest terms, how can you ever know you are not just fooling yourself? How can you ever be sure your own biases, assumptions, and expectations are not subtly determining what you believe you are discovering in a dream? How can you be sure you are not just finding what you want to find?

Considered in the light of the foregoing story, this could be called "the Odyssian fallacy": a dream interpretation that fails to recognize and account for the influence of the interpreter's own beliefs, interests, and desires. Every attempt to interpret a dream is subject to the criticism that it is committing the Odyssian fallacy; every claim about the meaning of a particular dream is open to the charge that the alleged "meaning" is in fact an unwitting projection of the interpreter's own assumptions and prejudices. Indeed, history is filled with examples of misinterpreted dreams, and modern psychologists like Freud and Jung are frequently and justifiably criticized for their failure to recognize as fully as they might have the undue influence of their personal biases and prejudices on their interpretive practices.[8] In view of this troubling history, it would be hard to argue that the Western cultural tradition has made much progress over the past three thousand years in dealing with the problem of self-deception in dream interpretation.

The ultimate logical extension of the Odyssian fallacy is to deny that dream interpretation can ever be anything other than personal projection. Whether dreams have meaning in themselves or not, interpreters will never know because they can never be certain they have eliminated all the potentially distorting influences of their own expectations. Dream interpretation, in this line of thinking, is doomed to failure from the very beginning. It is reduced to the status of reading Rorschach ink blots, of interest perhaps in revealing aspects of the interpreter's personality, but of no legitimacy whatsoever as a means of producing trustworthy knowledge.[9]

This may appear to end the discussion. I would suggest it is rather the beginning of a new discussion. The pessimism elicited by a full appreciation of the Odyssian fallacy can be relieved at least in part by what I would call "Penelope's response." After twenty years of hoping, dreaming, weeping, and praying for her husband's safe return, Penelope knows as well as anyone the tempting allure of wish-fulfilling fantasy. She knows how easy it is to see what you want to see and believe what you want to believe. And yet Penelope still hopes that her wishes *really will* come true. Despite her sharp awareness of the ever-present danger of self-deception, Penelope maintains a passionate faith that one day her deepest desires will really and truly be fulfilled. Penelope's caution, skepticism, and wariness in defense of this faith are legendary, and even Odysseus is moved to exclaim in amazement and frustration (in Book 23, when Penelope plays the bed trick on him) that she never stops testing, probing and questioning whether she can really believe what she is seeing. Odysseus is right, Penelope has become a supremely skeptical person—yet she has also become a supremely faithful person. She has not allowed her skepticism to overwhelm her with despair, but neither has she let her faith carry her off into vain fantasy. She has learned to live with the vibrant tension between a powerful skepticism and an equally powerful faith; she has learned to hold these two passions together in all their creative dynamism. This, I imagine, is Penelope's response to the Odyssian fallacy: Dream interpretation is always difficult but never impossible. Our desires always threaten to deceive and mislead us, yet the vital fact remains that some dreams, "those that come through solid polished horn, may be borne out, if mortals only know them."

In this spirit, I propose the following four principles for the interpretation of dreams. These principles may be employed in any context in which dreams are interpreted, and I believe they provide a coherent and trustworthy basis for determining the validity of different interpretations and distinguishing better ones from worse ones. Most important, these principles give interpreters specific methodological guidance in dealing with the danger of self-deception.

1. *The dreamer knows best what his or her dream means.* Only the dreamer has direct access to all the images and feelings in the dream, and only the dreamer is familiar with all the memories and associations making up the dream's broader context. This does not necessarily mean that the dreamer's own view on the dream's meaning is the only legitimate one; dreamers are often unaware of many significant dimensions of their dreams. But this principle does imply that the dreamer's perspective must be accounted for. It further implies that interpreters should be concerned if their claims about a dream's meaning deviate too far from what the dreamer says the dream means. This again is where Odysseus failed—his condescending words "my dear, how can you choose to read the dream differently?" express a hermeneutic attitude that fails to acknowledge and respect the dreamer's point of view.
2. *A good interpretation will account for as many of the dream's details as possible.* I call this the principle of internal coherence. An interpretation that brings together more of the various elements of a dream will be better than an interpretation that only refers to a few isolated pieces. Naturally, problems arise if interpreters try to force all the details of a dream into a single fixed idea of what the dream means. But on the whole, the interpretation that accounts for the most details is the best interpretation. A corollary of this principle is that any interpretation should be considered suspect which fails to account for a key detail in the given dream. The exact number of geese in Penelope's dream, twenty, the significance of which countless interpreters have neglected to recognize, is an example of this. Indeed, it often happens in dream interpretation that what initially seems to be a random and unimportant element—the color of a tree, the shape of a character's face, the layout of a house—turns out to be remarkably vital piece of the dream's overall meaning.
3. *A good interpretation will make as many connections as possible between dream's content and the dreamer's waking life.* This is the principle of external coherence, and it is

grounded in the fact that dreams are usually created out of images, ideas, and feelings from the dreamer's daily existence. A good interpretation identifies the connections between those waking-life sources and the various symbolic strands of the dream. Sometimes the connections relate to experiences from the previous day; sometimes they involve events from farther in the past; and sometimes they refer to anticipated events in the future. Indeed, many dreams weave all three temporal strands together. For example, Penelope's dream is directly connected to her present (waking up to find the geese actually outside in hallway), yet it harkens back to her distant past (the twenty years since she last saw her husband), while also envisioning a possible future (a joyful reunion with him). The principle of external coherence asks how well any proposed interpretation has contextualized the given dream in the full temporal span of the dreamer's life and how well it accounts for the waking world origins of the dream's imagery.

4. *A good interpretation will be open to new and surprising discoveries and will look beyond the obvious (what is already known) to find the novel and the unexpected (what is not already known).* This is the most effective methodological strategy for addressing the danger of self-deception. If the interpreter admits to *not knowing* what exactly will come of the process, if she or he stays open to the possibility that startling new meanings may emerge, the potentially malign influence of personal assumptions and expectations will be greatly reduced (if never absolutely eliminated). I share Jung's view on this point: "So difficult is it to understand a dream that for a long time I have made it a rule, when someone tells me a dream and asks for my opinion, to say first of all to myself: 'I have no idea what this dream means.' After that I can begin to examine the dream."[10]

These four principles—privileging the perspective of the dreamer, focusing on the details, identifying connections to waking life, and being open to surprise—constitute what I regard as a postcritical hermeneutics of dreaming. It would take a much lengthier chapter to discuss the many ways of applying these principles in psychotherapy, anthropology, historical research, and other interpretive arenas, so I will simply say that if interpreters keep the four principles in mind, they will be well prepared to meet whatever distinct methodological difficulties they encounter in their fields of study.

In closing, I must acknowledge the paradoxical nature of illustrating my approach in the way I have, with a retelling of an old story about a fabricated dream—a fiction within a fiction within a fiction. What could make a reader more skeptical about an author's argument? Well, how about ending with one of the author's own dreams? In March of 2000, when I was anxiously working to organize the American Academy of Religion conference panel at which I presented the essential argument of this chapter, I had a short but quite vivid dream. In the dream I am with Kurt Cobain, the singer-guitarist from the Seattle rock band Nirvana who killed himself with a shotgun in 1994. In my dream he is alive and well, in a classroom with me and several college students at the university where I teach. I feel a strong desire somehow to weave Kurt into the conference panel—I need his creative energy, yet I fear his self-destructive unpredictability.

I awoke from the dream with that tension fresh and vivid in my mind. I hope this chapter has provoked some of that same tension in you.

Notes

1. See Jane White-Lewis, chapter 10, this volume; Clara Hill, *Working with Dreams in Psychotherapy* (New York: Guilford Press, 1996); Alan Siegel, *Dreams That Can Change Your Life* (Los Angeles: Jeremy Tarcher, 1990); Walter Bonime, *The Clinical Use of Dreams* (New York: DeCapo Press, 1988); Marion Cuddy and Kathryn Belicki, "The Fifty-Five Year Secret: Using Nightmares to Facilitate Psychotherapy in a Case of Childhood Sexual Abuse," in *Among All These Dreamers: Essays on Dreaming and Modern Society,* ed. Kelly Bulkeley (Albany: State University of New York Press, 1996).
2. Homer, *The Odyssey,* trans. Robert Fitzgerald (Garden City: Anchor Books, 1963), 19.575, 603–640.
3. Defenders of this basic line of interpretation include F. M. Combellack, "Three Odyssean Problems," *California Studies in Classical Antiquity* 6 (1973): 17–46; Bernard Fenik, *Studies in the Odyssey,* in *Hermes Einzelschriften,* no. 30 (Franz Steiner Verlag GMBH, 1974); John H. Finley, Jr., *Homer's Odyssey* (Cambridge: Harvard University Press, 1978); C. Emlyn-Jones, "The Reunion of Odysseus and Penelope, *Greece and Rome* 31 (1984): 1–18; Sheila Murnaghan, *Disguise and Recognition in the Odyssey* (Princeton: Princeton University Press, 1987); M. A. Katz, *Penelope's Renown* (Princeton: Princeton University Press, 1991); R. B. Rutherford, *Homer's Odyssey: Books XIX and XX* (Cambridge, England: Cambridge University Press, 1992); and Nancy Felson-Rubin, "Penelope's Perspective: Character from Plot," in *Reading the Odyssey: Selected Interpretive Essays,* ed. Seth L. Schein (Princeton: Princeton University Press, 1996). Katz has usefully summarized modern scholarly debate on this section of *The Odyssey* into three groups. One group takes an "Analytic" approach, arguing that the combination of at least two different story traditions in Book 19 is the cause of the narrative inconsistencies and contradictions. Another group uses an "Aesthetic" perspective to argue that the importance of plot structure made it inevitable that plausible character development in Book 19 (particularly regarding Penelope) would suffer as a by-product. The third group draws on "Psychological" thinking to seek deeper motivations in the characters that would help to account for otherwise problematic or inexplicable events in Book 19. My approach in this essay is, in Katz's categorization, psychological. However, I come to very different conclusions from those offered by the other primary exponents of the psychological view and I thereby avoid the biggest problems that critics have identified in their treatments of this scene.
4. 11.439 ff.
5. Book 19, 364 ff. It is worth noting that just before stepping aside from Eurycleia and the beggar Penelope leaves her guest with this mournful thought: "Odysseus will not come to me; no ship will be prepared for you. We have no master quick to receive and furnish out a guest as Lord Odysseus was. Or did I dream him?" (313–317).
6. The twenty years are mentioned at 2.196, 13.102, 16.235, 19.256, and 19.547.
7. For a more fully developed analysis of this passage, see "Penelope as Dreamer: A Reading of Book 19 of *The Odyssey,*" in *Dreaming,* vol. 8, no. 4 (1998): 229–242. In this article I go on from this point to discuss the implications this interpretation of Penelope's dream has for understanding her seemingly capricious decision to hold the contest of the bow the following morning (at the very end of Book 19) and the strange longings felt by Penelope and Odysseus during their "shared dream" the night before the contest (at the very beginning of Book 20).
8. See Frederick Crews, ed., *The Unauthorized Freud: Doubters Confront a Legend* (New York: Penguin, 1998) and Richard Noll, *The Aryan Christ: The Secret Life of Carl Jung* (New York: Random House, 1997).
9. See J. Allan Hobson, *Dreaming as Delirium: How the Brain Goes Out of Its Mind* (Cambridge: MIT Press, 1999), p. 93.
10. "On the Nature of Dreams," in Carl Jung, *Dreams,* trans. R. F. C. Hull (Princeton: Princeton University Press, 1974), p. 69.

Section III

METHODS

14

Western Dreams about Eastern Dreams

Wendy Doniger

1. What can we learn about dreams from the myths of other cultures?

It is often argued that quantum physics confirms Zen Buddhism, that our own "modern" ideas were prefigured by "Oriental" mythologies. This may or may not be so, but I do not think it is a useful path to follow. Instead, I would argue that some of the insights of non-Western mythologies do indeed bear striking resemblances to some of the most abstract formulations of modern science, but only because the same basic human mind is searching for a limited set of metaphors with which to make sense of the same basic human experiences, be the expressions Eastern or Western, "factual" or imaginative. This is the bridge that justifies our attempts to gain insights about our dreams from the stories that other cultures tell about their dreams.

2. What relevance does our understanding of lucid dreams, on one hand, and orgasmic dreams, on the other, have for the interpretation of myths about sexual dreams?

Stephen LaBerge has summarized the growing literature on what are called lucid dreams, which take place "when we 'awaken' within our dreams—without disturbing or ending the dream state—and learn to recognize that we are dreaming while the dream is still happening."[1] In addition to demonstrating that such dreams do occur, LaBerge goes onto argue that they can be made to occur. He cites, first, a passage from Hervey de Saint-Denys:

> I dreamt that I was out riding in fine weather. I became aware of my true situation, and remembered the question of whether or not I could exercise free will in controlling my actions in a dream. "Well now," I said to myself, "this horse is only an illusion; this countryside that I am passing through is merely stage scenery. But even if I have not evoked these images by conscious volition, I certainly seem to have some control over them.' I

> decide to gallop, I gallop; I decide to stop, I stop. Now here are two roads in front of me. The one on the right appears to plunge into a dense wood; the one on the left leads to some kind of ruined manor; I feel quite distinctly that I am free to turn either right or left, and so decide for myself whether I wish to produce images relating to the ruins or images relating to the wood.[2]

This is also a classical mythological image; the challenge of controlling a horse functions as a metaphor for free will and the harnessing of the senses in Plato, the Upanisads, and many other texts throughout the world. Here the image of controlling the horse expresses for Saint-Denys his ability to control his own dreams.

For LaBerge, "This brings up two questions regarding control of lucid dreaming. The first is, how much is possible? . . . The second question regarding dream control involves what kind is desirable."[3] This is a problem on which the mythology of dream narratives, particularly orgasmic dream narratives, sheds some light.

On one hand, orgasmic dreams seem to be significantly different, in physiological terms, from lucid erotic dreams:

> Wet dreams may result from genital stimulation and reflex ejaculation. . . . Wet dreams would be the result of actual erotic sensations accurately interpreted by the dreaming brain. In other words, first comes the ejaculation, then comes the wet dream. Apparently, the opposite normally holds for lucid dream orgasms. The erotic dream comes first, resulting in orgasm "in the brain." However, in this case, the resulting impulses descending from the brain to the genitals are evidently too inhibited to trigger the genital ejaculatory reflex. So, reflex dreams are only wet in the dream.[4]

In lucid erotic dreams, by contrast, there is some physiological change, but not as much as in a genuine, nonlucid wet dream. A woman named "Miranda" dreamed, in a lucid dream, that she was flying, found an attractive man, made love with him, and experienced an orgasm. "She said the dream orgasm had been neither long nor intense, but was quite definitely a real orgasm." In the laboratory experiments, measurements of vaginal blood flow and heart rate "Provided the first objective evidence for the validity of Miranda's reports (and, by extension, those of others) of vividly realistic sex in lucid dreams."[5] And a man who had a lucid orgasmic dream reported, "Although I found I had not actually ejaculated, I still felt the tingling in my spine and I marvelled at the reality that the mind could create."[6]

The mental intensity of nonejaculatory erotic dreams is still more complex than this evidence implies: "Men whose spinal cords have been shattered through injury, so that there is no longer any nervous connection between their brains and their lower bodies, still have sexual dreams in which they experience all the feelings and sensations of orgasm. The basis of this experience is not in their isolated lower bodies. It is wholly within their brains."[7] In other words, this man, incapable of a physiological orgasm, had a vivid lucid dream of orgasm.

Thus, as LaBerge points out, "In some respects, lucid dream sex has as powerful an impact on the dreamer's body as the real thing. . . . What happens in the inner world of dreams—and lucid dreams, especially, can produce physical effects on the dreamer's brain no less real than those produced by corresponding events happening in the external world."[8] We are left, therefore, with a paradox: The lucid orgasmic dream produces erection, excitement (often said to be more mentally intense than in a real orgasm), but no significantly heightened heartbeat and no actual ejaculation. Is it, therefore, more or less real than a wet dream?

An orgasmic wet dream is physically real; a real orgasm has taken place, inside and outside the body of the dreamer, and it seems at first to have happened more or less as it would have taken place had the dream partner been physically present. In another sense, however, the orgasmic dream is emotionally unreal; one has had a fantasy of an experience that cannot be entirely real without a partner. The semen is a biological fact, but it is proof only of the fantasy. Unlike other "things" that the hero brings back from the dream world, the semen cannot prove the physical existence of the person who caused it to be present in the dream—the lover from the other world. Like the dream itself, semen is "emitted" by the dreamer in one of the basic processes of illusory creation.

Another way to approach this problem is to return to the question of control, for one cannot control an orgasmic dream as one can control a lucid dream. The element of control brings the lucid dream closer to the *mental* waking world but, there being less physiological response, farther from the *physical* waking world. Indian philosophical texts tell us a great deal about the control of lucid dreams, and Indian mythological texts tell us a great deal about the experience of orgasmic dreams. LaBerge attempts to apply the Oriental dream-control techniques of yogis and shamans to Western goals of improving one's life or even, indeed, one's lifestyle. But this cannot be done.

The yogis' goals and assumptions differ from ours; their gods are not our gods. On one hand, they are not trying to get ahead in the world of *samsara* (material life and rebirth); they are trying to leave it (as the texts that LaBerge cites show). They do not use dream techniques for the sorts of things that yuppies want to have; no Hindu would name a sexy perfume Samsara, as Guerlain has done.[9]

Yet yogis are not control freaks; on the contrary, the key to all of their meditational techniques is the cultivation of a complete emptying out of oneself, a complete passivity, so that God, or the force of the universe, takes over. This approach is closer to the old Alcoholics Anonymous slogan—"Let go and let God"—than it is to any self-help creed. So, too, in the "Oriental" stories of shared dreams, the mutuality is always conceived of as passive, and the dreamer is at the mercy of the lover; these are myths of surrender, not myths of conquest. For both of these reasons, therefore, the control achieved in yogic dreams would never be applied to orgasmic dreams, since yogis would not want to have an orgasmic dream, and since orgasmic dreams are, in stories at least, passive.

But these are merely symptoms of the underlying, far more basic problem: that the healing techniques of India are designed to heal what Indians think of as the human person, more precisely to produce what Indians think of as a good (or normal, or healthy, or realized—choose your own ideal) person. And such a person is someone embedded in an Indian social system, someone whose expectations of relationships with parents, children, spouse, and everyone else are very different from our own. Ideas such as "individual" and "maturity" would have been utter nonsense to the authors of the textbooks on yogic techniques. It is therefore problematic—not impossible, perhaps, but certainly more problematic than is usually acknowledged—for a Westerner to achieve an Eastern enlightenment.[10]

3. What can Hindu mythology tell us about the problems inherent in our attempts to study someone else's dreams?

I have attempted elsewhere[11] to approach this problem through the use of a story that occurs in the great Sanskrit compendium of dream narratives, the *Yogavasistha,* a philosophical treatise composed in Kashmir sometime between the tenth and twelfth centuries C.E.

The myth is the story of a hunter who meets a sage who has entered another man's body and lodged in his head:

> One day a hunter wandered in the woods until he came to the home of a sage, who became his teacher. The sage told him this story:
>
> > In the old days, I became an ascetic sage and lived alone in a hermitage. I studied magic. I entered someone else's body and saw all his organs; I entered his head and then I saw a universe, with a sun and an ocean and mountains, and gods and demons and human beings. This universe was his dream, and I saw his dream. Inside his head, I saw his city and his wife and his servants and his son.
> >
> > When darkness fell, he went to bed and slept, and I slept too. Then his world was overwhelmed by a flood at doomsday; I, too, was swept away in the flood, and though I managed to obtain a foothold on a rock, a great wave knocked me into the water again. When I saw that world destroyed at doomsday, I wept. I still saw, in my own dream, a whole universe, for I had picked up his karmic memories along with his dream. I had become involved in that world and I forgot my former life; I thought, "This is my father, my mother, my village, my house, my family."
> >
> > Once again I saw doomsday. This time, however, even while I was being burned up by the flames, I did not suffer, for I realized, "This is just a dream." Then I forgot my own experiences. Time passed. A sage came to my house, and slept and ate, and as we were talking after dinner he said, "Don't you know that all of this is a dream? I am a man in your dream, and you are a man in someone else's dream."
> >
> > Then I awakened, and remembered my own nature; I remembered that I was an ascetic. And I said to him, "I will go to that body of mine (that was an ascetic)," for I wanted to see my own body as well as the body which I had set out to explore. But he smiled and said, "Where do you think those two bodies of yours are?" I could find no body, nor could I get out of the head of the person I had entered, and so I asked him, "Well, where *are* the two bodies?"
> >
> > The sage replied, "While you were in the other person's body, a great fire arose that destroyed your body as well as the body of the other person. Now you are a householder, not an ascetic." When the sage said this, I was amazed. He lay back on his bed in silence in the night, and I did not let him go away: he stayed with me until he died.
>
> The hunter said, "If this is so, then you and I and all of us are people in one another's dreams." The sage continued to teach the hunter and told him what would happen to him in the future. But the hunter left him and went on to new rebirths. Finally, the hunter became an ascetic and found release.[12]

As we read the story of the hunter and the sage, we become confused and are tempted to draw charts to figure it all out. It is not clear, for instance, whether the sage has entered the waking world or the sleeping world of the man whose consciousness he penetrates, and whether that person is sleeping, waking, or, indeed, dead at the moment when we meet the sage. But as the tale progresses, we realize that our confusion is neither our own mistake nor the mistake of the author of the text; it is a device of the narrative, constructed to make us realize how impossible and, finally, how irrelevant it is to attempt to determine the precise level of consciousness at which we are existing. We cannot do it, and it does not matter. We can never know whether we have become trapped inside the minds of people whose consciousness we have come to share.

Inside the dream village, the new householder (*ne* sage) meets another sage, who enlightens him and wakes him up. Yet although he is explicitly said to awaken, he stays where he is inside the dream; the only difference is that now he knows he is inside the dream. Now he becomes a sage again, but a different sort of sage, a householder sage, inside the dreamer's dream. While he is in this state, he meets the hunter and attempts to instruct him. But the hunter misses the point of the sage's saga: "If this is so . . ." he mutters, and he goes off to get a whole series of bodies before he finally figures it out. The hunter has to experience everything for himself, dying and being reborn;[13] he cannot learn merely by dreaming, as the sage does.[14]

This story can teach us many things. On one hand, it may provide a wonderful example of a lucid dream, to encourage us in our attempts to find out more about our own lucid dreams. But, on the other hand, it may serve as a caveat, a warning of the possible dangers of attempting to get into other people's heads to understand their dreams. Since dreams are often the fulcrum of our whole unconscious personality, to apply *someone else's lever* at this point may uproot far more than we intended; it may tear out not only the roots of our own particular life but the deeper roots that our society has implanted in us, roots that are also, by this time, deeply imbedded in the unconscious. This may catapult us into an entirely different world—and, as the story of the hunter demonstrates, it is not always as easy to get out of such a world as it is to get in.

Notes

This chapter is taken in large part from an invited address presented at the Seventh International Conference of the Association for the Study of Dreams, Chicago, June 28, 1990.

1. Stephen LaBerge, *Lucid Dreaming: The Power of Being Awake and Aware in Your Dreams* (New York: Ballantine Books, 1985).
2. Hervey de Saint Denys, *Dreams and How to Guide Them* (London: Duckworth, 1982), cited in LaBerge, *Lucid Dreaming,* p. 116.
3. LaBerge, *Lucid Dreaming,* p. 117.
4. Ibid., p. 95.
5. Ibid., p. 91.
6. Ibid., p. 93.
7. Oswald, cited by Charles Rycroft, *The Innocence of Dreams* (New York, Pantheon, 1979), p. 111.
8. LaBerge, *Lucid Dreaming,* pp. 93, 97.
9. See Wendy Doniger O'Flaherty, *Dreams, Illusion, and Other Realities* (Chicago: University of Chicago, 1984), passim.
10. For further discussion of the problems inherent in cross-cultural interpretations of symbols, see Wendy Doniger, "When a Lingam is Just a Good Cigar," in the "Festschrift for Alan Dundes," edited by L. Bryce Boyer, forthcoming in a special issue of *The Analytic Quarterly.*
11. See Wendy Doniger O'Flaherty, *Other People's Myths: The Cave of Echoes* (New York: Macmillan, 1988).
12. *Yogavasishtha-Maha-Ramayana* of Valmiki, ed. W. L. S. Pansikar, 2 vols. (Bombay, 1918), 6.2.136–157.
13. See the story of the hundred Rudras and the wild goose in chapter 5 of O'Flaherty, *Dreams.*
14. O'Flaherty, *Other Peoples' Myths,* pp. 7–10.

15

The Dream of Scholarship

Some Notes on the Historian of Mysticism as a Dreaming Creative

Jeffrey Kripal

In a sense, creativity is practical dreaming.
. . . penile erection is an invariable feature of REM sleep.

—*James Hughes, Altered States: Creativity Under the Influence*[1]

In the following chapter I wish to make (which is not to say establish) three points. First, I would like to suggest, with a very large chorus of other thinkers, that dreaming is, potentially at least, a creative activity and, a bit more originally, that the dream is commonly tapped as a creative state in the humanities, particularly in religious studies, and especially in that subfield of religious studies that we might designate as the history of mysticism, that is, the historical, social and psychological study of altered states of consciousness as these are recorded or, better I think, "deposited"[2] in texts.

Second, I would like to argue that this same scholarly dreaming bears any number of connections to artistic creativity and its analogous states of dissociation, suffering, possession and trance: The historian of mysticism, if you will, is also often an artist who suffers, dissociates, enters various forms of consciousness, and produces a cultural product out of all of this, partly to heal to himself or herself, partly simply for the joy of creating. In truth, then, what I am addressing here is actually broader than the dream itself. I am more interested in what we might call dreamlike states and the psychosexual processes that seem to form both them and the more usual "dream."

Finally, I would like to suggest that the erotic dimensions of dream creativity are as apparent in the history of mysticism and its study as they are in any other area of creative activity. Most baldly and physiologically put, it is a physical and easily observable fact that the male dreamer is inevitably erect, an observation that gives witness in an unusually clear way to the sexual base (which is not to say end) of the hallucinatory qualities of the dream and, just as often, I think, the religious vision. If, in other words, nocturnal dreams and religious visions are neurologically similar processes—and I think they are—then the night dream's demonstrable connection to an ithyphallic sleeping body may tell us something important about the visionary and the psychology of the visionary process. Although the latter point is quite beyond proof or falsification, since the nature of mystical texts removes them (and us as readers) from the physical bases of the experiences which they deposit, the often explicitly erotic content of these same texts gives more than a little probability to my admittedly speculative thesis.

In an attempt to give a bit more substance to all of this, I will proceed through three brief studies of three very different connoisseurs of the mystical, one artist and two academics: the American Beat and Buddhist poet Allen Ginsburg (1926–1997), the French Islamicist Louis Massignon (1883–1962), and the Romanian-American historian of religions Mircea Eliade (1907–1986).[3] I will approach each of these sleeping male bodies as a dreaming creative.[4]

The Blakean Vision

In 1948 Allen Ginsburg was twenty-two and a college student at Columbia University.[5] Since he was subletting an apartment from a Columbia theology student, he was also subletting a not insignificant library of theological and philosophical books, among them many works of Western mystical literature: Blake, Yeats, John of the Cross, Plato, and Plotinus in particular. Ginsburg was particularly drawn to Blake. And a little masturbation. Lying in his bed, in what his biographer Michael Schumacher describes as "a sort of dull postorgasmic blankness resulting from his having read Blake's poetry while he was idly masturbating,"[6] Ginsburg stared out his window onto East Harlem and experienced a *satori* or enlightenment event that would change his life. Specifically, he heard a voice reciting Blake's "Ah Sunflower":

> Ah Sunflower! weary of time
> Who counts the steps of the sun.
> Seeking after that sweet golden clime
> Where the traveller's journey is done. . . .

But it was a strange voice, for although it was clearly his voice, somehow it was also just as clearly Blake's, speaking to him through the long corridors of eternity. Ginsburg's consciousness now shifted and he could, with Blake, see eternity in time, this time, not in the famous grain of sand but in the much larger gray Harlem sky and its rooftops: "In one shudder of illumination," Schumacher writes, "Allen reached the understanding that poetry was eternal: A poet's consciousness could travel timelessly, alter perception, and speak of universal vision to anyone attaining the same level of consciousness."[7] In the poet's mind at least, Blake and Ginsburg had shared the same consciousness, mediated through the visionary poetry on the page. Words were alchemy. Texts could transform. A kind of hermeneutical union was thus effected between Ginsburg the young aspiring poet and Blake the very dead visionary.

Ginsburg responded to this momentous, if utterly bizarre, event in two ways. The first thing he tried was to communicate the experience directly to unsympathetic listeners, that is, to people who had not had similar experiences and were not particularly keen to hear about them. More specifically, Allen climbed out onto the fire escape of the apartment building, tapped on his neighbors' window, and tried to tell the two women living next door that "I've seen God!" The women were not impressed. They slammed the window in his face. Next he tried to call his analyst on a public pay phone. Perhaps he would appreciate what had happened. The psychiatrist refused to accept the charges or talk to him.

Ginsburg's third response was far more successful. He went back to his room's theological library and began paging through other visionary texts: "I immediately rushed to Plato and read some great image in the *Phaedrus* about horses flying through the sky, and rushed over to Saint John and started reading fragments . . . and rushed to the other part of the bookshelf and picked up Plotinus about The Alone—the Plotinus I found more difficult to interpret. But I immediately doubled my thinking process, quadrupled, and I was able to read almost any text and see all sorts of divine significance in it."[8] A few days later he had a similar experience in—where else?—a bookstore. He sensed that everyone in the bookstore somehow knew the same cosmic consciousness, so utterly at peace with itself, so eternal, but that they preferred to hide it from themselves so that they could go about their daily banalities. Perhaps, however, this was for the better, he reasoned, as, should they all decide to give their immediate attentions to it at once, daily life as we know it would no doubt collapse.[9] The mystical was somehow everywhere and in everything, and yet its full force was quite incompatible with the mundane workings of social life. Still, the memory could remain without too much violence. And it did, guiding Ginsburg's poetry and art for the next fifteen years.

What happened here? And more specifically, how was it related to the reading and interpretation of mystical and poetic texts? And what are we to make of the event's obvious (auto)erotic context? Before I try to address such questions, let us look at two examples of a similar creative process in the practice of the history of mysticism.

The Waking Dream and the Tantric Twilight

Ginsburg is by no means alone in his vocation-determining altered states of consciousness. Similar patterns can often be found in the lives of historians of religion as well. Consider, for example, the case of Mircea Eliade. By his own confession, Eliade did not have "a mystical vocation"[10] within an isolated monastery, ashram or hermitage, for it was his "destiny" to live paradoxically, "to exist concurrently in 'History' and beyond it. . . ." Such a both-and existence, a philosophical analog to Ginsburg's Blakean "eternity-in-time" perhaps, was in Eliade's case "camouflaged in biographical incidents and creations of a cultural order,"[11] that is, in the synchronous events of his life course and in the texts, both scholarly and literary, that he produced in such abundance on that same course. It was Eliade's experiences in India that helped teach him this basic truth about himself and his world, and particularly his romantic encounters there with his Indian teacher's sixteen-year-old daughter (he was kicked out of the house and the student-teacher relationship for the affair[12]) and a young woman he met in a Himalayan ashram named "Jenny." With the latter he practiced some form of sexual yoga until they were caught and he had to leave the ashram.[13] As with Ginsburg, but in a different cultural mode, the erotic and the mystical were of a single piece here, united paradoxically in Eliade's own appropriation of

Indian Tantra and its divinization of the body and the physical world. Unlike the *Upanishads* and the tradition of Vedanta, whose doctrines Eliade knew but found lacking,[14] Tantric yoga sought to transform one's psychophysiological experience of the world through bold, alchemical-like physical disciplines and sacramental rituals of a deeply sensual, and sometimes sexual, nature. It was here, in the concrete engagement with the tradition and the world through the authenticity of his own "lived experience" (the Romanian category of *traire*), that Eliade sought his understanding and creativity.[15] Sergiu Al-George aptly describes this Tantric-yogic matrix of the scholar's thought as "the realm of symbolic thought and experience," "the fantastic sphere of his consciousness," and "the experience of ambiguity and paradox,"[16] and insists that these same Indian beginnings are "laden with the prestige of origins, which must be understood in the full initiatory sense as an opening to a life cycle, to a new ontological status."[17] To understand Eliade's later oeuvre, in other words, one must begin here, "from this primordial element in his cultural destiny."[18]

We might also speculate that Eliade came to his vocational choice to create culture through his dreams as well, for Eliade clearly believed in the role of premonitorial dream-visions in deciphering one's destiny: "I believe that in such dreams, which I can sometimes recall very clearly, one is being given an autorevelation of one's own destiny."[19] Similar themes appear in his literary works and were not lost on his readers. Sergiu Al-George, the Romanian scholar of Indian languages and philosophy, for example, had this to say about Eliade's novel *The Forbidden Forest* (Al-George had been sent to prison for reading it): "The reading of that book not only helped me acquire an existentialist philosophy, but the very act of my reading it intervened in a disruptive way in the unfolding of my life . . . the philosophy which I deduced from that book permitted me to meet all the subsequent events with the sentiment that above their directly concrete significance, they can and must be understood as having a superior significance, a coherence and harmony with the whole."[20] In the figure of Stefan, the hero of the novel, Al-George had discovered a figure who could accept his "fate," not as an absurdity to bemoan or suffer but as a meaningful pattern signaled by striking coincidences and synchronous signs to embrace as one's vocation or destiny.[21]

Certainly altered states of consciousness, including dream states, were also central to Eliade's self-understanding and early work on yoga, for they taught him "the reality of experiences that cause us to 'step out of time' and 'out of space.'"[22] These he would later "camouflage" in his literary writings and particularly in his novella *The Secret of Doctor Honigberger.*[23] Consider, for example, the following passage in the novella, on the "waking sleep" of a young man studying Indological works and trying to practice the techniques of yoga he found described therein:

> I really don't know how it happened, but after some time I woke up sleeping, or, more precisely, I woke up in sleep, without having fallen asleep in the true sense of the word. My body and all my senses sank into deeper and deeper sleep, but my mind didn't interrupt its activity for a single instant. Everything in me had fallen asleep except the clarity of consciousness. I continued to meditate on fire, at the same time becoming aware, in some obscure way, that the world around me was completely changed, and that if I interrupted my concentration for a single instant, I too would quite naturally become part of this world, which was the world of sleep.[24]

Whether such an account, and many others like it, are "pure fiction" or are accurate, if "literary," reflections of Eliade's own yogic experiences is difficult to say. Eliade's camouflaging technique prevents us from every truly knowing. Art and life merge imperceptibly here. Still, it seems relatively clear that such sleeping experiences convinced Eliade of the reality of those states described in the yogic traditions and so gave him a way to sympathetically enter their world and its seemingly strange doctrines. Drawing on the conviction born in these states and working out of his discovery of his own *coincidentia oppositorum,* Eliade would use, however consciously, these experiences as models to write about the Tantric yogin in his doctoral thesis and later, in his more theoretical books, about the nature of religious experience in general.

In his famous *Yoga: Immortality and Freedom* (the published version of his dissertation begun in India), for example, Eliade wrote about Tantric yoga and its own "conjunction of opposites." Expressed both symbolically and ritually through sexual union, such a state effects a "non-conditioned existence"[25] in which one becomes conscious that "the ultimate nature of the phenomenal world is identical with that of the absolute."[26] According to Eliade, a similar "paradox of opposites" is found at that base of every sacred form.[27] Such a notion, which he had "realized" or at least sought after in his own Tantric experiments, he would later employ as an overarching methodological principle in his morphology of religious forms, evident in such works as *The Sacred and the Profane* and *Patterns in Comparative Religion.* His early work (and experience) of Tantric yoga and his later morphology of religious forms, in other words, were united through the common category of the *coincidentia oppositorum.*[28]

The same pattern of combining opposites into a greater (Tantric) whole occurs in his well-known self-description of his creative process as alternating between "nocturnal" and "diurnal" modes of consciousness. Whereas his literary works participated in the nocturnal modes of creative imagination, night (and no doubt dream), the scholarly or academic works flowed from his diurnal, linear or rational thought processes. But Eliade was clear that it was the whole work that counted. The dialectic between the two modes—the *coincidentia*—was central to both his health and his creativity as a writer. And to the Tantric use of language, for both the day and the night, or better, that liminal moment between them, finds a unique linguistic incarnation in Tantric *sandha-bhasa* ("intentional speech," often translated from an alternate form as "twilight [*sandhya*] language [*bhasa*]"), that mystical use of language which refers simultaneously to a sexual form and a mystical state or doctrine. As Eliade describes it in his own dissertation become book:

> The *sandha-bhasa* . . . seeks to . . . project the yogin into the "paradoxical situation" indispensable to his training. The semantic polyvalence of words finally substitutes ambiguity for the usual system of reference inherent in every ordinary language. And this destruction of language contributes, in its way too, toward a "breaking" the profane universe and replacing it by a universe of convertible and integrable planes.[29]

This, I would suggest, is precisely what Eliade was trying to do in his own way through his literary/nocturnal and academic/diurnal modes of being, which met and transcended themselves here, in the twilight of the Tantric creative.

The Dream Conversion

Perhaps even more striking is the case of the French Islamicist Louis Massignon (1883–1962). The son of a prominent Parisian sculptor and engraver Fernand Massignon (known under his pseudonym Pierre Roche), Massignon was always something of an artist himself, attuned to the signs of both human consciousness and the natural world. He thus made it something of a habit to apologetically share in print with his fellow historians of religions the strange instances of his own "premonitorial dreams"[30] and what he called his "intersigns," those striking moments in life when external events seem to coincide perfectly with his internal state and its questions and so act as confirming guides on one's vocational path. (The idea is very close to Jung's notion of "synchronicity," not to mention Eliade's ideas about "destiny" and the reading of one's mundane life through coincidence and sign as the narrative of a meaningful script.) Massignon, like his father, sculpted life into meaning.

More unusual still was his conviction that a tenth-century Sufi, al-Hallaj (the subject of his dissertation and lifelong *magnum opus*), had communicated with him and helped effect his conversion back to Roman Catholicism within a series of altered states, hallucinatory experiences, and dreams that he suffered in the spring of 1908 in Iraq.

The story is a long one, complicated and mired in historical, political, and psychological questions. But it is also a well-documented event, by both Massignon and his interpreters, and it is particularly rich in dreamlike states and erotic subtexts.[31] The conversion occurred (or more accurately began, since it would take weeks to play itself out) on a steamship on the Tigris River. It was May 1, and Massignon had just been arrested as a French spy and was under surveillance. He was also being terrorized by some men, who were threatening to kill him before the next morning. To make matters even more dramatic, this threatened, accused foreigner was in the throes of a seemingly irresolvable moral crisis over his homosexuality (which had played more than a small role in his arrest) and also may have been suffering from malaria or, at the very least, serious heat exhaustion.

For any or, more likely, all of these reasons, Massignon's behavior became extremely erratic, if not to say bizarre, over the next few days. He pointed a gun at the captain and then at his own head. He swallowed two lit cigarettes. When the boat stopped near the ancient ruins of Ctesiphon on the evening of May 2, Massignon, fearing for his life, tried to escape but was captured again. Back on the steamer the next day, May 3, utterly exhausted and morally distraught over "four and a half years of amorality,"[32] Massignon tried to commit suicide with a small knife for some unspecified "horror"[33] he felt about himself, a barely veiled reference to his homosexual tendencies, about which he would speak with such candor later in his life. The self-inflicted wound on his chest, however, was superficial and was easily treated by the steamer's doctor, a Dr. Essad.

Still, the crisis was hardly over. Later the same day, the despairing Massignon, bound hand and foot in the captain's cabin, was suddenly struck down by what he would later call "the lightning of revelation."[34] There are numerous passing references to this event in his writings. The most beautiful and certainly the fullest account occurs in his piece "Visitation of the Stranger: Response to an Inquiry about God":

> The Stranger who visited me, one evening in May before the Taq, cauterizing my despair that He lanced, came like the phosphorescence of a fish rising from the bottom of the deepest sea; my inner mirror revealed Him to me, behind the mask of my own features. . . . The Stranger who took me as I was, on the day of His wrath, inert in His hand like the gecko of the sands, little by little overturned all my acquired reflexes, my precautions, and my deference to public opinion.[35]

What is significant for our purposes is the event's unmistakable connection to a moral crisis and, more specifically, to Massignon's conscience tortured over his homosexuality. The possibility that the cigarettes he ingested may have in fact been hashish cigarettes and that he may have also been given opium by the steamer's doctor to calm him down are also worth considering, as they may have played a small role in the genesis of the mystical experience.[36] But however we want to analyze the chemical or sexual causal factors of the experience, one thing is unmistakably clear: It changed his life forever and came to dominate his consciousness as he gave more and more of his life to the study of Sufi mysticism, to the life of al-Hallaj (whom he believed had been present at the visitation), and to innumerable political and religious causes aimed at Christian-Muslim dialogue and community building. This was the pole-event around which everything else revolved.

This was a pole, however, erected within a series of dream states, many of them of a distinctly suffering type. When, for example, the young Frenchman finally fell asleep after being threatened by the men on the steamship, his mind was still haunted by "impure desires."[37] And even after the visitation of the Stranger, dreams of guilt, moral horror, and the loss of identity continued to visit him during the nights of May 3 and 4. He kept his eyes closed, we are told, for two solid days: "I kept silent, the eyes closed (from horror and shame), feigning mutism, trying to pass for a fool."[38] Finally back at Baghdad, his eyes still shut tight, he was taken to the civil hospital on May 5, where he continued to be pursued "by nothingness" as a "series of terrible mental images continued to pass before my retinas against a background of Hallajian flames [*sur un fond de flames hallagiennes*]"[39]: Even within, or better, behind his suffering, Massignon saw fiery beauty. He would not awake until May 8, but not before the Presence visited him again as he clung to a beloved name (almost certainly that of Luis de Cuadra, a Spanish aristocrat, fellow Islamicist and lover who had recently killed himself) until he could surrender this person to God as well. When Massignon finally awoke on the morning of the eighth, the ordeal was over. The pardon had been granted, the conversion effected.

Pondering his conviction that it was al-Hallaj himself who helped effect the conversion and who was somehow present that terrible but beautiful day in May, Massignon would later write of "a distortion of Space *and* Time" that had occurred, a kind of warping of history back on itself.[40] And he intentionally underlined that "and," for he knew and proclaimed that the single most significant presence of his life was a man who has been dead for over nine hundred years: "I do not pretend that the study of his life has yielded to me the secret of his heart, but rather it is he who has fathomed mine and who fathoms it still."[41] The researched had become the researcher, the "reader of hearts" who knew Massignon across the centuries and now guided his life. Like Allen Ginsburg, Louis Massignon had known a hermeneutical union with a dead mystic through an altered state of consciousness akin to dream suffused with erotic meanings.

Discussion: Dreams, Destiny and the Creative Process

What seems important for our purposes is the indubitable fact that, whatever we might think of Ginsberg's postorgasmic eternity-in-time vision, Eliade's paradoxical Tantric state sought in sexual yoga and realized to some extent in a waking dream state, and Massignon's dramatic conversion back to Roman Catholicism and from his own homosexuality, these individuals considered such events foundational to their lives and, just as important, to their creativity as writers and thinkers.

Nor are such men alone in their "dreams of scholarship" and art.[42] I suspect that we could go on for some time listing dozens of other cases, and certainly we would have to evaluate each of these differently. What, for example, should we do with Frithjof Schuon, the philosopher of religion and premier theorist of the perennialist school of the study of mysticism? How many of his readers know that he painted a number of his dream-visions, many of them involving the vaginas of naked Christian Madonnas and Native American goddess figures, and then ritualized these in his own southern Indiana religious community within a sacred ritual dance (he would stand naked in the center, wearing a feather crown, as female devotees danced bare-breasted around him) before legal charges and sexual scandal closed the group down?[43] Once again, altered states of consciousness, the mystical, the academic, and the erotic flow in and out of one another in highly instructive ways here.

For my own part, I do not see how we can begin to assess the twentieth-century study of mysticism without taking such states seriously (which is not to say uncritically). But it is important to point out here that such dreams and altered states of consciousness are seldom enough. That is to say, the creative process, at least in the humanities, involves much more than a shifting of consciousness or a temporary rapture, however delightful or terrifying. It also involves hard and usually banal work, the conscious manipulation of ideas and images and questions, interaction with professional peers and critics, and, most of all, active interpretation. The dream-state does not and cannot stand alone. It needs a script through which to work, a cultural universe through which to express itself, an interpretation in which to live. Creativity is thus always dialectical, not just a perfect dream but, more likely, a dream to perfect. This, I would suggest, is how we might read these forms of cultural creativity—as cultural and eminently constructive transformations of dream-states.

It is this creative aspect of dreams, dreamlike states, and erotic modes of being, so central to so many Western intellectuals, that I would like to put on the table, as it were, for discussion. Or perhaps a bed, and all that that simple English word carries for us, would be a better and more fruitful site of questioning. "To go to bed." To enter into an altered state of consciousness that is too familiar. To dream and see visions. To have sex (as if we ever possess "it"). It is there that our creations often begin in a kind of absurd, seemingly senseless series of images, acts, symbols, and physiological states. "Poetry is made in bed like love," André Breton once wrote.[44] So too are we.

Notes

1. James Hughes, *Altered States: Creativity Under the Influence* (New York: Watson-Guptill, 1999).
2. My choice of the term will become obvious shortly. Briefly, however, I prefer this term because it suggests that the subjective mystical experiences of authors are carried or contained somehow by, through and in their texts, and that these same experiential deposits can catalyze similar or analogous experience-events in their sensitive readers. This is what I refer to and develop elsewhere as "hermeneutical mysticism," that is, the engendering of mystical states through the close reading and subjective interpretation of mystical texts. For much more on this, see my work *Roads of Excess, Palaces of Wisdom: Eroticism and Reflexivity in the Study of Mysticism* (Chicago: University of Chicago Press, 2001), i.

3. The sections on Eliade and Massignon are based on an earlier article, my "The Visitation of the Stranger: On Some Mystical Dimensions of the History of Religions," *CrossCurrents* 49/3 (Fall 1999).
4. I borrow the expression "creative" from Hughes, *Altered States.*
5. I am relying here on Michael Schumacher, *Dharma Lion: A Biography of Allen Ginsberg* (New York: St. Martin's Press, 1992), 94–99. My thanks to Amy Hungerford for pointing this text and passage out to me.
6. Ibid., 95.
7. Ibid.
8. Ibid., 96.
9. Ibid., 97.
10. Mircea Eliade, *Autobiography: Volume I, 1907–1937, Journey East, Journey West* (San Francisco: Harper & Row, 1981), 256.
11. Ibid., 257.
12. The teacher was Surendranath Dasgupta, at that time the world's leading authority on Indian philosophy. Eliade would later fictionalize the affair in his novel *La nuit bengali* (1950), translated by Catherine Spenser, in which he chose to use the daughter's actual name, Maitreyi. Maitreyi Devi, an accomplished poet and cultural figure in her own right, read the novel some forty years after the original romantic encounter and responded with her own Bengali novel, *Na Hanyate* (1974), literally "It does not die." Both novels, *Bengal Nights* and *It Does Not Die,* were recently republished by University of Chicago Press (1995).
13. Eliade, *Autobiography,* 198–200.
14. "Moreover, Vedanta had never held much attraction for me. I liked Tantric yoga because it had hammered out a technique of liberation in which life was not sacrificed, but was transfigured" (ibid., 187).
15. Sergiu Al-George, "India in the Cultural Destiny of Mircea Eliade," trans. Mac Linscott Ricketts with prefatory and concluding notes by J. W. Jamieson, *The Mankind Quarterly* (1978), 124.
16. Ibid., 134.
17. Ibid., 120.
18. Ibid.
19. Mircea Eliade, *Ordeal by Labyrinth: Conversations with Claude-Henri Rocquet* (Chicago: University of Chicago Press, 1982), 66.
20. Quoted in Al-George, "India in the Cultural Destiny of Mircea Eliade," 118–119.
21. I am following Jamieson's prefatory remarks on Al-George here in Ibid., 119.
22. Eliade, *Ordeal,* 49.
23. Ibid.
24. Mircea Eliade, *Two Strange Tales* (Boston: Shambhala, 1970), 98.
25. Mircea Eliade, *Yoga: Immortality and Freedom* (Princeton: Princeton University Press, 1969), 268.
26. Ibid., 269.
27. Eliade, *Autobiography,* 297.
28. Eliade says as much: "Nearly all the ideas that I expounded in the books published in French after 1946 are found *in nuce* in studies written between 1933 and 1939 [foremost among them his *Yoga*]" (*Autobiography,* 309).
29. Eliade, *Yoga,* 241.
30. Louis Massignon, "The Transfer of Suffering," in Herbert Mason, *Testimonies and Reflections: Essays of Louis Massignon* (Notre Dame: University of Notre Dame Press, 1989), 158.
31. For three fuller descriptions and analyses, see: Christian Destremau and Jean Moncelon, *Massignon* (Paris: Plon, 1994), chap. 3; Mary Louise Gude, *Louis Massignon: The Crucible*

of Compassion (Notre Dame: University of Notre Dame Press, 1996), chap. 2; Kripal, *Roads of Excess, Palaces of Wisdom,* chap. 2.

32. Quoted by Gude, *Louis Massignon,* 41.
33. Massignon, "An Entire Life with a Brother Who Set Out on the Desert: Charles de Foucauld," in Mason, *Testimonies,* 25.
34. Massignon, "Meditation of a Passerby on His Visit to the Sacred Woods of Ise," in Mason, *Testimonies,* 167.
35. Massignon, "Visitation of the Stranger," in Mason, *Testimonies,* 41.
36. Destremau and Moncelon, *Massignon,* 62.
37. Ibid., 58.
38. Quoted in ibid., 63; translation mine.
39. Quoted in Gude, *Louis Massignon,* 45.
40. Massignon, "The Transfer of Suffering," in Mason, *Testimonies,* 162.
41. Mason, "Preface," xix.
42. Perceptive readers probably have already asked themselves about my own dreams and their impact on my scholarship, and they would not be wrong to ask such reasonable questions. As, however, I have addressed such dreams and my interpretations of them at considerable length in *Roads of Excess, Palaces of Wisdom,* I will not repeat myself here.
43. See Hugh B. Urban, "A Dance of Masks: The Esoteric Ethics of Frithjof Schuon," in G. William Barnard and Jeffrey J. Kripal, eds., *Crossing Boundaries: Essays on the Ethical Status of Mysticism* (New York: Seven Bridges Press, 2001).
44. Quoted in J. Allan Hobson, *Consciousness* (New York: Scientific American Library, 1999), 229.

16

The New Anthropology of Dreaming

Barbara Tedlock

In recent years dream researchers have become sensitive to the differences between dream accounts and dreams. While dreams are private mental acts, which have never been recorded during their actual occurrence, dream accounts are public social performances taking place after the experience of dreaming. When dreamers decide, for whatever reason, to share a dream experience, they choose an appropriate time and place, a specific audience and social context, a modality (visual or auditory), and a discourse or performance form. While some clinicians and experiential dream workers operate with the fiction that when they hear or produce a sufficiently dramatic dream report they can recover the dream itself, as if entering into a "real dream life" (Mahrer 1989: 44–46), cultural anthropologists have turned their attention to the study of dream sharing as a communicative event (B. Tedlock 1987a).

Psychologists of both the psychoanalytic and the cognitive bents have, for the most part, read anthropology in order to compare the dreams of what have been categorized as "preliterate," "tribal," "traditional," or "peasant" peoples with the dreams of "literate," "urban," "modern," or "industrial" peoples. While cultural anthropologists made such comparisons in the past, today we have turned away from this labeling practice because of its use of typological time, which denies people living in other cultures "coevalness," or contemporaneity with ourselves (Fabian 1983). The use of typological time, which fictively places some people in an earlier time frame than ourselves, functions as a distancing device. An example of this practice is the assertion that there currently exist societies practicing "stone age economics." We cultural anthropologists also experience this temporal displacement ourselves, whenever we identify ourselves to our neighbors, hairdressers, or physicians as "anthropologists" only to find ourselves confused with "archaeologists," studying ancient stone tools, pyramids, and human remains. Instead of using typological time to create and set off an object of study such as "tribal dream typologies" (Hunt 1989: 87), cultural anthropologists today are interested in intersubjective time in which all of the participants involved are "coeval," that is, share the same time. The current focus on communicative processes in cultural anthropology demands that coevalness not only be created and maintained in the field but also be carried over during the write-up process. Thus, for example, Robert Dentan, while discussing the principle of contraries in which dreams indicate the opposite of what they seem, noted that practitioners of this type of dream interpretation include "such widely separated peoples as Ashanti, Malays, Maori, Buffalo (New York) Polish-American parochial schoolgirls, psychoanalysts, Semai and Zulu" (Dentan 1986: 33). In other words, at least some Americans share this principle of dream interpretation with people living in faraway, exotic places.

The change in research strategy away from treating so-called non-Western dreams as totally "other" but nonetheless fully knowable objects to be gathered, tabulated, and compared with our own "Western dreams," and toward paying attention to the problematics of dream representation, communication, and interpretation worldwide has occurred within anthropology for several reasons. First, cultural anthropologists have come to distrust survey research in which "data" is gathered for the purpose of testing Western theories concerning universals in human psychology. Thus, for example, Calvin Hall's (1951, 1953) cross-cultural content analysis, in which statistical assertions about dream patterns within particular ethnic groups or genders are the goal, have been critiqued by anthropologists (B. Tedlock 1987a; Dentan 1988a). There are several reasons for this, including the fact that sample surveys aggregate respondents who are deeply distrustful of the researcher with those who are not, as if suspicion made no difference whatsoever in the validity of their replies (Scheff 1986). Further, a comparativist focus on the extractable contents of a dream report not only omits important phenomena such as pacing, tones of voice, gestures, and audience responses that accompany dream narrative performances, but is also an expression of the culture of alphabetic literacy and is thus culture-bound (Crapanzano 1981; B. Tedlock 1987a; Dentan 1988a).

Another reason for the abandonment of content analysis by anthropologists is that our formal training in linguistics encourages us to reject the basic assumption of aggregate statistical research, namely, that meaning resides within single words rather than within their contexts (Dentan 1988a).[1] This critique rests on a basic axiom of semantics, known as the premise of nonidentity, which states that the word is not the object. Dream narratives are not dreams, and neither narrating nor enacting dreams can ever recover dream experiences. Furthermore, dream symbols taken in isolation can be misleading if the researcher has not spent at least a year observing and interacting within the culture in order to gather enough contextual details to make sense of local knowledge and produce a "thick description" of that culture (Geertz 1973; Dentan 1988b: 38).[2] Thus, rather than interpreting the language of dream narratives in semantico-referential, context-independent terms, it is more appropriate to utilize context-dependent, or pragmatic, meaning (Silverstein 1976).

Because of these considerations anthropologists no longer set out to elicit dream reports as ethnographic objects to be used as raw data for comparative hypotheses (e.g., Lincoln 1935; Schneider and Sharp 1969). Instead, we now go into the field for extended periods of time with broad sets of research interests; for example, the religion and worldview of a particular society, the performance of healing, or the construction of self and personhood. By living within the community we learn not only the language but also how to interact appropriately, and, perhaps most important, we are present for various formal and informal social dramas.[3] Sooner or later we cannot help but be present when a dream is narrated within a family or to a practicing shaman or some other dream interpreter. If this type of event or social drama attracts our attention, we make notes about it in our field journals and we may later record other such occurrences on audio- or videotape. Once we have translated such texts we may ask the narrator, who may or may not be the dreamer, questions about the meaning, significance, and use of the dream account.

This shift in research strategy from directly eliciting dozens of fixed objects (dreams) to studying naturally occurring situations (dream sharing, representation, and interpretation) is part of a larger movement within anthropology in which there has been a rapidly growing interest in analyses focused on practice, interaction, dialogue, experience, and performance, together with the individual agents, actors, persons, selves, and subjects of all this activity (Bourdieu 1978; D. Tedlock 1979; Ortner 1984). Three recent doctoral dissertations in anthropology clearly display this shift from the dream as an object to the context surrounding the personal experience and cultural uses of dreaming (Desjarlais 1991; Roseman 1990; Degarrod 1989). Robert Desjarlais, during his fieldwork in Nepal with the Yolmo Sherpa, noted a large degree of agreement among individuals concerning the meaning of dream imagery and found what he called "an implicit 'dictionary' of dream symbolism," which individuals relied on most frequently in times of physical or spiritual distress (Desjarlais 1991: 102–117). Thus, for example, dreaming of an airplane, bus, or horse indicates that one's spirit has left the body and that one will soon fall ill, while dreaming of a new house or clothes, snow failing on the body, consuming sweet white foods such as milk, and watching the sun setting or the waxing of the moon all indicate future good health.

In this dream interpretation system, like many others, the experience of dreaming is believed to have a close, even causal, connection with the future life of the dreamer. (See also Bruce 1975, 1979; Laughlin 1976; Herdt 1977; Kilborne 1978; Kracke 1979; Basso 1987; B. Tedlock 1987b; Dentan 1983; Degarrod 1989; Hollan 1989; McDowell 1989.) However, it is important to remember that such interpretations are often provisional, that not all people in a given society place their faith in such interpretations, and that in some societies only certain individuals are believed to be able to experience prophetic or precognitive dreams (Devereux 1956; Meggitt 1962; Charsley 1973; Jackson 1978; Dentan 1983; Merrill 1987). Nevertheless, prophetic dreams and visions have often triggered anticolonial revolts (Wallace 1959; Dentan 1986). But lest we fall into the comfortable assumption that prophetic dream interpretation systems are characteristically found in "tribal," "non-Western," or "nonindustrial" societies, and only rarely in "modern," "Western," "industrialized" societies (Hodes 1989:7–8), cultural anthropologists who have undertaken substantial fieldwork within American society have found that middle-class dreamers admit to having experienced dreams of the prophetic or precognitive sort in which they obtain information about future events (Collins 1977: 46, 49, 58–59; Hillman 1988: 134; Dombeck 1989: 89). Furthermore, the popular Western conception of dreams as predictors of misfortune or success, together with the anecdotal literature on "psychic dreams," indicates that this form of dream interpretation is far from rare in Western societies (Stevens 1949; Ullman, Krippner and Vaughan 1973; Staff 1975; Tolaas 1986, 1990; Persinger 1988; Persinger and Krippner 1989).

Labeling certain dream experiences "prophetic" or "precognitive," however, does not explain how these and other dream experiences are used both individually and culturally within a society. In order to learn about the actual use of dreaming, researchers cannot simply gather examples of different types of dreams by administering a questionnaire but must instead interact intensively for a long period of time. Thus while Desjarlais (1991) quickly discovered the implicit "dictionary" of dream symbolism among the Sherpa, it took him some time as an apprentice shaman to learn the precise way in which these dream symbols served as symptoms and signifiers both reflecting and shaping distress. Likewise, Marina Roseman (1986), through her active participation as a singer within an all-female chorus in Temiar society, learned the precise manner in which local dream sharing through song connects the musical and medical domains of knowledge and practice. In this Malaysian society, spirit guides teach dreamers songs by singing them phrase by phrase, and dreamers learn songs during their dreams by repeating the songs phrase by phrase. This dream-teaching relationship is echoed in public performance when a male medium sings a song phrase that is then repeated by a female chorus. In time Roseman grasped the fact that dream songs varied by the spirit guide source, creating formal musical genres with characteristic textual content and vocabulary, melodic and rhythmic patterns, dance movements, and trance behavior. Not only do these genres vary individually, but they also vary regionally and historically. During her twenty months of fieldwork she taped hundreds of these dream-song performances, together with intricate dream narratives and interpretations (Roseman 1986, 1990).

Lydia Degarrod (1989), like Roseman and Desjarlais, recorded the majority of her dream materials within a natural setting rather than by arranging formal interviews. During her research among the Mapuche Indians of Chile she gathered dream accounts and various interpretations of these narratives from several members of two families who were coping with serious stress caused by witchcraft and illness (Degarrod 1990). Through dream sharing and interpreting, the afflicted members of the families were able to express their anxieties and externalize their illness, and other family members were able to participate directly in the healing of their loved ones. Degarrod hypothesized that these types of family interventions were possible due to the nature of both the communal dream sharing and interpreting system, which allowed for the combination of elements from different individual's dreams to be related through intertextual and contextual analysis, and the general belief that dreams facilitate communication with supernatural beings.

By studying dream sharing and the transmission of dream theories in their full social contexts as communicative events, including the natural dialogical interactions that take place within these events, anthropologists have realized that both the researcher and those who are researched are engaged in the creation of a social reality that implicates both of them. Even though cultural anthropologists have long subscribed to the method of participant observation, it still comes as a shock when they discover how important their participation is in helping to create what they are studying (LeVine 1981). Thus, for example, Gilbert Herdt reported his surprise at discovering the therapeutic dimension of his role in New Guinea as a sympathetic listener to his key consultant, who shared with him erotic dreams taking place in menstrual huts, which he could not communicate to anyone within his own society (Herdt 1987: 73–74). Likewise, the importance to anthropology of the psychodynamic process of transference, which is to say the bringing of past experiences into a current situation with the result that the present is unconsciously experienced as though it were the past (Freud 1958; Bird 1972; Loewald 1986), has only recently been fully realized and described for anthropology. Waud Kracke (1987a), during his fieldwork with the Kagwahiv Indians of Brazil during 1967 to 1968, kept a diary containing his personal reactions, dreams, and associations. In a sensitive essay discussing these field responses, Kracke not only analyzes his personal transference of his own family relationships to certain key Kagwahiv individuals but also his cultural transference of American values to Kagwahiv behavior patterns. Other cultural anthropologists have not only recorded their dreams and associations in their field diaries but have also told their dreams to members of the society in which they were working for the purpose of having them interpreted (Bruce 1975; Jackson 1978; B. Tedlock 1981; Stephen 1989).

When anthropologists have paid close attention to their own dreams during their fieldwork, they have found that dream experiences have helped them to integrate their unconscious with a conscious sense of personal continuity in this totally new, even threatening, situation. Laura Nadar, for example, reported that during her research among Zapotec Indians in Mexico, the amount of her nocturnal dreaming, as well as her ability to remember dreams, multiplied several times over her usual behavior and that her dreams dealt almost exclusively with her experiences as a child and young adult back home in the United States. "Not only my dreams, but also my general emotional state appeared to be more related to pre-Zapotec experiences than anything else" (Nadar 1970: 11). And although she did not feel herself to be equipped professionally to analyze why her dreams were more directly related to experience outside of the field situation, she states that "it was not because I was emotionally neutral about the people I was studying" (ibid.: 111–112). It is as though her dreams were reminding her not to lose herself completely, not to become possessed by Zapotec "otherness." Her dreams reassured her that she was indeed still the same person she was as a child, that there was a continuity within her self, in spite of her strong feelings to the contrary.

A juxtaposition of earlier and recent life events in the dreams of fieldworkers is also a common experience. A study by Barbara Anderson (1971) of fifteen American academics living in India reports a major change in dream content, moving from an initial retreat to earlier life events toward the establishment of a "secondary identity" that allows dreams with mixed but clearly distinct American and Indian elements. In the first month of fieldwork she and her fellow academics reported dreaming of people from their childhood—old neighbors and school friends—whom they had not thought about in years. During the second month, current family members entered their dream life, but shyly and from a great distance; for example, one man's wife talked with him from a doorway. It was not until a good deal later that their dream worlds included a wider spectrum of personages and backdrops with Indian settings in which their spouses, siblings, and children mingled together with Indians. Anderson suggests that these dreams are the resolution of the serious identity crisis that accompanies mixed cultural affiliation.

Karla Poewe, a Canadian anthropologist of German extraction who published her memoir of fieldwork in West Africa under the pseudonym Manda Cesara (1982: 22), reported a dream in which she found herself in a position where she and a group of other people had to make a decision between fascism and freedom. For some reason many people found themselves standing in line to join the will of the government, while she chose to swim free of the crowd singing "I want freedom." An official approached her and said, "A very important person wants to see you," and he took her to the front of a line of people into a place off to one side. There she had to wait again and, while waiting, saw a child who had also chosen freedom. The child was playing with a cuddly animal that disappeared in the bushes. She did not want to lose the child, but it looked around furtively then slid through the shrubbery to freedom. As she continued waiting, a gorgeously dressed elderly woman came by and stood before the mirror, saying how absurd it was to emphasize dress. The dreamer then moved away from the crowd with the realization that freedom lay beyond the shrubs, not in this line of waiting people, and she awoke. Later, as she established her second cultural identity, her dreams, like those Barbara Anderson reported, changed to include mixed but clearly distinct American and African elements.

Remembered dream images can also serve as a mirror reflecting back to the cultural anthropologist a secure sense of self-integrity and identity. Not all people are equally suitable to serve as "mirrors," however. For some people it seems to be only in the eyes of their own countrymen, or even themselves, that they can find a mirror. Thus, Polish anthropologist Bronislaw Malinowski reported in his posthumously published field diary: "Today . . . I had a strange dream; homo-sex, with my own double as a partner. Strangely auto-erotic feelings: the impression that I'd like to have a mouth just like mine to kiss, a neck that curves just like mine, a forehead just like mine (seen from the side)" (Malinowski 1967:12). Typically, mirror or double images in dreams represent an attempt to restore, retrieve, or bolster a threatened sense of self through the mechanisms psychologists have labeled "projection" and "identification" (Devereux 1978: 224).

Malinowski's field diaries shocked many people because this self-proclaimed father of participant observation, the key methodology still used today in cultural anthropology, exposed his remarkable lack of participation in, and even respect for, the culture he described. He revealed his distaste for Trobrianders, with whom he lived for four years. The lack of Trobriand features in his reported dreams are particularly disturbing. In the diaries, which cover two separate one-year periods, 1914–15 and 1917–18, he mentions and briefly reports twenty dreams (ibid.: 12–13, 66, 70, 71, 73, 78, 80, 82, 116, 149, 159, 191, 202, 203, 204, 207, 208, 255, 290, 295). The settings of these dreams were usually in Poland, and the people who appeared most frequently were his mother and boyhood friends, including a girlfriend he expressed guilt about having abandoned. While two of the dreams included colonial officers, none as set within the Trobriand culture, nor did any include a single indigenous person. Apparently, Malinowski did not successfully establish a "secondary identity" in the field, which would have allowed for dreams with mixed but clearly distinct Polish and Trobriand elements.

In *Sex and Repression in Savage Society,* a book with the expressed purpose of critiquing both the Oedipus and dream interpretation theories of Sigmund Freud, Malinowski claims that, unlike other non-Westem peoples, the Trobrianders "dream little, have little interest in their dreams, seldom relate them spontaneously, do not regard the ordinary dream as having any prophetic or other importance, and have no code of symbolic explanation whatsoever" (Malinowski 1927: 92). This surprising account sounds rather like the situation today in bourgeois middle-class Western society. However, reading on a bit further in the text, we find a five-page discussion of the premonitory dreams of fishermen and kula traders, the use of dreams by ritual specialists to initiate novices and to advise their community, dreams in which women's dead kinsmen inform them of their pregnancy, and the sending of dreams by magical means to cause others to fall in love with one (ibid.: 92–96).

It appears that Malinowski's greatly exaggerated claim of a lack of Trobriand interest in dreams originates from his anxiety to establish the Trobrianders as exempt from repression. If indeed this were the case, it would weaken the supposed universality of

Freud's Oedipus complex. However, Malinowski began with the faulty premise that, in Freudian theory, "the main cause of dreams is unsatisfied sexual appetite." He then reasoned that the absence of psychological repression among Trobrianders accounts for the noticeable lack of erotic material in their dreams, which in turn explains their lack of concern with dreams in general. But this scarcity of eroticism in the manifest content of dreams may, of course, bear the opposite interpretation. If anything, freedom from repression should be indicated by the presence of sexual elements, since wishes that appear undistorted at the manifest level must not have been subject to a remarkable amount of censorship. Thus, the absence of sexual elements suggests disguise, which presupposes repression.

While it is true that the majority of cultural anthropologists have been unwilling to discuss dream material, except incidentally and in passing, there have always been individuals who are not antipsychological in the clear manner in which Malinowski was. The renowned American anthropologist Robert Lowie, for example, kept a personal dream journal for nearly fifty years (from 1908 to 1957), and he was preparing an essay about his dream experiences when he died. Shortly thereafter, his wife published his essay in the prestigious international journal *Current Anthropology.* Lowie was, in his own words, a "chronic and persistent dreamer" who also often heard voices or saw visions when he was lying with his eyes half-closed. He remarks that during his later years his dreams helped him greatly in understanding visionary experiences of the Native Americans with whom he worked. According to him, the difference between himself and "an Eskimo shaman who has heard a meaningless jumble of sounds or a Crow visionary who has seen a strange apparition is that I do not regard such experiences as mystic revelations, whereas they do. But I can understand the underlying mental and emotional experiences a good deal better than most other ethnologists can, because I have identical episodes every night and almost every day of my life" (Lowie 1966: 379).

French anthropologist Michel Leiris, during the 1931 to 1933 Dakar-Djibouti expedition to the Dogon and Ethiopians, recorded not only the doings of various African subjects and the strained relationships between the European members of the research team but his own dreams. Thus, his diary entry for October 10, 1931 reads as follows: "Hard to sleep, for the others as for me, since we're possessed by the work. All night, dreams of totemic complications and family structures, with no way to save myself from this labyrinth of streets, tabooed sites and cliffs. Horror at becoming so inhuman. . . . But how to shake it off, get back in contact? Would have to leave, forget everything" (Clifford 1986: 31). His September 1, 1932 diary entry opens: "Very bad night. First insomnia, then, very late, a little sleep. A dream of Z [his wife], a dream I get some mail, which makes me feel better. Then suddenly, the smell of the herbs I've had scattered around my room enters my nostrils. Half dreaming. I have the sensation of a kind of swirling (as if reddening and turning my head I were doing the *gourri* dance characteristic of trance) and I let out a scream. This time I'm really possessed" (Leiris 1934: 358; English translation Clifford 1986: 44). Here desire for his wife is transformed, by the odor of African herbs, into possession. And it just so happens, as his diary also reveals, that at the time he was erotically infatuated with the beautiful daughter of the charismatic leader of the Zar possession cult he was busy documenting.

Another early cultural anthropologist, Alice Marriott, after she had been in the field for some time with the Kiowa of western Oklahoma, began having dreams with dozens of tepees mixed together with other dream elements. After experiencing this dream numerous times the tepees slowly became clearer, then larger and larger, until they swarmed around her and danced with a drum beating time to their movements. Finally, an ancient and totally blind Kiowa holy man had a dream about Marriott in which his power spirit stood on one side of her and an important religious bundle stood on the other side. He interpreted his dream as an indication that he should talk with her about the Kiowa religion. However, when other Kiowa holy men caught wind of his intention, they forbade him to teach her the religion. So, although she had exchanged what most members of the tribe considered "power dreams" (what anthropologists have labeled "culture pattern dreams") with a holy man, she was blocked from gaining further religious knowledge (Marriott 1952: 74–87).

More recently, Australian anthropologist Michael Jackson, who did extensive research in the early 1970s among the Kuranko of northeast Sierra Leone, reported some of his own dreams and carefully noted the differences between a native interpretation and his own. About a month after commencing his fieldwork and the day before he made his first formal inquiries about dreams, Jackson reported a dream of his own. In the first episode he found himself in a bare room, reminiscent of one of the classrooms at the District Council Primary School in a town where he had first met his field assistant. A corrugated iron door opened and a book was passed into the room by an invisible hand or by some other invisible agency. The book hung suspended in midair for several seconds, and he identified a single word in bold type on its cover: "**ETHNOGRAPHY.**" He had the definite impression that the book contained only blank pages. In the second episode he found himself again in the same room and again the door opened. "I felt a tremendous presence sweep into the room. I felt myself lifted up bodily and, as if held in the hands or by the power of a giant, I was taken out of the room. The hand and arms of the giant exerted such pressure against my breast that I could not breathe easily. I was borne along aloft, still being squeezed. At this point I awoke in fear from the dream" (Jackson 1978: 120).

According to Jackson, the dream manifested many of his anxieties at that time, most notably his concern that he would not be able to carry out the necessary research for his thesis and his dependence on his field assistant, who was not only instructing him in the language but who was mediating all his relationships. He also admitted to feeling what he described as a mild form of paranoia, which consisted of feelings of vulnerability, loneliness, and ignorance.

The following day he made a scheduled trip to a nearby village where he met a Kuranko diviner who knew something of dream interpretation and recounted his dream to him. The diviner was puzzled and discussed the dream with other elders who were present. They asked Jackson whether the giant flew up into the sky with him and whether or not he had been placed back on the ground. When these questions were answered, the diviner announced the meaning of the dream: It signified that, if Jackson were a Kuranko, he would be destined to become a chief. The diviner added, "I do not know about you because you are a European, but for us the book means knowledge, it came to reveal knowledge." So, despite this diviner's caveat that he might not be able to interpret a European's dream correctly, his elucidation of the meaning of the dream was consistent with orthodox Kuranko formulations in which a book signified knowledge; being in a strange place among strange people denoted good fortune in the near future; being in a high place indicated the imminent attainment of a prestigious position; and flying like a bird signified happiness and prosperity.

Where the diviner's interpretation differed from Jackson's own interpretation was both at the level of exegesis and in the diviner's conviction that the dream presaged future events rather than revealing present anxieties. Nevertheless, Jackson reports that these assurances helped him to allay his anxieties and that he felt that the diviner's treatment of the dream was not simply a reflection of a set of standardized interpretative procedures. Instead, it was consciously or unconsciously the outcome of sympathetic attention to Jackson's position as a stranger in his society.

In 1976 when my husband, Dennis Tedlock, and I had traveled to highland Guatemala to undertake a year of fieldwork with Quiche-Mayans, we also found ourselves, early in our stay, consulting a diviner about our own disturbing dreams. In the first month of field research, on the same night, we each dreamed about Hapiya, one of our Zuni Indian consultants, who, when we first saw him, was in the hospital recuperating from a gallbladder operation. I dreamed that I read his obituary in the *Gallup* [New Mexico] *Independent,* which reported that he had entered the hospital on October 6 and that he had been eighty seven when he died there. (Both his age and the date of his hospital admission were wrong.) Meanwhile Dennis was dreaming that he was going over the transcript of a written text with Hapiya and that Hapiya had said that two of the lines were saying exactly the same thing (a typically Mayan, rather than Zuni, form of semantic coupleting). Dennis, who awakened abruptly from his dream with the horrible feeling that he had been with a man who was already dead, awakened me in order to share his dream. I then narrated my own dream about Hapiya.

The next morning we told our dream narratives to our consultant, Andres Xiloj, who also turned out to be a trained dream interpreter. As soon as we finished narrating our dreams, he immediately replied: "Yesterday, or the day before, he died. At first it seemed that he was in agony, ready to die, but when you [Barbara] said you dreamed he was already deceased, I knew it to be so." Xiloj then commenced a formal calendrical divination by asking us for the correct date of the hospital admission. It was January 22, which he then determined to have been *Kib' N'oj* (Two Thought) on the Mayan calendar. He spread out his divining paraphernalia and counted out groups of seeds, arriving at *Hob' Kame* (Five Death), and said: "Yes, it happened that he was alleviated a little when he arrived at the hospital, but later his sickness became more grave."

At this point we described the situation in the hospital, where Hapiya had survived an operation, but then, for some inexplicable reason, had simply been abandoned, left alone in a room with the window open. Since this action was interpreted by his family as the staff's decision to simply let him die, they forced entry into his room and massaged him, returning his breath to him, and sent for a Zuni medicine man. The healer performed the traditional sucking cure, removing deer blood and hair from Hapiya's throat so that he could once again talk.

Xiloj continued with an interpretation of our amplified account, saying "What happened to this man was not a simple sickness and was not sent by God. It is the act of a man; because of some business or other things he has done with his neighbor the man was put to rest."

We told Xiloj that Hapiya spoke of having an enemy who wanted to kill him, and he concluded, "The one who envied him is already incarcerated, he doesn't walk the face of the earth, but is in purgatory where he is being punished for his deeds. This man died before this sickness but his deed remained for Hapiya to receive."

These two dreams revealed our anxiety and guilt over leaving our previous fieldwork commitment to start up new fieldwork elsewhere. Also, as of that time we did not know whether Hapiya was dead or not (it turned out that he was dead), but Xiloj's dream interpretation helped us deal with what we feared was the death not only of a person we had come to deeply respect and love, but also of our own first fieldwork. We were unaware of just what we had communicated about ourselves when we shared our troubling dreams with Xiloj.

One thing was certain, though, and that was that we were going far beyond the telling of our dreams as a token of friendship, a technique that George Foster utilized in his dream research in Mexico. In an essay entitled, "Dream, Character, and Cognitive Orientation in Tzintzuntzan" (Foster 1973), he explained that he obtained his data by volunteering his own dreams, as a gesture of amity and openness, which rewarded him with comparable personal disclosures from his informants. He suggests this procedure to other investigators as a useful eliciting tool that can produce excellent field data. While it is true that the dream narratives he collected were far richer than the brief statements of the manifest content of typical dreams collected by earlier anthropologists such as Jackson Lincoln (1935), Foster, in keeping with his procedure of using his own dreams only as a field tool, neglected to record any of them in his publications. It is as though his own dream life were unimportant and, further, that the dreams he chose to relate to his subjects in no way influenced which dreams they in turn selected to share with him.

In our own situation, since we were not sharing dreams as part of a preconceived field strategy, there was quite a different turn of events. Shortly after telling our Zuni dreams to Xiloj we were seen visiting outdoor non-Christian shines on several occasions, thus revealing our intense curiosity about Mayan spirituality. Later, when I fell ill with what I self-diagnosed as pneumonia, Xiloj divined the ultimate cause of my illness to lie in our offenses before the earth deities and informed us that we would both die. It seems that what we thought were innocent visits to the shrines had in fact annoyed not only the human *ajq'ij* (daykeepers) who were praying there but also the deities. We had thoughtlessly entered the presence of the sacred shrines without even realizing that we must be ritually pure before doing so.

Later, when we asked Xiloj for more details about the people who were praying at these shrines, specifically how they were trained and initiated, he replied that the best way to find out was to undertake an apprenticeship. When we asked him whether he would in fact be willing to train us, he chuckled and said, "Why, of course." During this four and a half months of formal training, timed according to the Mayan calendar, we were expected to narrate all of our dreams in order for him to interpret them. Thus, dream sharing, instead of being our methodology for recording a ethnographic subject's dreams, became Xiloj's way of instructing and reinforcing us in our training as well as a way of checking on our spiritual, or psychic, progress. So the dreams that we ended up gathering were our own. Only occasionally and mostly for pedagogical reasons did we hear any of Xiloj's dreams. It was not until after our initiation that we were brought dreams by various Mayan individuals for interpretation.

Twenty days into our apprenticeship I dreamed, sometime in the night between the *Wajxakeb'* (Eight Deer) and *B'elejeb' Q'anil* (Nine Yellowripe) on the Mayan calendar, that I was diving in a spot off Catalina Island that looked like my favorite scuba location, where I had gathered abalones nearly fourteen years earlier. I was passing through some dark plants and saw a shaft of light coming down through the water ahead, showing me a cave with a floor covered with seashells. Suddenly an enormous fish emerged from the cave. I was scared because I thought it was a shark, but then I realized that it was a dolphin, and I surfaced.

Xiloj counted the Mayan calendar through then said, "It seems this is the family, ancestors, these are the ones who are giving the sign that the work you two are accomplishing here, and the permissions, are going to come out all right, are going to come out into the light. It is a woman who has died who came to give this notice, this sign. This dream that the fish came out over the water means the work, it's going to come out well. The light fell into the water." (This is a literal translation from a tape-recording.)

> I replied, "Yes, the dolphin went up also."
>
> "And the work is going to mate with you, to come out into the light. But I don't know if it was your mother or your grandmother who came to give the sign."
>
> "What about the cave?"
>
> "The cave is the tomb of the mother or grandmother who has died. Is your mother still living?"
>
> "Yes, but my grandmothers are both dead."
>
> "Then it's your grandmother who came."
>
> "And the shells in the cave?"
>
> "The shells are not shell, but—all kinds were found there?"
>
> "Yes.
>
> "Then these are the red seeds, the crystal [the key contents of the sacred divining paraphernalia we would be receiving at our initiation]."
>
> "And the dark plants?"
>
> "The plants are like the shade. When one is in the shade the ground is somewhat dark. When one goes out into the sun, then everything is clear."

At this point Dennis told his dream of this same night,

> "I saw a blue-jay and put my hand out to invite it to come. The bird came and rubbed its breast against my fingers [here he gestured demonstrating that his hand was closed with his fingers in a horizontal position]. The next moment I found the bird on a blanket in front of me on its back, as if sick, and I gave it a piece of bread. When I next looked, it was gone."
>
> "The bird means that it seems that you are going to have an offspring. The birds, when dreamed of, are offspring one is going to have. But the offspring is as if sick; on being born, it is sick. Here, when we dream that we take hold of a bird, any kind of bird, and we put it in the pocket, or we put it inside the shirt, now we know we are going to have an offspring."

Dennis then related his second dream of the previous evening. "I was being followed by a large deer with enormous antlers when I encountered, by the right side of the road, another deer, also with large antlers, seated on the ground. When I passed this deer, it got up, but, though it had first seemed like one deer, it was now two. The left deer had the left set of antlers and the right deer had the right. The two of them, side by side [their sides touching], followed me.

"B'elejeb' Q'anil (Nine Yellow), what is this?" After a long silence, Xiloj looked at Dennis and said, "What this dream means, what these deer are, here is the Holy World. Yes, it is the World. *Ch'uti Sab'al* (Little Declaration Place), and *Paja'* (At the Water), and *Nima Sab'al* (Big Declaration Place). The three. And these three places are already

following the two of you. If you leave here, they will go with you, they won't let you go without them, they'll go on appearing to you. Two of the deer are already united, since I've already been going to *Paja'* (the One Place shrine) and I started going to *Ch'uti Sab'al* (the Eight Place shrine) yesterday. The third deer is farther away because I still haven't gone to *Nima Sab'al* (the Nine Place shrine). That will come on *B'ele-jeb' Kej* (Nine-Deer)."

After this dream, while Dennis was in a hypnagogic half-waking state called *saq waram,* or "white sleep" in Quiche, two small yellow sparks appeared before him in succession.

Xiloj began muttering to himself then said aloud, "These sparks are the light of the World. The World already knows you two are going to accept what you're hearing. The sparks, the light is now being given to you. Right now it's tinged with yellow, but as we go along it will clarify."

These dreams pleased Xiloj, since they occurred on the very evening when he had first visited the shrines at Ch'uti Sabal in order to present us to the Mundo as apprentices. At the time he had looked for bad omens, in both the natural world and in his own dreams, indicating that our training would not work out well. Not only did he fail to find negative omens, but we had, unknowingly, produced positive ones, indicating that the ancestors (the dolphin) and the shrines (the deer) were willing to accept us. As time went by we began to have dreams with more and more Mayan cultural elements, including religious images and mountain spirits as well as Mayan individuals, including Xiloj. Xiloj, in turn, also had dreams that included both us and cultural items from our society which we had brought into the field with us. Some of these dreams revealed strong currents of anxiety as well as transference and countertransference between ourselves and Xiloj. Finally, on *Wajakeb' B'atz'* (Eight Monkey), or August 18, 1976, we were initiated together with dozens of other novices at the shrines Xiloj had been visiting on our behalf until then. After our initiation we were consulted as dream interpreters by Mayan people, and we have continued to pay attention to our dreams, to record and interpret them in the way we were taught, in accordance with the Quiche Mayan calendar. (See D. Tedlock 1990.)

Conclusion

Anthropologists no longer set out to elicit dream reports as though they were ethnographic objects that might be arranged, manipulated, and quantified like items of material culture. Rather than making typological or statistical comparisons between the dreams found in so-called Western versus non-Western societies, cultural anthropologists have turned their attention to studying dream theories and interpretation systems as complex psychodynamic communicative events. By studying dream sharing and the transmission of dream theories in their full social contexts, anthropologists have realized that both the researcher and the subject of research create a social reality that links them in important ways.

Today fieldworkers are participating within native contexts and learning not only the local cultural uses of dream experiences but also paying attention to their own dreams. This latter practice has helped them to become aware of their unconscious responses to the people and culture they are attempting to understand and describe. In time, perhaps, cultural anthropologists, like psychoanalysts, will develop the necessary skill and training to listen to emotional dream communications of others as well as to their own feelings (Kracke 1978). For, as Rosalind Cartwright and other dream lab researchers have suggested, dreams play an important part in mastering new affective experiences and assimilating them into one's self-schemata (Cartwright 1977: 131–133; Palombo 1978). This particular form of self-mastery would seem to be an important undertaking, not only for psychoanalysts but for anthropologists who use participant observation as their key research methodology.

Notes

1. An exception to this general situation in cultural anthropology today is the work of Thomas Gregor (1981 and chapter 7 in this volume).
2. "Thick description" is an ethnographic concept originated by Clifford Geertz (1973) that refers to the slow gathering of hundreds of contextual details in order to make sense of local categories of reality.
3. My use of the phrase "social drama" here is different from Victor Turner's formal concept of social dramas as "units of aharmonic or disharmonic process, arising in conflict situations" (Turner 1974: 37). Dream sharing as a social drama may be an harmonic, aharmonic, or disharmonic process and it rarely arises in conflicted situations.

References

Anderson, Barbara G. 1971. "Adaptive Aspects of Culture Shock." *American Anthropologist* 73: 1121–1125.

Basso, Ellen B. 1987. "The Implications of a Progressive Theory of Dreaming," in *Dreaming.* Ed. Barbara Tedlock, pp. 86–104. Cambridge: Cambridge University Press.

Bird, Brian. 1972. "Notes on the Transference: Universal Phenomenon and Hardest Part of Analysis." *Journal of the American Psychoanalytic Association* 20: 267–301.

Bourdieu, Pierre. 1978. *Outline of a Theory of Practice.* Richard Nice, trans. Cambridge: Cambridge University Press.

Bruce, Robert D. 1975. *Lacandon Dream Symbolism: Dream Symbolism and Interpretation,* vol. 1. Mexico: Ediciones Euroamericanas.

———. 1979. *Lacandon Dream Symbolism: Dictionary, Index and Classifications of Dream Symbols,* vol. 2. Mexico: Ediciones Euroamericanas.

Cartwright, Rosalind D. 1977. *Night Life: Explorations in Dreaming.* Englewood Cliffs, NJ: Prentice-Hall.

Cesara, Manda (pseudonym of Karla Poewe). 1982. *Reflections of a Woman Anthropologist. No Hiding Place.* New York: Academic Press.

Charsley, S. R. 1973. "Dreams in an Independent African Church." *Africa* 43(3): 244–257.

Clifford, James. 1986. "New Translations of Michel Leiris." *Sulfur* 15: 4–125.

Collins, Kathleen May. 1977. " Secret Desires in Social Contexts: An Anthropological Approach to Dreams." M.A. thesis in anthropology, University of Illinois, Chicago.

Crapanzano, Vincent. 1981. "Text, Transference, and Indexicality." *Ethos* 9: 122–148.

Degarrod, Lydia Nakashima. 1989. *Dream Interpretation among the Mapuche Indians of Chile.* Ph.D. diss. in anthropology, University of California, Los Angeles.

———.1990. "Coping with Stress: Dream Interpretation in the Mapuche Family." *Psychiatric Journal of the University of Ottawa* 15(2): 111–116.

Dentan, Robert Knox. 1983. *A Dream of Senoi.* Special Studies Series, Council on International Studies, State University of New York. Amherst: State University of New York at Buffalo.

———. 1986. "Ethnographic Considerations in the Cross-Cultural Study of Dreaming, in *Sleep and Dreams.* Edited by Jayne Gackenbach, pp. 317–358. New York: Garland.

———. 1988a. "Butterflies and Bug Hunters: Reality and Dreams, Dreams and Reality." *Psychiatric Journal of the University of Ottawa* 13(2): 51–59.

———. 1988b. "Lucidity, Sex, and Horror in Senoi Dreamwork." In *Conscious Mind Sleeping Brain*. Ed. Jayne Gackenbach and Stephen LaBerge, pp. 37–63. New York: Plenum Press.

Desjarlais, Robert. 1991. "Samsara's Sadness: Sherpa Shamanism and the 'Calling of Lost Souls.'" Ph.D. diss. in anthropology, University of California, Los Angeles.

Devereux, George. 1956. "Mohave Dreams of Omen and Power." *Tomorrow* 4(3): 17–24.

———. 1978. *Ethnopsychoanalysis. Psychoanalysis and Anthropology as Complementary Frames of Reference.* Berkeley: University of California Press.

Dombeck, Mary-Therese Behar. 1989. "Dreams and Professional Personhood. The Contexts of Dream Telling and Dream Interpretation among American Psychotherapists." Ph.D. diss. in anthropology, University of Rochester.

Fabian, Johannes. 1983. *Time and the Other: How Anthropology Makes its Object*. New York: Columbia University Press.

Foster, George M. 1973. "Dreams, Character, and Cognitive Orientation in Tzintzuntzan." *Ethos* 1: 106–121.

Freud, Sigmund. 1958 [1914]. "Remembering, Repeating, and Working Through." *Standard Edition* 12: 145–156. London: Hogarth.

Geertz, Clifford. 1973. "Thick Description: Toward an Interpretive Theory of Culture," in *The Interpretation of Cultures,* pp. 3–30. New York: Basic Books.

Gregor, Thomas. 1981. "A Content Analysis of Mehinaku Dreams." *Ethos* 9: 353–390.

Hall, Calvin S. 1951. "What People Dream About." *Scientific American* 184(5): 60–63.

———. 1953. *The Meaning of Dreams.* New York: Harper & Row.

Herdt, Gilbert H. 1977. The Shaman's 'Calling' among the Sambia of New Guinea." *Journal de la Societe des Oceanistes* 33: 153–167.

———. 1987. "Selfhood and Discourse in Sambia Dream Sharing," in *Dreaming.* Ed. Barbara Tedlock, pp. 55–85. Cambridge: Cambridge University Press.

———. 1988. "Dream Work and Field Work: Linking Cultural Anthropology and the Current Dream Work Movement," in *The Variety of Dream Experience.* Ed. Montague Ullman and Claire Limmer, pp. 117-141. New York: Continuum.

Hodes, Matthew. 1989. "Dreams Reconsidered." *Anthropology Today* 5(6): 6–8.

Hollan, Douglas. 1989. "The Personal Use of Dream Beliefs in the Toraja Highlands." *Ethos* 17(2): 166–186.

Hunt, Harry T. 1989. *The Multiplicity of Dreams: Memory, Imagination, and Consciousness.* New Haven: Yale University Press.

Jackson, Michael. 1978. "An Approach to Kuranko Divination." *Human Relations* 31: 117–138.

Kilborne, Benjamin. 1978. *Interpretations de reve au Maroc.* Claix: La Pens6e Sauvage, Bibliotheque d'Ethnopsychiatrie.

Kracke, Waud. 1978. "A Psychoanalyst in the Field: Erikson's Contributions to Anthropology," in *Childhood and Selfhood. Essays on Tradition, Religion, and Modernity in the Psychology of Erik H. Erikson,* pp. 147–188. Lewisburg, PA: Bucknell University Press.

———. 1979. "Dreaming in Kagwahiv: Dream Beliefs and their Psychic Uses in an Amazonian Culture." *Psychoanalytic Study of Society* 8: 119–171.

———. 1987a. "Encounter with Other Cultures: Psychological and Epistemological Aspects." *Ethos* 15(1): 58–81.

———1987b. "'Everyone Who Dreams Has a Bit of Shaman': Cultural and Personal Meanings of Dreams—Evidence from the Amazon." *Psychiatric Journal of the University of Ottawa* 12(2): 65–72.

Laughlin, Robert M. 1976. *Of Wonders Wild and New. Dreams from Zinacantan. Smithsonian Contributions to Anthropology,* no. 22. Washington D.C.: Smithsonian Institution Press.

Leiris, Michel. 1934. *L'Afrique fantome.* Paris: Plon (Terre Humaine).

LeVine, Sarah. 1981. "Dreams of the Informant about the Researcher: Some Difficulties Inherent in the Research Relationship." *Ethos* 9: 276–293.

Lincoln, Jackson S. 1935. *The Dream in Primitive Cultures.* Baltimore: Williams & Wilkins.

Loewald, Hans. 1986. "Transference-Countertransference." *Journal of the American Psychoanalytic Association* 34(2): 275–288.

Lowie, Robert. 1966. "Dreams, Idle Dreams." *Current Anthropology* 7(3): 378–382.

Mahrer, Alvin R. 1989. *Dream Work in Psychotherapy and Self-Change.* New York: W. W. Norton.

Malinowski, Bronislaw. 1927. *Sex and Repression in Primitive Society.* New York: E. P. Dutton.

———. 1967. *A Diary in the Strict Sense of the Term.* Stanford: Stanford University Press.

Marriott, Alice. 1952. *Greener Fields.* Garden City: Dolphin Books.

McDowell, John Holmes. 1989. *Sayings of* the *Ancestors. The Spiritual Life of the Sibundoy Indians.* Lexington: University Press of Kentucky.

Meggitt, Mervyn J. 1962. "Dream Interpretation among the Mae Enga of New Guinea." *Southwestern Journal of Anthropology* 18: 216–220.

Merrill, William. 1987. "The Raramuri Stereotype of Dreams," in *Dreaming.* Ed. Barbara Tedlock, pp. 194–219. Cambridge: Cambridge University Press.

Nadar, Laura. 1970. "Research in Mexico," in *Women in the Field: Anthropological Experiences.* Ed. Peggy Golde, pp. 97–116. Chicago: Aldine.

Ortner, Sherry B. 1984. "Theory in Anthropology since the Sixties." *Comparative Studies in Society and History* 26(l): 126–166.

Palombo, Stanley R. 1978. *Dreaming and Memory: A New Information Processing Model.* New York: Basic Books.

Persinger, M. A. 1988. "Psi Phenomena and Temporal Lobe Activity," in *Research in* Parapsychology. Ed. L. A. Henkel and R. E. Berger, pp. 121–156. Metuchen, NJ: Scarecrow.

Persinger, M. A. and Stanley Krippner. 1989. "Dream ESP Experiments and Geomagnetic Activity." *Journal of the American Society for Psychical Research* 83: 101–116.

Roseman, Marina. 1986. "Sound in Ceremony: Power and Performance in Temiar Curing Rituals." Ph.D. diss. in anthropology, Cornell University.

Roseman, Marina. 1990. *Healing Sounds: Music and Medicine in Temiar Ceremonial Life.* Berkeley: University of California Press.

Scheff, Thomas J. 1986. Towards Resolving the Controversy over 'Thick Description.'" *Current Anthropology* 27: 408–410.

Schneider, David M. and Lauriston Sharp. 1969. *The Dream Life of a Primitive People: The Dreams of the Yir Yoront of Australia.* Anthropological Studies, no. 1. Washington, D.C.: American Anthropological Association.

Silverstein, Michael. 1976. "Shifters, Linguistic Categories, and Cultural Description," in *Meaning and Anthropology.* Ed. Keith Basso and Henry Selby, pp. 11–55. Albuquerque: University of New Mexico Press.

Staff, Vera S. 1975. *Remembered on Waking: Concerning Psychic and Spiritual Dreams and Theories of Dreaming.* Crowborough, Sussex: Churche's Fellowship for Psychical and Spiritual Studies.

Stephen, Michele. 1989. "Dreaming and the Hidden Self: Mekeo Definitions of Consciousness," in *The Religious Imagination in New Guinea.* Ed. Gilbert Herdt and Michele Stephen, pp. 160–186. New Brunswick: Rutgers University Press.

Stevens, William Oliver. 1949. *The Mystery of Dreams.* New York: Dodd, Mead.

Tedlock, Barbara. 1981. "Quiche Maya Dream Interpretation." *Ethos* 9: 313–330.

———. 1987a. *Dreaming: Anthropological and Psychological Interpretations.* Cambridge: Cambridge University Press.

———. 1987b. "Zuni and Quiche Dream Sharing and Interpreting," in *Dreaming,* pp. 105–131. Cambridge: Cambridge University Press.

Tedlock, Dennis. 1979. "The Analogical Tradition and the Emergence of a Dialogical Anthropology." *Journal of Anthropological Research* 35: 387–400.

———. 1990. *Days from a Dream Almanac.* Urbana: University of Illinois Press.

Tolaas, Jon. 1986. "Vigilance Theory and Psi. Part 1: Ethnological and Phylogenetic Aspects." *Journal of the American Society for Psychical Research* 80: 357–373.

Tolaas, Jon. 1990. "The Puzzle of Psychic Dreams," in *Dreamtime & Dreamwork*. Ed. Stanley Krippner, pp. 261–270. Los Angeles: Jeremy P. Tarcher.

Turner, Victor. 1974. "Social Dramas and Ritual Metaphors," in *Dramas, Fields, and Metaphors,* pp. 23–59. Ithaca: Cornell University Press.

Ullman, Montague, Stanley Krippner, and Alan Vaughan. 1973. *Dream Telepathy.* New York: Macmillan.

Wallace, Anthony C. 1959. "Cultural Determinants of Response to Hallucinatory Experience." *AMA Archives of General Psychiatry* 1: 74–85.

17

How Metaphor Structures Dreams

The Theory of Conceptual Metaphor Applied to Dream Analysis

George Lakoff

What Is Metaphor?

It was discovered in the late 1970s that the mind contains an enormous system of general conceptual metaphors—ways of understanding relatively abstract concepts in terms of those that are more concrete. Much of our everyday language and thought makes use of such conceptual metaphors. This chapter claims that the system of conceptual metaphor that functions in ordinary thought and language is also used, first, to provide plausible interpretations of dreams and, second, to generate dreams.

But before I turn to the discussion of dreams, I should spend a bit of time explicating in detail what I mean by "conceptual metaphor."

Conceptual Metaphor

Imagine a love relationship described as follows:

Our relationship has hit a *dead-end street.*

Here love is being conceptualized as a journey, with the implication that the relationship is *stalled,* that the lovers *cannot keep going the way they've been going,* that they must *turn back* or abandon the relationship altogether. This is not an isolated case. English has many everyday expressions that are based on a conceptualization of love as a journey, and they are used not just for talking about love but for reasoning about it as well. Some are necessarily about love; others can be understood that way:

Look *how far we've come.*
It's been *a long, bumpy road.*
We can't *turn back* now.
We're at a *crossroads.* We may have to *go our separate ways.*
The relationship isn't *going anywhere.*
We're spinning our wheels.
Our relationship is *off the track.*
The marriage is *on the rocks.*
We may have to *bail out* of this relationship.

These are ordinary, everyday English expressions. They are not poetic, nor are they necessarily used for special rhetorical effect. Those like *Look how far we've come,* which are not necessarily about love, can readily be understood as being about love.

As a linguist and a cognitive scientist, I ask two commonplace questions:

1. Is there a general principle governing how these linguistic expressions about journeys are used to characterize love?
2. Is there a general principle governing how our patterns of inference about journeys are used to reason about love when expressions such as these are used?

The answer to both is yes. Indeed, there is a single general principle that answers both questions. But it is a general principle that is neither part of the grammar of English nor the English lexicon. Rather, it is part of the conceptual system underlying English: It is a principle for understanding the domain of love in terms of the domain of journeys.

The principle can be stated informally as a metaphorical scenario:

The lovers are travelers on a journey together, with their common life goals seen as destinations to be reached. The relationship is their vehicle, and it allows them to pursue those common goals together. The relationship is seen as fulfilling its purpose as long as it allows them to make progress toward their common goals. The journey is not easy.

There are impediments, and there are places (crossroads) where a decision has to be made about which direction to go in and whether to keep traveling together.

The metaphor involves understanding one domain of experience, love, in terms of a very different domain of experience, journeys. More technically, the metaphor can be understood as a mapping (in the mathematical sense) from a source domain (in this cases, journeys) to a target domain (in this case, love). The mapping is tightly structured. There are ontological correspondences, according to which entities in the domain of love (e.g., the lovers, their common goals, their difficulties, the love relationship, etc.) correspond systematically to entities in the domain of a journey (the travelers, the vehicle, destinations, etc.).

To make it easier to remember what mappings there are in the conceptual system, Johnson and I (Lakoff and Johnson 1980) adopted a strategy for naming such mappings, using mnemonics that suggest the mapping. Mnemonic names typically have the form: X IS Y, where X is the name of the target domain and Y is the name of the source domain. In this case, the name of the mapping is LOVE IS A JOURNEY. When I speak of the LOVE IS A JOURNEY metaphor, I am using a mnemonic for a set of ontological correspondences that characterize a mapping, namely:

The Love-as-Journey Mapping

- The lovers correspond to travelers.
- The love relationship corresponds to the vehicle.
- The lovers' common goals correspond to their common destinations on the journey.
- Difficulties in the relationship correspond to impediments to travel.

It is a common mistake to confuse the name of the mapping, LOVE IS A JOURNEY, for the mapping itself. The mapping is the set of correspondences. Thus, whenever I refer to a metaphor by a mnemonic like LOVE IS A JOURNEY, I will be referring to such a set of correspondences.

The LOVE-AS-JOURNEY mapping is a set of ontological correspondences that map knowledge about journeys onto knowledge about love. Such correspondences permit us to reason about love using the knowledge we use to reason about journeys. Let us take an example. Consider the expression "We're stuck," said by one lover to another about their relationship. How is this expression about travel to be understood as being about their relationship?

"We're stuck" can be used of travel, and when it is, it evokes knowledge about travel. The exact knowledge may vary from person to person, but here is a typical example of the kind of knowledge evoked. The capitalized expressions represent entities in the ontology of travel, that is, in the source domain of the LOVE IS A JOURNEY mapping given above.

Two TRAVELERS are in a VEHICLE, TRAVELING WITH COMMON DESTINATIONS. The VEHICLE encounters some IMPEDIMENT and gets stuck, that is, becomes nonfunctional. If they do nothing, they will not REACH THEIR DESTINATIONS. There are a limited number of alternatives for action:

- They can try to get it moving again, either by fixing it or getting it past the IMPEDIMENT that stopped it.
- They can remain in the nonfunctional VEHICLE and give up on REACHING THEIR DESTINATIONS.
- They can abandon the VEHICLE.

The alternative of remaining in the nonfunctional VEHICLE takes the least effort but does not satisfy the desire to REACH THEIR DESTINATIONS.

The ontological correspondences that constitute the LOVE IS A JOURNEY metaphor map the ontology of travel onto the ontology of love. In so doing they map this scenario about travel onto a corresponding love scenario in which the corresponding alternatives for action are seen. Here is the corresponding love scenario that results from applying the correspondences to this knowledge structure. The target domain entities that are mapped by the correspondences are capitalized:

Two LOVERS are in a LOVE RELATIONSHIP, PURSUING COMMON LIFE GOALS. The RELATIONSHIP encounters some DIFFICULTY, which makes it nonfunctional. If they do nothing, they will not be able to ACHIEVE THEIR LIFE GOALS. There are a limited number of alternatives for action:

- They can try to get it moving again, either by fixing it or getting it past the DIFFICULTY.

- They can remain in the nonfunctional RELATIONSHIP and give up on ACHIEVING THEIR LIFE GOALS.
- They can abandon the RELATIONSHIP.

The alternative of remaining in the nonfunctional RELATIONSHIP takes the least effort but does not satisfy the desire to ACHIEVE LIFE GOALS.

This is an example of an inference pattern that is mapped from one domain to another. It is via such mappings that we apply knowledge about travel to love relationships.

Metaphors Are Not Mere Words. What constitutes the LOVE-AS-JOURNEY metaphor is not any particular word or expression. It is the ontological mapping across conceptual domains, from the source domain of journeys to the target domain of love. The metaphor is not just a matter of language but of thought and reason. The language is secondary. The mapping is primary, in that it sanctions the use of source domain language and inference patterns for target domain concepts. The mapping is conventional, that is, it is a fixed part of our conceptual system, one of our conventional ways of conceptualizing love relationships.

This view of metaphor is thoroughly at odds with the traditional view of metaphor. The traditional view includes the following claims:

1. Metaphors are linguistic expressions (as opposed to conceptual mappings).
2. Metaphors use words from one literal domain to express concepts in another literal domain, but there is no such thing as metaphorical thought or metaphorical reasoning where inference patterns from one domain are applied to another domain.
3. Metaphors are based on similarity: Words from one domain express similar concepts in other domains.
4. Metaphorical language is not part of ordinary, everyday, conventional language but rather part of poetic or especially rhetorical language.

All these claims are false. For example, if metaphors were merely linguistic expressions, we would expect different linguistic expressions to be different metaphors. Thus, "We've hit a dead-end street" would constitute one metaphor. "We can't turn back now" would constitute another, entirely different metaphor. "Their marriage is on the rocks" would involve still a different metaphor. And so on for dozens of examples. Yet we don't seem to have dozens of different metaphors here. We have one metaphor, in which love is conceptualized as a journey. The mapping tells us precisely how love is being conceptualized as a journey. And this unified way of *conceptualizing* love metaphorically is realized in many different *linguistic* expressions.

In addition, we saw above that inference patterns from the travel domain can be used to reason about love. Hence, metaphorical reasoning does exist. As to similarity, there is nothing inherently similar between love and journeys, yet they are linked metaphorically. Finally, all of the metaphorical expressions we looked at in the LOVE IS A JOURNEY metaphor are ordinary, everyday expressions rather than poetic or especially rhetorical expressions.

It should be noted that contemporary metaphor theorists commonly use the term "metaphor" to refer to the conceptual mapping and the term "metaphorical expression" to refer to an individual linguistic expression (like *dead-end street)* that is sanctioned by a mapping. We have adopted this terminology for the following reason: Metaphor, as a phenomenon, involves both conceptual mappings and individual linguistic expressions. It is important to keep them distinct. Since it is the mappings that are primary and that state the generalizations that are our principal concern, we have reserved the term "metaphor" for the mappings rather than for the linguistic expressions.

In the literature of the field, capitalized phrases like LOVE IS A JOURNEY are used as mnemonics to name mappings. Thus, when we refer to the LOVE IS A JOURNEY metaphor, we are referring to the set of correspondences discussed above. The English sentence "Love is a journey," on the other hand, is a metaphorical expression that is understood via that set of correspondences.

Generalizations. THE LOVE IS A JOURNEY metaphor is a conceptual mapping that characterizes a generalization of two kinds:

1. Polysemy generalization: A generalization over related senses of linguistic expressions, e.g., *dead-end street, crossroads, stuck, spinning one's wheels, not going anywhere,* and so on.
2. Inferential generalization: A generalization over inferences across different conceptual domains.

That is, the existence of the mapping provides a general answer to two questions:

1. Why are words for travel used to describe love relationships?
2. Why are inference patterns used to reason about travel also used to reason about love relationships?

Correspondingly, from the perspective of the linguistic analyst, the existence of such cross-domain pairings of words and of inference patterns provide evidence for the existence of such mappings.

Novel Extensions of Conventional Metaphors. The fact that the LOVE IS A JOURNEY mapping is a fixed part of our conceptual system explains why new and imaginative uses of the mapping can be understood instantly, given the ontological correspondences and other knowledge about journeys. Take the song lyric

> We're driving in the fast lane on the freeway of love.

The traveling knowledge called upon is this: When you drive in the fast lane, you go a long way in a short time, and it can be exciting and dangerous. The general metaphorical mapping maps this knowledge about driving into knowledge about love relationships. The danger may be to the vehicle (the relationship may not last) or the passengers (the lovers may be hurt emotionally). The excitement of the love journey is sexual. Our understanding of the song lyric is a consequence of the preexisting metaphorical correspondence of the LOVE-AS-JOURNEY metaphor. The song lyric is instantly comprehensible to speakers of English because those metaphorical correspondences are already part of our conceptual system.

Motivation. Each conventional metaphor, that is, each mapping, is a fixed pattern of conceptual correspondences across conceptual domains. As such, each mapping defines an open-ended class of potential correspondences across inference patterns. When activated, a mapping may apply to a novel source domain knowledge structure and characterize a corresponding target domain knowledge structure.

Mappings should not be thought of as processes or as algorithms that mechanically take source domain inputs and produce target domain outputs. Each mapping should be seen instead as a fixed pattern of ontological correspondences across domains that may, or may not, be applied to a source domain knowledge structure or a source domain lexical item. Thus, lexical items that are conventional in the source domain are not always conventional in the target domain. Instead, each source domain lexical item may or may not make use of the static mapping pattern. If it does, it has an extended lexicalized sense in the target domain, where that sense is characterized by the mapping. If not, the source domain lexical item will not have a conventional sense in the target domain, but may still be actively mapped in the case of novel metaphor. Thus, the words *freeway and fast lane* are not conventionally used of love, but the knowledge structures associated with them are mapped by the LOVE IS A JOURNEY metaphor in the case of "We're driving in the fast lane on the freeway of love."

Imageable Idioms

Many of the metaphorical expressions discussed in the literature on conventional metaphor are idioms. According to classical views, idioms have arbitrary meanings. But within cognitive linguistics, the possibility exists that they are not arbitrary but rather motivated. That is, they do arise automatically by productive rules, but they fit one or more patterns present in the conceptual system. Let us look a little more closely at idioms.

An idiom like "spinning one's wheels" comes with a conventional mental image, that of the wheels of a car stuck in some substance—in mud, sand, snow, or on ice, so that the car cannot move when the motor is engaged and the wheels turn. Part of our knowledge about that image is that a lot of energy is being used up (in spinning the wheels) without any progress being made, that the situation will not readily change of its own accord, that it will take a lot of effort on the part of the occupants to get the vehicle moving again—and that movement may not even be possible.

The LOVE-AS-JOURNEY metaphor applies to this knowledge about the image. It maps this knowledge onto knowledge about love relationships: A lot of energy is being spent without any progress toward fulfilling common goals, the situation will not change of its own accord, it will take a lot of effort on the part of the lovers to make more progress, and so on. In short, when idioms have associated conventional images, it is common for an independently motivated conceptual metaphor to map that knowledge from the source to the target domain.

Mappings at the Superordinate Level. In the LOVE IS A JOURNEY mapping, a love relationship corresponds to a vehicle. A vehicle is a superordinate category that includes such basic-level categories as car, train, boat, and plane. Indeed, the examples of vehicles are typically drawn from this range of basic-level categories: car *(long bumpy road, spinning our wheels)*, train *(off the track)*, boat *(on the rocks, foundering)*, plane *(just taking off, bailing out)*. This is not an accident: In general, we have found that mappings are at the superordinate rather than the basic level. Thus, we do not find fully general submappings like A LOVE RELATIONSHIP IS A CAR; when we find a love relationship conceptualized as a car, we also tend to find it conceptualized as a boat, a train, a plane, and so on. It is the superordinate category VEHICLE, not the basic level category CAR, that is in the general mapping.

It should be no surprise that the generalization is at the superordinate level while the special cases are at the basic level. After all, the basic level is the level of rich mental images and rich knowledge structure. (For a discussion of the properties of basic-level categories, see Lakoff 1987, pp. 31–50.) A mapping at the superordinate level maximizes the possibilities for mapping rich conceptual structure in the source domain onto the target domain, since it permits many basic-level instances, each of which is information rich.

Thus, a prediction is made about conventional mappings: The categories mapped will tend to be at the superordinate rather than the basic level. Thus, one tends not to find mappings like A LOVE RELATIONSHIP IS A CAR or A LOVE RELATIONSHIP IS A BOAT. Instead, one tends to find both basic-level cases (e.g., both cars and boats), which indicates that the generalization is one level higher, at the superordinate level of the vehicle. In most of the hundreds of cases of conventional mappings studied so far, it has been borne out that superordinate categories are used in mappings.

There are, however, occasional cases where basic-level categories seem to show up in mappings, or where it is not clear whether a category should be considered basic-level. For example, anger is a basic emotion. Should it be considered a basic-level concept? There is no shortage of conceptual metaphors for anger: ANGER IS A HOT FLUID IN A CONTAINER, ANGER IS MADNESS, and so on. It is not clear whether anger should not be considered a basic-level category or a case where a basic-level category occurs in a mapping. Another case will be discussed below: In the IMPOTENCE IS BLINDNESS metaphor (observed by Freud), there is a submapping that TESTICLES ARE EYES. This certainly involves basic-level concepts. It is not clear what significance this has, if any, for the theory of metaphor. There is nothing in the general theory that requires mappings to be on the superordinate level. It is simply an empirical fact that they tend to occur that way. This tendency may just follow from the fact that mappings at the superordinate level do more conceptual work than mappings at lower levels. It could be that mappings tend to be optimized for information content but that occasional mappings at the basic-level occur for other reasons, for example, when there is an experiential basis for a mapping at the basic level but not at the superordinate level.

In the remainder of this chapter, when I speak of a "metaphor" or a "conceptual metaphor," I shall be referring to a mapping of the sort we have just discussed. With this example of a conceptual metaphor in place, let us turn to the relationship between conceptual metaphor and dreams.

Metaphor and Dreams

What I have to say about dreams is not entirely new. The basic point goes back to a remark of Freud's in *The Interpretation of Dreams,* in a discussion of dream symbolism: "this symbolism is not peculiar to dreams, but is characteristic of unconscious ideation . . . and it is to be found in folklore, and in popular myths, legends, linguistic idioms, proverbial wisdom and current jokes, to a more complete extent than in dreams." (Freud 1965, section VI.E., p. 386)

It is my job, as a linguist and a cognitive scientist, to study systematically what Freud called "unconscious ideation" of a symbolic nature. I specialize in the study of conceptual systems—the largely unconscious systems of thought in terms of which we think and on which ordinary everyday language is based. I do this largely on the basis of the systematic study of what Freud called "linguistic idioms."

What I and my colleagues have found, in a decade and a half of study, is that, as Freud suggested, we have systems of "unconscious ideation" of a symbolic nature. Part of this is a very large system of conceptual metaphor and metonymy, and I and my colleagues and students have been tracing out this system in extensive detail. Freud was right when he suggested that this system is even more elaborately used in ordinary "linguistic idioms" than in dreams.

Having worked out a very large part of this system for English, I would like to show in some detail how it functions in dreams. Interestingly enough, Freud and other dream analysts have not already done this. Neither Freud nor other psychoanalysts have been interested in working out the details of the system of mundane metaphoric thought, although they implicitly recognized the existence of such a mode of thought and have made use of it implicitly as part of dream interpretation. The job of working out the details of the metaphor system has fallen to linguists and cognitive scientists. Freud and many of his followers were interested more in sexual symbolism-metaphors of a tabooed nature. But what we find through the study of everyday language is that unconscious symbolic thought is, for the most part, not sexual or tabooed. Tabooed thought only rarely shows up in ordinary everyday conventional language. What I will be doing is thus something that other dream analysts have not already done. It is, if anything, the tame part of dream analysis—the study of how unconscious symbolic thought of the most ordinary non-tabooed kind shows up in dreams.

The purpose of this chapter is to provide a set of examples of commonplace dreams in which our ordinary system of metaphor mediates between overt content of the dream and the way we understand dreams as applying to our everyday lives. In the examples of dream interpretations that I will be discussing, conceptual metaphor plays the following role:

Let D	the overt content of the dream
Let M	a collection of conceptual metaphors from our conceptual system
Let K	knowledge about the dreamer's history and everyday life
Let DI	an interpretation of the dream in terms of the dreamer's life

That is, DI is the interpreted meaning of the dream, which the interpreter hopes he has accurately portrayed. The relationship between the dream and its interpretation is:

$$D \text{—} M \rightarrow I, \text{ given } K$$

Metaphors map the dream onto the meaning of the dream, given relevant knowledge of the dreamer's life.

D is what Freud called the "manifest content" of the dream, and DI is what he called the "latent content."

If this is correct, then the system of conceptual metaphor plays a critical role in the interpretation of dreams. However, it cannot be used in isolation, without knowledge of the dreamer's everyday life to yield a meaningful interpretation. This will become clear in the cases to be discussed below.

DI, the interpretation of the dream, can be understood in two ways.

The Weak Interpretation: DI is the meaning ascribed to the dream by an interpreter—either another party or the dreamer on conscious reflection.

The Strong Interpretation: DI is the hidden meaning of the dream to the dreamer.

The weak claim of this chapter is that our everyday system of conventional metaphor is employed whenever an interpreter interprets a dream. It is part of what defines a plausible interpretation. I believe I can demonstrate this beyond doubt.

But the stronger claim is more interesting: The metaphor system plays a generative role in dreaming—mediating between the meaning of the dream to the dreamer and what is seen, heard, and otherwise experienced dynamically in the act of dreaming. Given a meaning to be expressed, the metaphor system provides a means of expressing it concretely—in ways that can be seen and heard. That is, the metaphor system, which is in place for waking thought and expression, is also available during sleep, and provides a natural mechanism for relating concrete images to abstract meanings. The dreamer may well, of course, not be aware, upon waking, of the meaning of the dream since he did not consciously direct the choice of dream imagery to metaphorically express the meaning of the dream.

The stronger claim is harder to demonstrate, and I cannot demonstrate it by the methods of the linguist. At best I can make a plausible case for it by providing plausible interpretations—interpretations of what the dream can plausibly have meant to the dreamer, given the concerns of his everyday life.

Before we proceed, there are several points that need to be made. First, it is important to clarify what I mean by "unconscious" in the expression "unconscious conceptual system." Freud used the term to mean thoughts that were repressed but might in some cases be brought to consciousness. But the term "unconscious" is used very differently in the cognitive sciences. Most of the kinds of thought discussed in the cognitive sciences operate, like the rules of grammar and phonology, below a level that we could possibly have conscious access to or control over.

It is possible, through linguistic analysis, to discover what metaphors one uses in unconscious thought and to discuss them overtly. For example, you might discover that you think in terms of the LOVE IS A JOURNEY metaphor and then have a discussion about the way you have used the metaphor. But there is no way to get conscious control over all unconscious uses of that metaphor and other metaphors in your conceptual system. It is like discussing a rule of grammar or phonology consciously, without being able to control all the rules of your grammar and phonology in every sentence you speak. The system of metaphors, although unconscious, is not "repressed"—just as the system of grammatical and phonological rules that structure one's language is unconscious but not repressed. The unconscious discovered by cognitive science is just not like the Freudian unconscious.

Second, the interpretations I will be offering may well seem obvious or pedestrian. Indeed, that is their point. The everyday metaphor system characterizes the most normal and natural interpretations. My purpose is to say exactly why there are normal, natural interpretations of dreams. As a consequence, I will be starting where most dream analysts end. Most dream analysts are satisfied when they arrive at an intuitively plausible interpretation of a dream. I will be starting with intuitively plausible analyses and trying to show exactly what makes then intuitively plausible.

Third, as I said above, I cannot prove that the analyses I will be giving are the "right" ones, nor are they the only ones. What I claim to show is that they are yielded by the metaphor system given a choice of K, a selected portion of knowledge of the dreamer's everyday life. A different choice of relevant knowledge could produce a completely different interpretation.

Fourth, I assume that dreaming is a form of thought. Powerful dreams are forms of thought that express emotionally powerful content. Two of the main results of cognitive science are that most thought is unconscious and most thought makes use of conceptual metaphor. Dreams are also a form of unconscious thought that makes use of conceptual metaphor. As a form of thought, dreams can express content: desires, fears, solutions to problems, fantasies, and so on. If Freud was right in suggesting that something like repression exists, that there are some thoughts that we do not want to be aware that we are thinking, then the use of the unconscious metaphor system in dreams is a perfect way for the unconscious mind to hide thoughts from the conscious mind while nonetheless thinking them.

Fifth, since dreams are a form of thought, dreams make use of metaphor because thought typically makes use of metaphor. Since dreams are not consciously monitored, they do not make consciously monitored use of metaphor. Thus, the use of metaphor in dreams may seem to the conscious mind wild and incoherent.

Sixth, the imagery used in dreams is not arbitrary. It is constrained by the general metaphors used by the dreamer. The general metaphors are sets of correlations between source and target domains at the superordinate level. Dream imagery is chosen from the basic (and subordinate) level—that is, from special cases of superordinate categories characterized by the general metaphors.

For example, suppose the dream is about love. One of the metaphors for love will be used in the dream. If it is LOVE IS A JOURNEY, then the dream imagery will be about a particular kind of journey, say a car trip. Then the dream images might include a car, roads, bridges, bad weather, etc. Because metaphorical thought is natural, the use of images in dream thought is also natural.

Seventh, I therefore claim that dreams are not just the weird and meaningless product of random neural firings but rather a natural way by which emotionally charged fears, desires, and descriptions are expressed.

Incidentally, what I am claiming is consistent with the claim that dreams are set off by random neural firings in the brain stem. It is possible that a fixed, conventional metaphor system could channel random neural firings into a meaningful dream. In other words, if dreams turn out to be triggered by random neural firings, it would not follow that the content of dreams is random.

Eighth, dreaming is a process with open-ended possibilities for metaphorical expression. What those possibilities are is determined by the fixed, general metaphors in the conceptual system. The fixed metaphors are fixed correspondences across conceptual domains at the superordinate level. Those fixed correspondences make it possible for basic-level imagery to have systematic meaning. Since the possibilities for basic- and subordinate-level imagery are open ended, the fixed metaphorical correspondences allow for an open-ended range of possibilities in a particular dream. Dream construction is a dynamic process that makes use of the fixed metaphorical correspondences to construct the image sequences that occur in dreams.

Thus, there is a sense in which dreaming is like speaking. We have fixed rules of grammar and phonology that constrain what sentences we can construct and what they can mean. But the rules, being general, permit an open-ended range of special cases that fit the rules. Similarly, our metaphor system might be seen as part of a "grammar of the unconscious"—a set of fixed, general principles that permit an open-ended range of possible dreams that are constructed dynamically in accordance with fixed principles. To understand the system of metaphor is to understand those principles.

Ninth, I claim that deep and extensive knowledge of the dreamer's life is essential to pinpointing the meanings of dreams. Does that mean that dreams cannot have interpretations on their own, independent of what we know about the dreamer?

Well, yes and no. There is a certain well-demarcated range of typical emotional concerns in this culture: love, work, death, family, etc. It is a good bet that powerful dreams will be about one of those domains. That puts a constraint on what the target domains of metaphors are likely to be. Suppose each interpretation of a dream is about one of those domains. That means one can fix a single domain to be the target domain for all the metaphorical images used in the dream. The metaphor system allows each individual metaphorical image to have a wide range of interpretations. But if the dream is a long sequence of metaphorical images, then the choice of a single target domain limits the possibilities for interpretation of the whole collection of images. Thus, it might be possible to narrow the range of possible interpretations for a given dream without knowledge of the dreamer.

But even such a narrowed range of possibilities might be extremely large—so large that one could not even come close to imagining the range of possibilities. Two mechanisms make even such a narrowed range of possibilities very large. First, there is the range of specific instances of a general metaphor. That could be an extremely large range. Second, there is what Turner and I (1989) have called the GENERIC IS SPECIFIC metaphor schema. This is a schema that allows for an open-ended range of metaphorical correspondences across domains. The use of that schema will be described below. Its very use depends on detailed knowledge. These two mechanisms allow for such a broad range of possibilities that only detailed knowledge of the life of the dreamer can limit that range of possibilities to what the dream means to that dreamer.

It should be said, however, that the wide range of possibilities permits an individual dream to have multiple meanings for a dreamer, and I claim that especially powerful dreams commonly have multiple meanings.

In addition, because of the large range of possibilities permitted by the metaphor system, one person's dreams can have powerful meanings for other people. Other people's dreams hold for us the same fascination as myth and literature, the same possibility for finding meaning in our own lives. It is the operation of our metaphor systems that makes that possible.

The dream analyses to follow stress the importance of deep and extensive knowledge about the life of the dreamer. In each case, I have used a dream of someone I know very well, and it is only because I know the dreamer well that I feel confident of the interpretations.

The Blindness Dream

A man I will call Steve had the recurring dream that he had become blind: He would awaken his wife in the middle of night screaming out "I'm blind, I'm blind" hysterically, until his wife could wake him up, turn on the light, and show him that he could see.

Steve is a scrupulous, meticulous, and cautious academic who is always afraid that he does not know enough. In our everyday conceptual system, there is a metaphor that KNOWING IS SEEING, which appears in everyday expressions like:

> I see what you're getting at.
> His meaning was clear.
> You can't pull the wool over my eyes.
> This paragraph is a bit murky.
> What is your viewpoint?

Via this metaphor, "I can't see" maps onto "I don't know—and can't find out." Steve, in his dream, is expressing his constant fear: I'm ignorant, I'm ignorant.

But Steve's dream, as a powerful recurrent dream, is richer than that. Freud, in his interpretation of the Oedipus myth, observed that Oedipus' cutting out of his eyes was metaphorical castration, a metaphor that TESTICLES ARE EYES and IMPOTENCE IS BLINDNESS. By virtue of this metaphor, being blinded is a just punishment for a sexual transgression. It is because this metaphor is in our conceptual system that we understand Oedipus' punishment as being just. Incidentally, contemporary popular culture also has a manifestation of this metaphor in the folk theory that if you masturbate, you will go blind.

One of the banes of Steve's existence is the feeling that he lacks power and influence, and is therefore unable to get things for himself and others. Steve's recurring dream occurred several times just before he took on his first important administrative position, about which he feared that he would spend a lot of effort and not accomplish anything significant. We have common cultural metaphors that WORLDLY POWER IS SEXUAL POTENCY and POWERLESSNESS IS impotence.

Linguistic examples of this metaphor abound in everyday life. One of the most celebrated was Lyndon Johnson's remark about a political enemy whom he had the power to blackmail: "I've got his pecker in my pocket." Men threatening to get back at an enemy by rendering him powerless have been heard to say "I'll cut his balls off" or "I'll castrate him." Women who exert worldly power over men are regularly called "castrating bitches."

Via this metaphor, "I'm blind" in the dream expresses another of Steve's recurrent fears: "I'm powerless."

In addition, the dream has still further significance for Steve's life. Steve cannot have children because of a low sperm count. After years of trying to have children, Steve and his wife finally adopted children, and are happy and loving parents. Still, it was a traumatic experience in Steve's life not to be able to have biological children. Via the metaphor of IMPOTENCE IS BLINDNESS, when Steve cries out "I'm blind" he is expressing that trauma. Metaphorically, he is crying out "I'm impotent."

Steve's recurrent dream is powerful because it expresses three of the major fears and regrets in Steve's life. Metaphor is the mechanism that links the dream to what it means. What makes this dream extremely powerful is that it has not one metaphorical meaning but three simultaneous ones, via three different metaphors. Two of these metaphors are expressed in everyday language: Both KNOWING IS SEEING and WORLDLY POWER IS SEXUAL POTENCY are part of the largely unconscious system of metaphorical thought that underlies much of our everyday language. GENITALS ARE EYES and IMPOTENCE IS BLINDNESS has a very different status. It is an unconscious conceptual metaphor that is widespread in our culture but is taboo. Thus, there is no large set of everyday linguistic expressions that are comprehended via this metaphor. For example, "My eyes hurt" does not mean "My testicles hurt" and "He's blind" does not mean "He's impotent."

Yet the metaphor seems to be present nonetheless, and there is a good reason why it should be—it has the right kind of experiential basis to form a metaphor, namely, testicles are the same shape as eyes and losing one's eyesight renders one relatively powerless. The existence of such an experiential basis for the metaphor makes the metaphor natural. Apparently, the IMPOTENCE IS BLINDNESS metaphor, although taboo and unrealized in everyday language, is part of our conceptual systems. If it were not, the Oedipus myth would seem senseless since blindness, in the absence of such a metaphor, would not seem a just punishment for incest.

There are several theoretical morals that arise from this set of interpretations of the Blindness Dream:

First, Freudian symbolism (as when the eyes symbolize genitals) can have the status of a tabooed metaphor, which has no reflection in everyday linguistic expressions but is just as psychically real as other conceptual metaphors.

Second, tabooed metaphors (with no reflection in language), such as EYES ARE GENITALS and IMPOTENCE IS BLINDNESS, may combine with non-tabooed metaphors, such as WORLDLY POWER IS SEXUAL POTENCY, to jointly provide an interpretation of a dream. In short, much of Freud's symbolism is in the form of tabooed metaphors that are not segregated off by themselves but that instead can combine with everyday metaphors.

Third, there can be multiple interpretations of dreams, which are simultaneous and all of which are equally natural. It is natural for a powerful recurrent dream to have such multiple meanings.

At this point I would like to turn to perhaps the most famous example of dream interpretation in the Western world, Joseph's interpretation of Pharaoh's dream from Genesis.

Pharaoh's Dream

> In his dream, Pharaoh is standing on the riverbank, when seven fat cows come out of the river, followed by seven lean cows that eat the seven fat ones and still remain lean. Then Pharaoh dreams again. This time he sees seven "full and good" ears of corn growing and then seven withered ears growing after them. The withered ears devour the good ears. Joseph interprets the two dreams as a single dream. The seven fat cows and full ears are good years and the seven lean cows and withered ears are famine years that follow the good years. The famine years "devour" what the good years produce.

Millions of people, both Jews and Christians, have read this passage and understood Joseph's interpretation as making sense, that is, as being a natural and reasonable dream interpretation. The question I am raising is what makes Joseph's interpretation make sense and seem natural—so natural that no further discussion seems necessary. Even Freud, who cites the dream several times in *The Interpretation of Dreams,* sees no need to interpret it further.

It is my claim that this interpretation makes sense to us because of a collection of conceptual metaphors in our conceptual system—metaphors that have been with us since biblical times. The first metaphor used is: TIMES ARE MOVING ENTITIES. In this metaphor, there is an observer defining the present time standing, with the future in front and the past behind. Future times move toward him from the front; past times are in the rear moving away. Examples are:

> The time for action is here.
> The time for waiting has passed.
> The revolution is coming.
> Times flies.
> Time flows by.

This metaphor characterizes the "flow" of time, and a river is an appropriate special case of something that flows and that extends as far as the eye can see. Hence, a river is a common metaphor for the flow of time. The cows emerging from the river are individual entities (blocks of time—in this case, years) emerging from the flow of time and moving past the observer; the ears of corn are also entities that come into the scene.

The second metaphor used is ACHIEVING A PURPOSE IS EATING, where being fat indicates success and being lean indicates failure. Examples include:

> The league leaders fattened up on the last place team.
> He's starved for a win.
> I can taste victory.
> The sweet smell of success.
> He enjoyed the fruits of his labor.
> He's got a lot on his plate.

This metaphor is combined with the most common of metonymies: A PART STANDS FOR THE WHOLE, as in:

> We need a strong arm in right field.
> We've got a good glove at third base.
> Look at his new wheels.

Since cows and corn were typical of meat and grain eaten, each single cow stands for all the cows raised in a year and each ear of corn for all the corn grown in a year. The fat cows and corn stand for food in general, which in turn metaphorically symbolizes success via ACHIEVING A PURPOSE IS EATING. The fat cows and corn also symbolize years, via TIME IS A MOVING OBJECT. Thus, they jointly symbolize good years.

The final metaphor used is RESOURCES ARE FOOD, where using up resources is eating food. Examples include:

> I've got a gas guzzler.
> They've gobbled up all the wood available to the building trades.

The devouring of the good years by the famine years is interpreted as indicating that all the surplus resources of the good years will be used up by the famine years. The interpretation of both dreams is a composition of the same four parts: three conventional metaphors and one metonymy. The cow dream and the corn dream are both special cases of a single more general dream, where cows and corn are kinds of food.

What is of note here is that the analysis that I have given begins where Joseph's dream interpretation ends. The reason is that my analysis is an analysis of the interpretation, not of the dream. My purpose is to show why a given analysis of a dream makes sense to us. The answer is that metaphors and metonymies in our everyday conceptual system provide the link between the dream content and the interpretation.

Let us now return to analyses of dreams by people I know well.

The Bridge Dream

A man I will call Herb fell in love and moved in with his girlfriend. Moving in turned out to be a disaster. They simply could not live together without fighting. With great sadness, they decided to split up. That night he dreamed that they started out on a trip from Berkeley, when a fierce storm blew up, and as they reached the Richmond - San Rafael Bridge (across San Francisco Bay), the bridge blew away into the bay.

This dream uses two common conventional metaphors. The first is the Emotional Climate metaphor, in which interior emotions are exterior weather conditions. Thus, a happy person has a sunny disposition, happiness is light, while sadness and depression are dark. A special case of this is that EMOTIONAL DISCORD IS A STORM. Via this metaphor, the storm symbolized the emotional discord of the fighting involved in the lovers' breakup.

The other metaphor involved is LOVE IS A JOURNEY. Setting out on the journey corresponds to the long-term commitment made by the lovers when they moved in together. The washing out of the bridge, which made it impossible to continue the journey, corresponds to the ending of the love relationship. Without the bridge the journey could not continue.

The washing out of the bridge has a second meaning via another common metaphor, in which RELATIONSHIPS ARE LINKS BETWEEN PEOPLE. Here the falling away of the bridge indicates the end of the relationship link between the lovers.

The Flying Dreams

A man I will call David always does things to extremes, whether working or having fun. He tries to live as joyous and fulfilling a life as possible. He works as a lawyer, primarily on cases that he believes in, and spends very long hours, often for months at a time wearing himself out. He is also a musician who likes to play far into the night or go to late-night concerts and party for long hours. He loves the outdoors and will drive for many hours each way to go skiing for the weekend. He takes long vigorous walks and bike rides. He is generally happy, but when he exhausts himself, he gets gaunt and sick and depressed.

David has long had recurring dreams in which he was flying. In his early twenties, he would fly too high or fast or far in his dreams and get terrified. Then he took a chance and did something he had always wanted to do. He went to Paris, worked as a street singer, made a lot of friends, and had a wonderful time. At this point he had a flying dream in which he flew especially high and fast, got scared, feared crashing, landed on the shoulders of a friend, did a back flip in the air, and landed on his feet. Thereafter, his dreams of flying were pleasurable. He has been confident ever since that he would land on his feet.

The common metaphors involved are these:

ACTION IS SELF-PROPELLED MOTION
FREEDOM IS LACK OF CONSTRAINT
INTENSE ACTION IS FAST MOTION

Flying, in this metaphor, is a form of fast motion with no constraints but with the danger of falling and crashing, which signifies resulting harm. Metaphorically, flying is intense action with a sense of freedom—what David prizes most. The flying dreams accompanied periods of such intense action in the service of freedom—driving a taxicab in Boston after college, street singing in Paris, working as a lawyer for idealistic causes, putting together a band and making tapes and a video, going off on vigorous and exciting vacation trips.

In Paris, where he found the help of friends, the flying dream was extended by the metaphor of HELP IS SUPPORT—he landed on a friend's shoulders. Then he did a back flip (a form of playful showing off) and landed on his feet (signifying a safe result). Indeed, we have the idiom "to land on one's feet" in English, which works by the same metaphors.

The Classroom Dream

A woman I will call Karen dreamed that she was in the class of her favorite professor in college. He came over to her and said that she was not working and would fail the class.

Karen had recently married a professor who was a colleague of the professor in the dream. When she got married she quit a job she had hated and was not then working. She feared that her not working would lead to financial pressures that would cause the marriage to fail.

The metaphorical mechanism that links the dream and the knowledge to an interpretation is called the GENERIC IS SPECIFIC metaphor schema. It is a schema by which a general situation is understood in terms of one specific situation. Thus a General Case is understood in terms of what we will call Special Case 1. Because the General Case covers other special cases, another special case, call it Special Case 2, can also be understood in terms of Special Case 1. The result is a metaphorical analogy between Special Case 1 and Special Case 2.

Special Case 1 in the dream is a positive relationship with a professor in a course. The General Case is a positive relationship with a professor. Special Case 2 is a positive relationship with a professor in her marriage. The metaphorical analogy sets up a metaphorical correspondence:

- Karen's favorite professor in the dream is her current favorite professor—her husband.
- Working to assure success in class is working to assure success in her marriage.
- Failing in the class is failing in the marriage.

The dream expresses Karen's fear that her marriage will fail because she quit her job.

The Time Bomb Dream

A woman I will call Eileen dreamed that she was observing a mule having brain surgery. The mule's head was cut open and a time bomb was placed inside. The mule was then stitched up and ran off, becoming a beautiful, graceful horse. Eileen watches in terror as the horse prances gracefully with a time bomb in its head.

To comprehend this dream, the following information is necessary.

- Our cultural stereotype of the mule is that it is (1) stubborn, (2) sterile, and (3)clumsy by comparison with a horse.
- Eileen is in love with a man whom she wants to marry. She has a grown child by a former marriage, and at her age, with her biological clock ticking, she is not likely to have any children in her second marriage. This upsets her.
- She is also very determined about how she wants to live her life. She wants to pursue a particular career, and at her point in life she feels the clock is running out on her. She will have to start soon.
- Moreover, the way she had always assumed she would pursue a career conflicts with her plans for marriage. Indeed, a number of her plans and desires conflict with the marriage that she very much wants. Thus she is pursuing inconsistent desires.
- Eileen is a worrier, so much so that she has a history of anxiety attacks. For some years she was on medication to prevent such attacks, but she had been off the medicine for several months at the time of the dream. Just before the dream, she had an anxiety attack and wound up in an argument with her prospective husband about her conflicting desires. She fears further anxiety attacks.
- Eileen went into therapy four years before the dream, at a time when she was barely functioning because of the anxiety attacks. When she went into therapy she had just broken off a damaging long-term relationship and had difficulty dealing with men as well as functioning professionally. Through therapy, she reached a point where she could function well again. She established a good relationship with the man she wants to marry and was able to return to her professional goals.
- Eileen is also a former dancer, who takes joy in physical activity, especially in her regular aerobics class. She counts on physical activity to keep her healthy and stable. And her excellent physical shape makes her constantly aware that she is still capable of having children.

The mechanisms relating Eileen's dream to her life are the Great Chain of Being Metaphor Schema (Lakoff and Turner, 1989) and one of the major metaphors for ideas—IDEAS ARE OBJECTS IN THE MIND.

According to the IDEAS ARE OBJECTS metaphor, ideas move in the direction of their consequences. Thus, following an idea entails being led to its consequences. Ideas with inconsistent consequences are thus moving in opposite directions. They exert force on each other and are thus seen as in conflict.

The Great Chain metaphor schema makes use of a folk version of the Great Chain of Being, in which there is a hierarchy of beings, with humans at the top, higher animals below them, and lower animals, plants, and inanimate objects farther down. The metaphor schema is a mechanism by which human behavior is understood in terms of the behavior of forms of being lower on the chain. The metaphor works by metaphorically attributing to humans the distinguishing properties of beings lower on the chain. The being lower on the Great Chain is the mule; its distinguishing properties are stubbornness, sterility, and clumsiness (relative to horses).

Eileen was metaphorically a mule before therapy (an operation on her head), which enabled her to function well, to transform from a mule to a gracefully prancing horse. But she retains the inherent properties of a mule: stubbornness and sterility. She is stubborn about how she wants to live her life; sterile, in that she will not be having any children in her future marriage. The conflicting desires—her desire for marriage and her career aspiration—were restored to her through therapy, the operation on her head. But the desires conflict—they exert force on one another inside her head and have a potential to metaphorically explode. They constitute the time bomb in her head. The time bomb also symbolizes her biological clock and her career clock, and the possibility of explosion symbolizes the destruction of her hopes of having more children and of pursuing a career. The possible return of anxiety attacks symbolizes another kind of metaphorical explosion. Meanwhile, in joyful physical activity, functioning in a good relationship, and pursuing her career, she is the graceful horse—with a time bomb in her head!

The Puzzle Dream

A woman I will call Jane dreamed that she was invited to the home of an older Jewish couple of her acquaintance who welcomed her warmly. After a while she went into an adjoining room and, with her younger sister, began pulling pieces of a puzzle out of a plastic sheet and assembling them. The pieces were in the form of cups and saucers and kitchen utensils. Then she went into the kitchen with the older Jewish couple, and her sister went in the other direction and out of the dream.

Jane is half Catholic and half Jewish. Her Jewish father had converted to Catholicism and she was raised Catholic. She did not have a happy childhood; her parents were distant from her and had little understanding of her or sympathy for her. She felt her parents never accepted her. Jane has always wanted her parents to be understanding and supportive. She believes, from cases she has observed, that Jewish parents are more understanding and supportive of their children than Catholic parents.

Jane rejected the church in her late teens. Her younger sister, however, became a wholehearted Catholic: She is active in the church, she married a Catholic man, and she is raising her children in Catholic schools.

Jane has always felt confused about her ethnic identity. She has recently gotten involved with a Jewish man whom she is serious about marrying, and she has begun to experience the part of her that is Jewish in a positive way. She is still sorting out her ethnic identity. She is also trying to sort out her relationship to her sister.

In the dream, the older Jewish couple symbolizes an alternative set of parents with the other half of her ethnicity, accepting Jewish parents rather than critical Catholic parents. She has regressed to childhood, playing with toys with her sister. She is putting together the pieces of the puzzle of her identity. The pieces are cups and saucers and other kitchen utensils, which stand metonymically for the home. In going into the kitchen with the older Jewish couple, she is choosing a Jewish home. Her sister goes in the other direction, choosing a Catholic home.

The mechanisms of this dream interpretation are (1) the GENERIC IS SPECIFIC metaphor schema; (2) the PROBLEMS ARE PUZZLES metaphor; (3) the INSTRUMENTS STAND FOR ACTIVITY metonymy; and (4) the metaphor CHOOSING SOMETHING IS GOING TO IT.

The GENERIC IS SPECIFIC analysis works like this:
First specific case: the older couple
General case: Older couples
Second specific case: Jane's parents
Analogy: Jane's parents are the older couple

Since the older couple is Jewish and accepting of Jane, they represent parents who are Jewish and accepting of Jane.

In the dream, Jane is putting together the pieces of the puzzle. By the PROBLEMS ARE PUZZLES metaphor, she is trying to solve a problem. The puzzle pieces are domestic implements—cups and saucers and kitchen utensils. By the INSTRUMENTS FOR ACTIVITY metonymy, domestic implements stand for domestic life in general. In her life, she is obsessed with the problem of figuring out her identity as someone whose home life growing up failed her and who has rejected her parents' religion. Putting together the pieces of the home life puzzle corresponds to working out this consuming problem.

The final metaphor at work here is CHOOSING SOMETHING IS GOING TO IT; REJECTING SOMETHING IS MOVING AWAY FROM IT, as in expressions like:

I'll go for the Honda.
He almost bought that house, but then he backed off.
I wouldn't touch it with a ten-foot pole.

Jane's going into the room with the older Jewish couple symbolizes the choice of a Jewish domestic life, life with her prospective husband. Her sister's going in the opposite direction symbolizes her sister's choice of a Catholic family life.

Conclusion

Our conceptual systems contain an extensive system of conceptual metaphors that define correspondences across conceptual domains, typically from concrete spatial domains to more abstract domains. These conventional metaphors have the potential to link concrete imagery, especially visual imagery, to more abstract concepts.

Since the metaphor system is a fixed part of our unconscious system of concepts, conventional metaphors are always available to link concrete imagery to abstract meanings. And given abstract meanings, the metaphor system can act to constrain the choice of concrete imagery appropriate to express those meanings. As a result, the concerns of everyday life can be expressed via concrete imagery plus metaphors. Our system of conceptual metaphor makes it possible to express desires, fears, and descriptions of emotionally charged situations.

The metaphor system of English is now being studied systematically and scientifically. The result is a kind of dictionary of unconscious thought, the spelling out in detail of a large part of what I take Lacan (1977) to have meant by "the language of the unconscious."

The metaphor system of members of a culture can be thought of as having two parts: the everyday conventional metaphors, which, though unconscious, have reflexes in everyday language; and the tabooed metaphors, which, because of their tabooed nature, are not expressed in conventional language. Freud, because of his concern with sexuality and repression, was largely concerned with tabooed metaphors. I, because I am a linguist by profession, am largely concerned with the everyday metaphors that show up in ordinary language.

Because dream interpretation has largely been done by psychotherapists, the kinds of analyses I have discussed, although certainly noticed, have never been the subject of systematic and rigorous study. But now that linguistics and cognitive science have yielded an understanding of our everyday metaphor systems, it has become possible to apply that knowledge to dream interpretation in a systematic way.

The everyday, non-tabooed metaphors are every bit as important to the understanding of dreams as the tabooed ones. Some therapists have an instinctive understanding of how our everyday metaphor system operates in dreams. But many do not. When I read books on dream analysis by psychotherapists, I rarely find attention given over to those aspects of the meanings of dreams that depend on the everyday metaphor system.

The metaphor system is far from obvious. Those who want to make use of it in dream interpretation should probably get some training in how the system works. After all, if you are using the language of the unconscious, it might be useful to get a few grammar lessons and have a dictionary handy.

I would like to conclude by discussing what I am not claiming. I am not, for example, promoting a new form of dream therapy. I am certainly not claiming that metaphor analysis replaces other forms of dream work in therapy. The metaphor system will inevitably be used in any form of dream work, simply because we use that system whenever we think. But the metaphor system does not determine what form the dream work should take. For example, Fritz Perls introduced into gestalt therapy the technique of having the dreamer take on the role of every person and thing in the dream. In doing so, dreamers will almost without exception make some use or other of their everyday metaphor system, but the power of the therapeutic technique is not in the use of the metaphor system per se. As with poetry in a foreign language, you will need to use a dictionary, but the poetry is far more than what is in the dictionary.

References

Freud, Sigmund. 1965. *The Interpretation of Dreams,* trans. James Strachey. New York: Avon Books.

Kramer, Milton. 1991. "Dream Translation: A Nonassociative Method for Understanding the Dream." *Dreaming,* vol. 1, no. 2: 147–160.

Lacan, Jacques. 1977. *Ectits.* New York: Norton.

Lakoff, George, and Mark Johnson. 1980. *Metaphors We Live By.* Chicago: University of Chicago Press.

Lakoff, George. 1987. *Women, Fire, and Dangerous Things.* Chicago: University of Chicago Press.

Lakoff, George, and Mark Turner. 1989. *More Than Cool Reason.* Chicago: University of Chicago Press.

18

Dreams, Inner Resistance, and Self-Reflection

James J. DiCenso

A debate has dragged on for many years, and continues unabated, about the status of Freud's work and of psychoanalysis generally. The main issues concern evaluating psychoanalysis in terms of its claims to scientific status, and exploring related questions such as the falsifiability of its hypotheses or how psychoanalytic models and methods stand in relation to recent developments in physiologically based scientific psychology.

However, without wishing to minimize the significance of these concerns, the present analysis takes as its point of departure the tradition that comprehends psychoanalysis as essentially a development *within the human sciences.* My general approach, shared by a variety of theorists and practitioners, is that psychoanalysis seeks to give conceptual structure to domains of human experience that elude the methods and tools of "hard science." These domains include interpersonal and cultural dynamics, problems of ethics, and, most relevant for our present concerns, the realm of "inner experience." This latter is comprised of phenomena such as fantasies and dreams, which present themselves through introspection and recollection and necessarily appear in representational and narrativized forms. However, the present approach does not seek to release the propositions of psychoanalysis from accountability: It simply shifts the issue of evaluative criteria away from those of the natural sciences and toward those of the human sciences.

This is where the links between psychoanalysis and hermeneutics, established most lucidly and systematically by Paul Ricouer, become relevant.[1] To be sure, in hermeneutical approaches (and I include various postmodernist treatments of Freud under this general heading), evaluative criteria are less hard and fast, but perhaps more relevant to human experience and to concerns with self-understanding. The questions posed to psychoanalysis relate to its adequacy in explaining the subjective phenomena it describes, its ability to make sense of individual life issues and to offer therapeutic means of ameliorating personal distress. As a body of theoretical work, psychoanalysis is engaged in terms of its flexibility and translatability (rather than rigidly conceived "universality") in being applied to diverse individual and cultural phenomena[2] and its capacity for self-correction in light of new information and conceptual developments. Associated with hermeneutical schools of thought are interpretations of Freud's own writings that emphasize the interweaving of psychological, philosophical, and cultural analyses, producing a multifaceted discourse that can be engaged on a plurality of levels. The point here is not to encapsulate these works within an interpretive schema that prioritizes fact-gathering, physiological etiology, or statistical analysis. Rather, they are approached in terms of their capacity to illuminate aspects of the human condition (necessarily experienced within subjective and cultural interpretive frameworks) from diverse complementary angles.[3]

The *Interpretation of Dreams* exhibits these plurivocal qualities in several respects; like a great work of literature, its many facets engage the reader on various levels and serve to stimulate ongoing insight for those who are willing to work actively with the text (just as one must actively engage the phenomena of dreams). Thus, as Didier Anzieu points out, the structure of the book duplicates its subject matter, the dream.[4] That is, many of the analyses occur in layers, and ideas are built up and explicated in a variety of contexts, so that the reader is led back and forth along networks of associations that complement and alter one another. Both dreams and the book that seeks to disclose their meaning are complex communicative structures that require the work of deciphering and interpretation. In this vein, Anzieu also notes that the text "brings into play four distinct characters—the dreamer, the interpreter, the narrator and the theorist. . . ."[5] This proliferation of narrative voices indicates that Freud's arguments cannot be reduced to a single monological standpoint. Indeed, both dreams and the "Dream Book" reveal an otherness that speaks to us and yet remains elusive, always remaining somewhat beyond our conscious control and possession. This dimension of alterity exemplifies the psychoanalytic model of the personality as internally differentiated. It articulates the interactive and communicative processes (and the failures thereof) that constitute human subjectivity.[6] The dynamic interplay of perspectives engendered by this differentiated quality is essential to processes of self-reflection and possible self-transformation.

Having proposed that Freud's work can be engaged on numerous levels, it is nevertheless the case that it reveals a series of internal tensions. That is, the discernible levels of meaning are not always compatible or easily reconcilable with each other. Therefore, like much of Freud's work, *The Interpretation of Dreams* exhibits an ambivalent quality. It is poised between open and closed interpretive approaches, both of which seem to be necessary in order to avoid a collapse into a single extreme standpoint. As Serge Leclaire states of psychoanalytic technique, "it is vulnerable, on the one hand, to the degradation of a closed systematization and, on the other, to the anarchy of intuitive processes."[7] Ideally, then, psychoanalytic theory and practice maintain a dynamic balance between these tendencies, so that specific, necessarily limited interpretations form the touchstone from which additional counterinsights can emerge.

However, it often happens that attempts at systematization harden into "reductive," one-dimensional approaches to psychological phenomena. The models and explanations that ensue from this ossification attempt to reify latent meaning as a fully discernible, determinable foundation underlying the distortions of the manifest dream. This tendency appears, for example, in Freud's assertions concerning the primacy of wish fulfillment as the key to the hidden meaning of all dreams, and it is also evident in his attempts to establish definite childhood scenes behind fantasy life. Reductive tendencies actually become amplified in later editions of *The Interpretation of Dreams* where, under the influence of some of his disciples, Freud added material concerning "universal" symbolism that inevitably works in a codified manner to reveal sexual meaning. (These views are found in chapter VI, section E.) It is features such as this that lend themselves to the stereotypical views of psychoanalysis which have become prevalent. These instances of rigidity also make psychoanalytic theory vulnerable to those who take such totalizing, scientistic claims at face value, who isolate them from qualifying countertendencies within Freud's work, and who then seek to refute them on these limited terms.[8]

It is highly significant that Freud's work consistently exceeds the scope of one-dimensional interpretations of it, whether critical or laudatory. Indeed, Freud's writings provide internal antidotes to their own propensities toward positivism, reductionism, authoritarianism, and closure. One specific place where an ameliorating ambivalence appears is in the notion of *resistance,* defined by Freud as "whatever interrupts the analytic work."[9] For example, in psychoanalytic practice, the analyst observes the analysand's discourse for places of opacity, gaps, and dissimulations, and these provide indirect indications of unacknowledged problem areas in the individual's life. Attention to these places of resistance differs markedly from the initial hypnotic method, which, as Anzieu points out, served to reinforce Freud's "activistic and dominating" tendencies.[10] By virtually eliminating resistance, hypnosis makes therapeutic understanding more difficult, and possibly more random, because there are no emotional markers coming from the analysand's own behavior to indicate heightened intensity. As Laplanche and Pontalis note, initially, following the more interventionist hypnotic approach, "Freud tried to overcome this obstacle by insistence . . . and persuasion, but then he realized that resistance was itself a means of reaching the repressed and unveiling the secret of neurosis. . . ."[11] Therefore, awareness of places of resistance is crucial for allowing a dynamic engagement with unconscious material as it presents itself in the *interference* with a consciously directed narrative.

Resistance is the product of a disjunction between conscious and unconscious aspects of the personality, between what one recognizes and acknowledges about oneself and one's life and what one does not. It is the internal disjunction between these aspects of the self, symbolized by the revealing image of the *dream censor,* that engenders the labyrinthine formations, the compromises, evasions, and distortions, of the dream work. These occur as specific "mechanisms": condensation, displacement, considerations of representability, and secondary revision. In the dream, resistance becomes manifest in the form of intricate narratives that, with careful deciphering, can unfurl into unexpected and illuminating networks of meaning. In Jacques Derrida's words, "resistance must be interpreted; it has as much meaning as what it opposes [i.e., the psychoanalyst's assumption of knowledge]; it is just as charged with meaning and thus just as interpretable as that which it disguises or displaces. . . ."[12] These points indicate that the place of meaning is the dream work itself, not the posited substratum of the dream thoughts. As Laplanche and Pontalis put it, "it is the dream work, . . . and not the latent content, which constitutes the *essence of the dream.*"[13] This means that the "essence" of the dream is itself interstitial and unstable, occurring, as Ricoeur has illustrated, within a complex interplay of forces and meanings.[14]

✣ ✣ ✣

At this point, in order to develop a clearer understanding of how resistance is crucial to the production of meaning and to self-reflection, we need to examine a few features of Freud's basic topographical model. Freud frequently associates resistance with the entrenched attitudes of the ego, much as in the related notion of *defense.* Even as early as his letters to Wilhelm Fliess, Freud indicated that the ego habitually misinterprets dreams.[15] Later, in *The History of the Psychoanalytic Movement,* Freud makes a similar point. He refers to the problem of "systematization" in the thought of Alfred Adler, in which the dream material is, as he states, "viewed purely from the standpoint of the ego, reduced to the categories with which the ego is familiar, translated, twisted and . . . misunderstood."[16] Many subsequent psychoanalytic theorists and practitioners have elaborated on this problem of the "closed ego" in significant ways. From among these, I will simply mention the work of Cornelius Castoriadis. He links the ego with interiorized social norms so that it is understood as an agency of conformity that actually blocks off other potential aspects of the personality. In Castoriadis's words, "one of the objects of analysis is to free this flux [of unformed aspects of the self] from the repression to which it is usually subjected by an Ego that is a rigid and essentially social construct."[17] This problem of the ego, which links the question of self-reflection with that of social conditioning, is not explicitly formulated in *The Interpretation of Dreams.* However it is perhaps indirectly present in Freud's discussion of the psychical censorship as akin to political censorship.[18] In any case, Castoriadis's remarks, drawing on the psychocultural analyses of later Freudian works such as *Civilization and Its Discontents,* serve to supplement Freud's discussions of the ego as representing circumscribed awareness.

Again, it must be emphasized that Freud's work frequently reveals the coexistence of an awareness of the problem of ego-based impositions of meaning, with repeated instances where his own caveats seem to be forgotten. Freud's interpretive approach sometimes betrays the assumption of what Jacques Lacan would call "the subject supposed to know." That is, the analyst assumes the position of one possessing the keys to meaning, one who already knows in advance what will be found in the dream. On the part of the analyst, this approach feeds into the narcissistic ego's quest for order, control, and authority. On the part of the analysand, it responds to the need for definitive guidance coming from outside oneself that might allow one to abrogate the responsibility for therapeutic working-through. From both sides, the fantasy of the knowing master loses sight of resistance as something to be *worked with* rather than overcome.

One place where a tendency to impose interpretations may be evident is in the famous case of Dora. This analysis is particularly relevant because, as Anzieu points out, Freud's treatment "centred on two of Dora's dreams, thus making the case history a direct continuation of *The Interpretation of Dreams.*"[19] The Dora analysis may be seen to reflect unresolved reductionistic and authoritarian tendencies operative in Freud's technique. Richard Webster, for example, notes disdainfully of Freud that "in his case history of the attractive eighteen-year-old girl Dora, he responds to a dream in which she smelt smoke by pointing out that he himself is a heavy smoker, and goes on to interpret the dream as a cryptic allusion to her desire to be kissed by him."[20] In addition to this being a fairly obvious instance of Freud imposing his views on Dora, Webster sees this as an example of the analyst projecting his own fantasies onto the dream material, without sensitivity to the analysand's own situation and associations. Although I should say that I am not persuaded by most of the sweeping, one-sided criticisms made by Webster and other ideologically driven detractors of psychoanalysis, in this case the point alerts us to a persistent danger in psychoanalytic technique.

Fortunately, psychoanalysis contains resources that counteract its own tendencies toward closure and authoritarianism. Returning to Jacques Derrida's discussion of resistance, it is significant that he has taken up the ambiguity within this notion in order to bring out, in his words, the "resistance *of* psychoanalysis as we know it, a resistance to itself. . . ."[21] Derrida invokes the "French resistance" of World War II to convey associations of resistance with a liberating rather than merely a blocking force.[22] Understood thus, resistances *of* psychoanalysis appear in the manner in which Freud's technique rescues itself from potential closures of meaning by an internal fissuring and multiplication.

Additionally, and most important for the present discussion, Derrida points out that one of the concepts within *The Interpretation of Dreams* that explicitly resists totalization is the *dream navel*.[23] This concept first appears in a footnote to the centrally important dream of Irma's injection. After an extended analysis, Freud acknowledges his awareness that he has not been able to unravel the full spectrum of possible associations and meanings emerging from the dream narrative. In his words, "there is at least one spot in every dream at which it is unplumbable—a navel, as it were, that is its point of contact with the unknown."[24] Subsequently, Freud again invokes the dream navel, and tries to explicate it further by means of a variety of images. He refers to it as "a *tangle* of dream thoughts which cannot be unravelled," and states of these dream thoughts that they "*branch* out in every direction into the intricate *network* of our world of thought." Finally, Freud concludes with the well-known statement that "it is at some point where this *meshwork* is particularly close that the dream-wish grows up, like a *mushroom* out of its mycelium."[25] Even at first glance, what is most interesting here is the way in which Freud has undermined any possibility of establishing a fixed foundation of meaning for the dream narrative. The dream thoughts are posited as underlying the dream work and dream content, the related narrative. However, this substratum ultimately opens out into a "navel" that seem to be capable of description only in *imagistic* terms; thus Freud's exposition resorts to one of the mechanisms of the dream work itself. Moreover, readers are presented with such a plurality of images that they are drawn into more of a gaping abyss than a closed explanatory center. In the remainder of this chapter I illustrate that, while the concept of the dream navel as such appears infrequently, it condenses a significant network or meshwork of ideas and images that resonate throughout Freud's Dream Book. These related ideas indicate that internal resistance, as manifest in the dream narrative, can be a place where the closure of the ego is offset. Something in the nature of the unconscious, and in the dream, eludes the mastery of the egos of both the dreamer and the analyst. This point also speaks directly to issues of self-reflection and self-transformation, insofar as it indicates an internal source for *questioning oneself*.

Many of these issues appear in conjunction with Freud's analyses of another central dream, that of the Botanical Monograph, which I will use as a point of reference. The dream is extremely brief, and can be given in its entirety: "*I had written a monograph on a certain plant. The book lay before me and I was at the moment turning over a folded coloured plate. Bound up in each copy there was a dried specimen of the plant, as though it had been taken from a herbarium.*" (The dream is related in three slightly differing versions, *SE* IV: 165, 169, 282, of which I have given the second.) My intention here is not to add anything new in terms of directly interpreting this dream. Rather, I want to attend to the *manner* in which Freud's analyses take shape at intervals through the course of the book and to the many associated ideas that appear as this occurs. Freud's varying discussions of this dream exemplify qualities of his text that offset linearity and univocity.

The dream is first described and analyzed at length (on pp. 169–176) under the heading "Recent and Indifferent Material." In this section alone Freud provides a staggering variety of associations. He first notes, for example, the following: a book on plants he had seen in a shop window on the morning before the dream; his frequently forgetting to bring flowers for his wife, an instance of a parapraxis on the part of an associate, who also forgot to bring a bouquet for his wife on her birthday, that Freud saw as confirming his theories; Freud's own monograph on the coca plant and a related instance in which cocaine had been used as an anesthetic during an operation on his father for glaucoma; a daydream in which Freud's friend Fliess would operate on *him* for the same affliction; his encounter with a Professor Gärtner concerning a patient named Flora; and so forth. In a second wave of associations, focusing on the image of the dried specimen of the plant, Freud is led to further recollections from his school days, during which he had done rather poorly in botany; to the image of artichokes as his "favourite flowers," and to the insight that his wife, being the more generous of the two, frequently purchased these for him. He also recalls a comment from his friend Fliess, who had related in a letter that "I see the dream book lying finished before me and I see myself turning over its pages." Additionally, Freud's bibliophilic tendencies are mentioned, with associations concerning his one-sidedness and extravagance when it came to this passion. Finally, a scene from early youth is recalled, in which his father had given Sigmund and his sister a book of colored plates to pull to pieces.

Among the central underlying latent ideas that appear in these associations are two main antithetical chains of meaning, each with strong emotional overtones. On one hand, there are repeated instances of *guilt* and *self-doubt,* especially as related to Freud's relationships with his father, his wife, and his friend Fliess and to his career. On the other hand, there are multiple significations related to *ambition* and *self-justification* in relation to the same people and endeavors. At the level of theory, Freud introduces in this section two important ideas that will be further developed later in the text: that of links between significant latent thoughts and insignificant dream content connected by associative chains as in puns and riddles, and the related notion of *displacement* along associated paths.[26]

Further comments on the same dream appear fifteen pages later in a discussion of "Infantile Material." In this section, Freud informs us that he has not disclosed "the ultimate meaning of the dream" but that this is "intimately related to the subject of the childhood scene" (concerning exfoliating the book).[27] A second complete recounting of the dream and an additional analysis appears (at pp. 282–284) as a major example of the work of *condensation*. There Freud focuses on the terms "botanical" and "monograph" as highly condensed signifiers. Through association, these terms "led by numerous connecting paths deeper and deeper into the tangle of dream thoughts."[28] He also states that the terms "constituted 'nodal points' upon which a great number of the dream-thoughts converged."[29] In the course of this discussion, Freud also invokes Goethe's image of the weaver's masterpiece: "unseen the threads are knit together, and an infinite combination grows."[30] The notion of "nodal points," with its related images of depths, weavings, threads, and tangles, clearly extrapolates upon the more general concept of the dream navel. Both expressions refer to places of density in the dream that open up into a variety of associations and ranges of meaning.

Freud specifically uses the nodal points of *botanical* and *monograph* to discuss two key, related features of the dream work: condensation (in which multiple meanings are compacted into a single image) and over-determination (in which multiple factors and sources converge in the formation of the dream narrative). As Freud states, "the elements of the dream are constructed out of the whole mass of dream-thoughts and each one of those elements is shown to have been determined many times over in relation to the dream-thoughts."[31] Freud emphasizes that, in analysis, this densely imbricated over-determination calls for a corresponding process of over-interpretation.[32] The principle behind these notions is, basically, if you think you have completed an interpretation of a dream, look again and you will find something more. These ideas explicitly counteract positing a foundational or final meaning to dreams and convey the resistance to closure expressed in the image of the dream navel.

In the next section of *The Interpretation of Dreams,* dealing with "The Work of Displacement," the dream of the Botanical Monograph is introduced once again as an illustration. Freud adds to the complexity of his discussion of nodal points by arguing that "the dream is, as it were, differently centered from the dream-thoughts—its content has different elements as its central point."[33] In other words, a nodal or central point like "botanical" is a displacement of a totally different, but associated, focal point of the latent dream thoughts. Freud now adds a fresh aspect to his interpretation by describing this underlying emotional focus as related to "complications and conflicts arising between colleagues from their professional obligations."[34] Here again issues of fidelity, ambition, and guilt are indicated, but the *place* where the issues are enacted is shifted, in the dream work, to a more neutral location. There is a metonymic slippage from one center to another, so that each detected center is already decentered in relation to some other place of meaning that informs it. To convey this process, Freud introduces the notion of "*a transference and displacement of psychical intensities.*"[35] This characterizes the specifically emotional and value-laden dimension of this slippage; that is, the metonymic decentering allows overly troubling issues to surface in the disguise of innocuous images.

In the following section, "The Means of Representation," Freud further elaborates on this theme by introducing a notion reminiscent of Nietzsche, the "transvaluation of all psychical values." This describes a process whereby an underlying emotional issue of great intensity comes to be represented by an element in the dream, seemingly of little import, that reveals significant condensation.[36] In other words, emotional *intensity* translates into imagistic *density.* In this discussion, Freud makes the important point that the degree of emotional intensity has nothing to do with a correspondence with reality—it is not based on an external event or impression but on an internal psychical process.[37] This is significant because, if attended to, it steers interpretation away from causal explanation and toward the inner experience of the dreamer. Emotional intensity is personal and subjective, and not necessarily related to some obvious traumatic event. Much later in the text, under the heading "Affects in Dreams," the dream of the Botanical Monograph is mentioned yet again to illustrate this notion of transvaluation. As Freud puts it, "the thoughts corresponding to it consisted of a passionately agitated plea on behalf of my liberty to act as I chose to act and to govern my life as seemed right to me and me alone. The dream that arose from them has an indifferent ring about it."[38] What is also significant here is that, in each instance where Freud calls on this dream to illustrate a particular aspect of the dream work, some fresh insight into the meaning of the dream appears.

Almost a hundred pages later, Freud furthers the analysis. He notes that the dream work connects a central point of the dream-thoughts of great "*psychical* intensity" to elements of "*sensory* intensity" in the actual dream narrative.[39] How are these connections established by the dream work? As Freud states, the displacement onto seemingly trivial affairs occurs "owing to their being in what is often an artificially established connection with the central element. . . ."[40] Later, Freud clarifies the nature of these artificial connections by noting the example of "associations based on homonyms and verbal similarities. . . ."[41] Hence, to choose only one obvious example, the discussion with Professor Gärtner concerning the patient Flora allows the transference of emotionally significant issues appearing in their talk onto the nodal point "botanical."

The single brief dream of the Botanical Monograph, exhibiting so many associations and key features of the dream work, provides an excellent instance of the dream navel at work. The dream illustrates condensation, displacement, over-determination and over-interpretation, transvaluation, and associations along linguistic lines. As Freud repeatedly returns to this dream in a variety of different contexts, he brings out additional, multiple variations on its meaning. It is not only what is found in the dream but the text's own transmission of these insights that occurs in the form of what Ronald Barthes calls the "metonymic logic of the unconscious."[42] That is, the dream book is nonlinear and multidimensional, doubling back on itself so as to continually reillumine its material from fresh angles. Indeed, it has something of a "performative" quality; rather than simply presenting material and ideas, it engages the reader in a process of reflection and discovery.[43]

The notion of the dream navel as an irreducible point of resistance returns us to the constitutive insights of psychoanalysis, in which dreams are indicative of internal otherness. In several places in *The Interpretation of Dreams,* Freud's formulations resist flattening the unconscious into a determinable realm of basic drives and inscribed memories. For example, he states that "everything that can be the object of our internal perception is *virtual.*"[44] This indicates a dereification of the unconscious and a sense that all articulations thereof are partial and tentative. Freud also discusses the unconscious in terms that are akin to the Lacanian notion of the inexhaustible Real and the ultimately unknowable Kantian noumenal.[45] He states that "The unconscious is the true psychical reality; *in its inner nature it is as much unknown to us as the reality of the external world, and it is as incompletely represented by the data of consciousness as is the external world by the communications of our sense organs.*"[46]

These insights concerning a necessary remainder to any analysis or explanation do not simply leave us with an opaque sense of mystery; they do not simply indicate an unfathomable unconscious beyond our conscious grasp. Rather, within the context of the specific techniques and detailed analyses of *The Interpretation of Dreams,* Freud's acknowledgments of the dream navel provide an essential counterdynamic to the danger of systemic closure. We are pointed toward an ongoing interpretive process rather than toward a foundational theory that can harden into dogma. This opposition to closure, evidenced in Freud's texts, duplicates the same sort of meaningful inner resistance that characterizes dreams themselves.

Dream interpretation provides an occasion for an opening of human subjects to discourse that arises most intimately from within us and yet speaks in a difficult and different language. This difference compels us to stray beyond the familiar confines of our self-images and patterns of thinking. In this way, subjects are drawn out of a closed attitude and identity by an engagement with an alterity that resists easy assimilation. This fosters a reflective process in which, as Castoriadis puts it, "thought turns back upon itself and interrogates itself not only about its particular contents but also about its presuppositions and foundations."[47] This reflectiveness forms the basis for transformative self-critique, insofar as it serves to place in question the predominant, ingrained attitudes and assumptions of the ego, potentially allowing us to see and understand in alternate ways and from different standpoints. Because of this, dream interpretation can be seen as both a vehicle and a paradigm for an opening to alterity that has profound ethical implications.

Notes

1. Paul Ricoeur, *Freud and Philosophy: An Essay on Interpretation,* trans. Denis Savage (New Haven: Yale University Press, 1970).
2. For an excellent analysis of these issues, as well as an applied reinterpretation of psychoanalytic theory in a non-Western context, see Gananath Obeyesekere, *The Work of Culture: Symbolic Transformation in Psychoanalysis and Anthropology* (Chicago: University of Chicago Press, 1990).
3. I discuss these strategies for reading Freud's work at some length in *The Other Freud: Religion, Culture and Psychoanalysis* (London: Routledge, 1999).
4. Didier Anzieu, *Freud's Self-Analysis,* trans. Peter Graham (New York: International Universities Press, 1986), p. 512.
5. Ibid., p. 511.
6. See DiCenso, *The Other Freud,* pp. 130–131.
7. Serge Leclaire, *Psychoanalysing: On the Order of the Unconscious and the Practice of the Letter,* trans. Peggy Kamuf (Stanford, CA: Stanford University Press, 1998), p.16.
8. Obeyesekere's discussion of Grünbaum's work is exemplary in elucidating the assumptions and limitations of this positivistic type of critique. See *The Work of Culture,* pp. xxiii-xxv.
9. Sigmund Freud, *The Standard Edition of the Complete Psychological Works of Sigmund Freud,* translated under the general editorship of James Strachey, 24 vols. (London: Hogarth Press, 1953–74) (hereafter *SE*), vol.V, *The Interpretation of Dreams,* p. 517.
10. Anzieu, *Freud's Self-Analysis,* p. 251.
11. Jean Laplanche and J.-B. Pontalis, *The Language of Psychoanalysis,* trans. Donald Nicholson-Smith (New York: Norton, 1973), p.395.
12. Jacques Derrida, *Resistances of Psychoanalysis,* trans. P. Kamuf, P.-A. Brault, and M. Naas (Stanford: Stanford University Press, 1998), p. 13.
13. Laplanche and Pontalis, *The Language of Psychoanalysis,* p.125 (emphasis in original).
14. See, for example, Ricoeur, *Freud and Philosophy,* p .92.
15. Sigmund Freud, *The Complete Letters of Sigmund Freud to Wilhelm Fliess,* trans. J. M. Masson (Cambridge, MA.: Harvard University Press, 1985), p. 255; also see Anzieu, *Freud's Self-Analysis,* p. 226.
16. Sigmund Freud, *History of the Psychoanalytic Movement, SE,* vol. XIV, p .50.
17. Cornelius Castoriadis, *World in Fragments: Writings on Politics, Society, Psychoanalysis, and the Imagination,* ed. and trans. David Ames Curtis (Stanford: Stanford University Press, 1997), p. 128.
18. See *The Interpretation of Dreams, SE,* vol. IV, pp. 142–144.
19. Anzieu, *Freud's Self-Analysis,* p. 545.
20. Richard Webster, *Why Freud Was Wrong: Sin, Science and Psychoanalysis* (London: Fontana Press, 1995), p. 272. Webster neglects to substantiate his account with references to Freud's text; however, the relevant passages can be found in Freud, *Fragment of an Analysis of a Case of Hysteria, SE,* vol.VII: 73–74.
21. Derrida, *Resistances of Psychoanalysis,* p. viii (emphasis in original).
22. Ibid., p. 2.

23. Ibid., p. 14.
24. Freud, *The Interpretation of Dreams, SE,* vol. IV, p. 111, note 1.
25. Ibid., p. 525 (emphasis added).
26. Ibid., pp. 176–177.
27. *SE,* vol. IV, p. 191; Serge Leclaire has expanded on Freud's analyses in this regard, see *Psychoanalysing,* pp. 32, 37, 117.
28. Ibid., p. 282.
29. Ibid., p. 283.
30. Ibid., pp. 283–284.
31. Ibid., p. 283.
32. For a discussion of these concepts, see ibid., pp. 279, 353, 523.
33. Ibid., p. 305.
34. Ibid., p. 305.
35. Ibid., p. 307 (emphasis in original).
36. Ibid., p. 330.
37. Ibid., p. 329.
38. *The Interpretation of Dreams, SE,* vol. V, p. 467.
39. Ibid., pp. 561–562 (emphasis in original).
40. Ibid., p. 562.
41. Ibid., p. 596.
42. Roland Barthes, *Image, Music, Text,* trans. Stephen Heath (London: Fontana Press, 1977), p.141. Barthes illustrates, in his analysis of Jacob's struggle with the angel (Genesis 32:22–32), that similar qualities to those we have discerned in the dream narrative appear in religious texts. These likewise call for a type of reading that is multiple and open-ended.
43. Barthes states the matter as follows: "The problem, the problem at least posed for me, is exactly to manage not to reduce the Text to a signified, whatever it may be (historical, economic, folkloristic or kerygmatic), but to hold its *significance* fully open." Ibid., p. 141.
44. *The Interpretation of Dreams, SE,* vol. V, p. 611 (emphasis in original).
45. See DiCenso, *The Other Freud,* p. 44, for further discussion.
46. *The Interpretation of Dreams, SE,* vol. V, p. 613 (emphasis in original).
47. Castoriadis, *World in Fragments,* p. 267.

19

Turning Away at the Navel of the Dream

Religion and the Body of the Mother at the Beginning and End of Interpretation

Diane Jonte-Pace

There is at least one spot in every dream at which it is unplumbable—a navel, as it were, that is its point of contact with the unknown.

—*Sigmund Freud, The Interpretation of Dreams*

On November 19, 1899, about two weeks after the publication of *The Interpretation of Dreams,* Freud wrote impatiently to his friend Wilhelm Fliess in Berlin, "It is a thankless task to enlighten mankind a little. No one has yet told me that he feels indebted to me for having learned something new from the dream book and for having been introduced to a world of new problems" (Masson 1985: 387).* Although it took longer than two weeks for the world to realize that Freud had "enlightened mankind a little" with his "Dream Book," we now understand that he did indeed introduce to our century a "world of new problems."

This chapter examines just how Freud "enlightened mankind a little" and how he introduced to us a "world of new problems," some of which we have barely noticed in a century of readings. Freud's justly famous *Interpretation of Dreams* will provide a "specimen text" for this inquiry, somewhat like the "specimen dream" that Freud described and interpreted in the second chapter of his Dream Book. I describe and interpret two key moments in *The Interpretations of Dreams,* suggesting that a more visible framework for the volume (which is in many ways oedipal) is undercut by an interruptive counterthesis subverting the "master plot" (Brooks 1989): The limitations of the master plot are acknowledged both implicitly and explicitly. Freud's text not only provides a cartography for the "royal road to the unconscious" but simultaneously deconstructs its own cartography at sites Freud described as the beginning and the end of interpretation and that coincide with the encounter with religion and the maternal body.

The Road Trip of the Century: "Acheronta Movebo"

Devoting an entire chapter of his mid-twentieth-century biography of Freud to *The Interpretation of Dreams,* Ernest Jones applauds the volume as Freud's most important, best known, and most original work, the work that would bring him lasting fame. "By general consensus," he says, "*The Interpretation of Dreams* was Freud's major work, the one by which his name will probably be longest remembered" (1953: 384). Emphasizing the oedipal themes in the work, Jones states, "the description of the now familiar 'Oedipus complex,' the erotic and the hostile relations of child to parent, are frankly exposed" (384).

Jones is correct, of course, to emphasize the significance of the work. The impact of Freud's "Dream Book" on the twentieth century is indisputable. At the beginning of the twenty-first century we all "speak Freud," as Peter Gay has said (1999: 69), and, in large part, the book Freud called his "Dream Book" is responsible for this new language. Jones is correct as well to point out oedipal themes in the volume. Although Oedipus became a "complex" in Freud's work only in 1910, *The Interpretation of Dreams* was the text in which he first published the oedipal theory that, he often said, had been "revealed" to him.[1] And although Oedipus did not make an appearance until nearly halfway through the volume (*Standard Edition of the Complete Psychological Works of Sigmund Freud* [hereafter *SE*] 5: 261), Freud commented on "Oedipus dreams" in a section on "typical dreams" (*SE* 5: 398); he devoted several pages to an interpretation of Sophocles' play *Oedipus Rex;* and he quoted Sophocles' famous words, "many a man 'ere now in dreams hath lain with her who bare him" (*SE* 4: 264). Letters to Wilhelm Fliess during the years he was writing the book document his sense of the centrality of Oedipus in its argument. He first outlined the "Dream Book" to Fliess in a letter of March 1898, describing his intention to incorporate in the six chapters "comments on *Oedipus Rex,* the talisman fairy tale, and possibly *Hamlet.*" He added "I first must read up on the Oedipus legend—do not yet know where" (Masson 1985: 304).

Yet Freud introduced the book not with a motto from Sophocles' famous account of the tragic oedipal legend but rather with a reference to another legendary tale from the ancient world, Virgil's heroic saga of the founding of the city of Rome. On the frontispiece of *The Interpretation of Dreams* and again in its final pages (*SE* 5: 608), Freud quoted Virgil's words from *The Aeneid:* "*Flectere si nequeo superos, Acheronta movebo*" (If I cannot bend the Higher Powers, I will move the Infernal Regions).[2] Freud understood the passage as a reference to the path of repressed instinctual impulses (*SE* 5: 608 n. 1), and thus as a reference to repressed fantasies, oedipal and otherwise, in the unconscious. It is also a self-reflexive comment: By selecting this epigraph, Freud suggested that he, in his quest for the meanings of dreams, would plumb the deepest layers, the lowest regions of the underworld or unconscious. His oedipal master plot is, in a sense, contained within Virgil's famous evocation of the journey to the depths.[3]

The motif of ceaseless exploration of the "Lower Regions," by its reiteration at the beginning and end of the Dream Book, frames the volume, defining it as a heroic narrative of indefatigable quest. Freud emphasized this theme in the often-quoted sentence immediately following the Virgilian passage, defining dream interpretation as the "royal road." After "*Flectere si nequeo superos* . . ." he continued, "The interpretation of dreams is the royal road to a knowledge of the unconscious activities of the mind" (*SE* 5: 608). Freud identified the descent to the "underworld" in dreams and their interpretations as the royal road, inviting the reader on the "road trip" of the century.

While Freud would not have used the contemporary term "road trip," the metaphor of an arduous journey is one that he used quite consciously in this book. After a first chapter surveying the literature on dreams and a second offering his "specimen dream," he began the third chapter with these poetic words: "When, after passing through a narrow defile, we suddenly emerge upon a piece of high ground, where the path divides and the finest prospects open up on every side, we may pause for a moment and consider in which direction we shall first turn our steps" *(SE* 4: 122). The narrow defile, the path, and the steps are the classic elements of the ancient road trip, pilgrimage, or perilous journey.

Freud had written to Fliess just a few months before the publication of the Dream Book describing his intent to structure the volume as a fantasized journey through the wilderness. In a letter of August 6, 1899, he noted, "The whole thing is planned on the model of an imaginary walk. First comes the dark wood of the authorities (who cannot see the trees), where there is no clear view and it is easy to go astray" (*SE* 4: 122 n. 1, parens. in original). Other letters, such as one from July 22, 1899, anticipate the imagery of the "dark forests" of the first chapter: "most readers will get stuck in this thorny thicket (*Dornengestrüpp*)" (Masson 1985: 362–363).[4]

Wittgenstein has called psychoanalysis a "powerful mythology" (1966); Harold Bloom has referred to Freud as "the dominant mythologist of our time" (1995: 113). References to Freud's myth-making, if not attempting to discredit psychoanalysis, usually refer to the theory of instincts that Freud himself called "our mythology" (*SE* 22: 95). Yet Freud is a mythologist in another sense as well. He draws upon the classic narratives and myths of Western culture to weave his own arguments.

By referring to his text as a dark forest, the well-read, middle-aged Freud was drawing a parallel between his book and another epic that begins in a dark wood in midlife. Dante's masterful *Divine Comedy,* which, like Freud's text, draws heavily on Virgil's *Aeneid,* starts with the following words: "In the middle of the journey of our life I came to myself within a dark wood (*una selva oscura*) where the straight way was lost" (1:1). Dante's "*selva oscura*" is the same sort of dark wood in which one loses one's way in Freud's text. Freud was consciously patterning his Dream Book on Dante's epic as well as on Virgil's.[5] Dante and Virgil describe road trips, royal roads, heroic quests along the path toward truth. But theirs are Roman or Christian road trips, which Freud's is not, and this is a crucial difference. Freud must "take another road," "*tenere altro viaggio*" (I: 91), to quote Dante again. This other road is a subversive, non-oedipal pilgrimage of sorts.

At the beginning of the last chapter of *The Interpretation of Dreams,* Freud reminded his readers of the journey they had accomplished and warned of the ordeals and dangers still to come: "It will be well to pause and look around, to see whether in the course of our journey up to this point we have overlooked anything of importance. For it must be clearly understood that the easy and agreeable portion of our journey lies behind us. Hitherto . . . all the paths along which we have traveled have led us towards the light—towards elucidation and fuller understanding. But as soon as we endeavor to penetrate more deeply into the mental processes involved in dreaming, every path will end in darkness" (*SE* 5: 511). These dire warnings of darkness and obscurity at the end of the journey, however, give way to a set of clear instructions on how to overcome the obstacles to understanding the dream, a description of where interpretation begins.

The Beginning of Interpretation

Interpretation begins, he stated, at a point of resistance revealed by changes in the dreamer's reiteration of the dream: "If the first account given to me by a patient is too hard to follow, I ask him to repeat it. In doing so he rarely uses the same words. But the parts of the dream which he describes in different terms are by that fact revealed to me as the weak spot in the dream's disguise" (*SE* 5: 515). Describing these "weak spot(s) in the dream's disguise" as the point at which interpretation can begin, Freud used a significant metaphor: These dream sites "serve my purpose just as Hagen's was served by the embroidered mark on Siegfried's cloak. That is the point at which the interpretation of the dream can be started." He continued the metaphor: "The trouble taken by the dreamer in preventing the solution of the dream gives me a basis for estimating the care with which its cloak has been woven" (*SE* 5: 515).

What are the metaphoric meanings of Siegfried's woven cloak, Hagen's purpose, and the embroidered mark in Freud's interpretive project? While the Virgilian resolve to "move the Infernal Regions" provided the larger narrative framework for *The Interpretation of Dreams,* Freud introduced with these references another heroic tale as metaphor for the more precise work of the interpreter: The Germanic saga the *Song of the Niebelungen,* best known to Freud and his contemporaries in its Wagnerian form, with its great adversaries Siegfried and Hagen. Hagen was the legendary slayer of Siegfried, who could be wounded at only one spot. Hagen was able to slay the hero, Freud's editor explained in a footnote, because, by trickery, he persuaded the woman who "alone knew where the spot was" to indicate the "vital point" (*SE* 5: 515 n. 2) with an embroidered mark on the cloak. The dream is thus like Siegfried's woven cloak: The part of the dream where interpretation can begin, marked by variations in words, is analogous to the embroidered mark indicating the site of vulnerability. Threads are woven and embroidered into dream cloaks and dream signs; interpretive swords cut through woven threads.

Religion is not far from the surface of this text: A heroic Aryan/Christian/Germanic Siegfried is slain by a stereotypically Jewish antihero, Hagen. Marc Weiner describes Siegfried's Aryan symbolism and Hagen's Jewishness in Wagner's drama: Siegfried "constitutes a metaphor for the salvation of Germany's future, a salvation based upon racial exclusion available to the fatherland . . . while Hagen's body is a physiological-metaphorical warning to a Germany that refuses to recognize the biological dimension of the purported Jewish threat" (1995: 310). In Freud's metaphor, Hagen's purpose, slaying the heroic Siegfried, is analogous to Freud's purpose, interpreting the dream. Dream interpretation is metaphorically likened to the Jewish antihero's act of killing the hero. It is an act of knowing, with religious resonance, wherein Jewish interpreters like Freud, with knowledge of secret marks and signs, can perceive hidden desires below "cloaked" surfaces. It implies a position of ultimate power. Through his knowledge of secret marks and signs, the Jewish dream interpreter has power like Hagen's power—even the power of death—over Germanic Christians.

In his use of this metaphor Freud reverses a historical reality: While the mark exposing the Jewishness of the male Jew—the cloaked or clothed mark of circumcision—would give to Germanic anti-Semites the power of life and death over Jews, Freud's hermeneutic exposes what is beneath the woven cloak of the dream, giving power to the Jewish dream interpreter. This metaphor also reverses the structure of one of Freud's own well-known narratives involving another Jew on another road. Freud's disillusionment at his father's "unheroic conduct" (also recounted in *The Interpretation of Dreams*) in the face of the anti-Semitic taunt "Jew, get off the pavement!" (*SE* 4: 197) is countered directly and replaced with its opposite in this narrative of the skilled Jewish interpreter on the royal road who understands the meaning of the embroidered mark on Siegfried's woven cloak. Here the Jew, master of the royal road, has power, knowledge, authority: Unlike Freud's father, he need not leave the pavement in resignation or defeat. If one Jew on the road loses his hat and his place on the path, this new version of the story gives knowledge and power to the Jew who is now master of the royal road. It is no accident that Freud constructed support for his argument through metaphors drawn from Germanic tales in which ambiguous signs expose secret meanings recognizable only to knowledgeable Jewish interpreters. He does not mention explicitly his Jewish identity in these remarks on the "point where interpretation begins," nor does he describe the widespread anti-Semitic assumptions that made Hagen appear Jewish, degenerate, villainous, and terrifying (Weiner 308), but to Freud and his readers, the associations would have been obvious. Weiner clarifies this point: "Wagner never included the word *Jude* in his words for the stage because he didn't need to; the corporeal features deemed obvious signs of the Jew in his culture would have made the anti-Semitic nature of his representations of purportedly Jewish characteristics self-evident in his time" (13).

Freud's own sense of dream interpretation as a Jewish project is ubiquitous throughout the book and the contemporaneous letters. His frequent references to *The Interpretation of Dreams* as "the Egyptian dream book" or "the Ancient Egyptian Dream Book" in letters to Fliess (Masson 1985: 366, 368) evoke the biblical tale of Joseph, the Jewish interpreter of dreams for the Egyptian pharaoh (Gen. 40–41). On August 6, 1899, for example, he wrote to Fliess: "With the most cordial greetings and thanks for your cooperation in the Egyptian dream book" (Masson 1985: 366). Similarly, he asked later that month (August 27): "What would you think of ten days in Rome at Easter (the two of us, of course), if all goes well, if I can afford it and have not been locked up, lynched, or boycotted on account of the Egyptian dream book?" (Masson 1985: 368). A footnote in *The Interpretation of Dreams* corroborates these associations: "It will be noted that the name Josef plays a great part in my dreams . . . My own ego finds it very easy to hide itself behind people of that name since Joseph was the name of a man famous in the Bible as an interpreter of dreams" (*SE* 5: 484 n. 2). His symbolic references to Christians and Jews are not far from the surface of the text.

The heroic royal road trip is subverted or diverted in subtle ways by Freud's metaphors. Not only can interpretation kill, but the interpretive road trip is neither a Roman nor a Christian road trip, but a Jewish one: A traveling or wandering Jew maps the royal road and reads the hidden signs. Freud's explicit references to himself as Ahasverus, the eternal, wandering Jew, come from later years, but I think the image lies behind this text as well. Freud states, in a letter to his son Ernst, a few days before leaving Vienna for London in May 1938, shortly after the *Anschlüss:* "I sometimes compare myself to old Jacob who, when a very old man, was taken by his children to Egypt . . . Let us hope that it won't also be followed by an Exodus from Egypt. It is high time that Ahasverus came to rest somewhere" (E. Freud 1992: 298).[6] The heroic adventurer on the royal road ends his years as a wandering Jew seeking a place of rest.

There is another important dimension to the subversion of the royal road in Freud's text: In the mythic associations used to present his theory, Freud's own interpretive identity shifts from the role of hero to the role of antihero or villain. Freud's role is an oppositional one: The Virgilian motto discussed above is actually spoken by Juno, the great goddess who is opposed to Aeneas' heroic quest to establish the city of Rome. In the Virgilian quote, Freud identifies with Juno, the opponent of the heroic adventurer Aeneas, and, in the metaphor enlivening the text, with Hagen, the slayer of the heroic Siegfried. Although he had written to Fliess in February 1900, "I am by temperament nothing but a *conquistador,* an adventurer" (Masson 1985: 398), and although he identified in many ways with Oedipus, the heroic solver of riddles, he took, at the same time, an ambivalent stance toward heroic figures, deconstructing his own master plot at the very beginnings of interpretation.[7]

The Ends of Interpretation

We noted above that Freud twice quoted Virgil's "*Flectere si nequeo superos,*" once at the beginning and once at the end of the "dream book," framing the volume as a trip on the royal road. This doubling of the royal road is both mirrored and negated in a double reference to the *end of interpretation.* The first reference to the end of interpretation appeared in a footnote early in the volume: Freud stated, "There is at least one spot in every dream at which it is unplumbable—a navel, as it were (*unergründlich, gleichsam einen Nabel*), that is its point of contact with the unknown (*mit dem Unerkannten*)" (*SE* 4:111, n. 1). This "unplumbable" point of contact with the unknown, this dream navel, reappears much later in the volume: there are points, Freud argued, at which the hero must turn aside, the interpreter must look away. He stated (*SE* 5: 525):

> There is often a passage in even the most thoroughly interpreted dream, which has to be left obscure [*man muss oft eine Stelle im Dunkel lassen*];[8] this is because we become aware during the work of interpretation that at that point there is a tangle [*Knäuel*] of dream-thoughts which cannot be unraveled [*der sich nicht entwirren will*] and which moreover adds nothing to our knowledge of the content of the dream. This is the dream's navel [*der Nabel des Traums*], the spot where it reaches down into the unknown [*Unerkannten*].

Freud continued this paragraph with a different metaphor for dream thoughts. In this case, dream threads are infinitely branching, rather than tangled: "the dream thoughts to which we are led by interpretation cannot, from the nature of things, have any definite endings; they are bound to branch out in every direction into the intricate network [*netzartige Verstrickung*] of our world of thought. It is at some point where this meshwork [*Geflecht*] is particularly close that the dream-wish grows up, like a mushroom out of its mycelium" (*SE* 5: 525). Regardless of the ever-branching pattern of meshworks or networks in the dream thoughts, however, some dreams are impenetrable; some unknowns unknowable; some tangles unravelable.

What leads Freud to turn away at the "navel of the dream"? What is the "unknown" that he finds unfathomable, impenetrable, or "unplumbable"? His own imagery is evocative. The "navel" of the dream, the spot where it "reaches into the unknown," evokes the human navel, the bodily mark of the passage through the maternal genitals and into the world. If the interpretation of the dream began at the point of the embroidered mark, where Hagen slew Siegfried, then the interpretation must end at another mark, the birthmark, the scar that marks the site of the connection to, and separation from, the mother. It is the site of connection to and separation from the mother that Freud cannot interpret by following the "royal road" to the "lower regions": Freud's turning aside at the "navel of the dream" is, in a sense, an acknowledgment of the limitations of the heroic paths of figures like Oedipus and Aeneas. The point at which interpretation must end is both navel and knot, birthmark and tangle of threads. Navel [*Nabel*] and tangle [*Knäuel*] both interrupt the saga of the *Niebelungen,* or the journey of the hero.

Freud's references to the intricate "network," "meshwork," or "tangle of dream thoughts which cannot be unraveled" are as evocative as his reference to the "dream navel." Like Homer, who interrupts the saga of Ulysses' road trip with the narrative of Penelope's woven and unwoven tapestry, Freud recounts a story of roads interrupted by threads, weavings, and tangles. As we have seen, his remarks on the beginnings of interpretation involve woven cloths, dream cloaks, and embroidered marks; his comments on the ends of interpretation involve unwoven tangles of threads and words, points at which dream thoughts become networks or meshworks of threads. The rhetoric of thread, knot, and weaving is dense.

What is this unravelable tangle that brings about the end of interpretation? According to Derrida, Freud's tangles can be unraveled by following the threads: "it is all a matter of knowing how to pull threads, pull on the threads, according to the art of the weaver" (1998: 15). One thread leads to women's work and women's genitals: Freud identified weaving as women's invention, developed to cover the genitals out of shame over the absence of the phallus (*SE* 22: 132).[9] Another thread in Freud's texts takes us to a similar destination: Twenty years after the publication of *The Interpretation of Dreams,* Freud wrote a short essay (published posthumously after yet another twenty years had passed) about another tangle of threads. In "Medusa's Head," Freud explicitly identifies the tangle. The unravelable tangle in "Medusa's Head," and, I maintain, the tangle in *The Interpretation of Dreams,* is the hair that covers the "dangerous" genitals of the mother: "Medusa's head takes the place of a representation of the female genitals . . . it isolates their horrifying effects from their pleasure-giving ones" (*SE* 18: 274). This tangle is also one at which the hero must turn away: Perseus, the heroic slayer of the Medusa, cannot look directly at her face lest he be paralyzed.[10]

Like Perseus, Freud averted his eyes from the psychoanalyst's task of interpretation when the task involved unraveling the threads that led to the mother's body. Freud's words represent an acknowledgment of the limitations of the oedipal master thesis. He turned away at the tangle of maternal hair and at the navel, the site of the scar that memorializes the loss of the mother through the cutting of the cord that once linked infant to mother, for he knew that the oedipal road, the royal road, although it theorizes an erotic reunion with the mother, could not take him to this uncanny destination. Indeed, this navel, which is a point of contact with the "unknown" [*Unerkannten*], which "has to be left obscure" (*SE* 5: 525), may in fact be the same "Great Unknown" [*Grosse Unerkannten*] Freud identified with Death in a dream interpretation a few pages earlier (*SE* 5: 472).

It may be relevant to note that Freud's footnote on the "unplumbable navel" of the dream is situated within his interpretation of the "specimen dream," the famous dream of Irma's injection that introduces the interpretive method of the "Dream Book." In

Freud's associations to the dream, he found three women: "I had been comparing my patient Irma with two other people. . . . If I had pursued my comparison between the three women, it would have taken me far afield" (*SE* 4: 110, 111 n. 1). The three women he does not pursue are Irma (who was in reality, at the time Freud dreamed this significant dream, near death because of surgical malpractice on the part of Freud's friend, Fliess), a friend of Irma's, and Freud's wife. Freud backed away from an interpretation of these three women, saying that he "had a feeling that the interpretation of this part of the dream was not carried far enough to make it possible to follow the whole of its concealed meaning" (SE 4: 111 n. 1). Freud ventured, in other texts and other decades, into the dangerous territory of female triads. In his essay "The Theme of the Three Caskets," three women are closely associated with death, the absence of God, and the fantasy of immortality (Jonte-Pace 1996). Here, however, he can only turn aside, looking away from the uncanny navel, in a gesture that repeats his acknowledgment of the limitations of the oedipal perspective.[11]

If the navel and the tangle are both references to the body of the mother and to death, then both signal the "end of interpretation," the place where the *telos,* the "end" (goal) of interpretation, gives way to the "end" (abandonment) of interpretation. From an oedipal perspective, Freud should not turn away from the fantasy of the mother's body. But the navel and the tangle do not invite or entice: In Freud's words, they produce "horror" or "*Grauen*" (*SE* 18: 274). Elsewhere, less fettered by attachments to royal road maps, he attempted hesitant unravelings of these tangled threads, exploring tentatively the dream's "point of contact with the unknown." These efforts are not unrelated to his attempts to plumb other "unknowns" and to solve other riddles, such as mortality, immortality, the afterlife, the psyche of the Jew, and the anxiety of the anti-Semite (Jonte-Pace 2001).

In his "Dream Book" then, Freud invites the reader to accompany him on a journey that, at first glance, appears to be a regal excursion to the unconscious to discover oedipal wishes and desires. But the beginning and end of interpretation enact detours in the oedipal journey. At the beginning of interpretation, woven threads mark the point at which Jewish dream interpreters are metaphorically identified with slayers of legendary heroes. At the end of interpretation we encounter insurmountable obstacles, at which the body of the mother lies hidden behind the navel of the dream and the tangle of dream thoughts. These tangles and obstacles are hints of Freud's awareness of the limitations of the oedipal paradigm. He weaves a subversive counterthesis within the larger narrative framework by drawing metaphoric connections between the methods of the (Jewish) dream interpreter and the actions of the antihero who slays Siegfried.

Freud's double articulation in *The Interpretation of Dreams* of the famous Virgilian passage "*si nequeo superos*" as an expression of masterplot and royal road is thus countered by his double acknowledgment of the limits of interpretation in the two passages on the "navel of the dream" and by his account of Siegfried's murder as a metaphor for the method of dream interpretation. Although the Dream Book maps the royal road, the master plot is subtly subverted both at the point where interpretation begins and at the "point of contact with the unknown," the navel of the dream where interpretation must end. Freud's intention to "enlighten mankind a little" with his Dream Book was a desire to communicate the map to a royal road that was in many ways oedipal. We now know the general contours of that topography quite well. What we have not fully explored is the "world of new problems" (Masson 1985: 387) that Freud hinted at in references to embroidered marks, woven cloaks, and tangled threads where the *ends* of interpretation are interwoven with and interrupted by the *end* of interpretation, and where the royal road meets religion and the maternal body.

Notes

* An earlier version of this paper was delivered at the meetings of the American Academy of Religion. The date of delivery was November 20, 1999, almost exactly one hundred years after Freud's impatient letter.

1. See Jonte-Pace (2001) for a discussion of Freud's vocabulary of "revelation."
2. *Aeneid* 7: 312. Freud leaves the passage in Latin. This translation, in the footnote to Freud's text, is provided by the editor of the *Standard Edition,* James Strachey.
3. Virgil's words have a complex history in Freud's intellectual trajectory and a complex history of interpretation in the literature on psychoanalysis. As early as 1896 Freud had announced to Fliess his plan to use the line as a motto for introducing a different text, an essay on symptom formation: "the psychology of hysteria will be preceded by the proud words '*Introite et hic dii sunt*' . . . the symptom formation by '*Flectere si nequeo superos Acheronta movebo*'" (Masson 1985: 205). (The "Introite" passage ["Enter, for the gods dwell here as well"], a quote from Aristotle's "De Partibus Animalium," 1:5, was a popular one among the early psychoanalysts: Carl Jung carved it on the lintel above his front door.) Three years later Freud mentioned Virgil's words specifically as his motto for *The Interpretation of Dreams* where he stated that it was not his first choice: Fliess had nixed a passage from Goethe that he had earlier selected (Masson 1985: 361). In addition, he used it in 1909 in one of his lectures at Clark University (editor's note, *SE*: 5: 608). Bakan provocatively interprets the "*flectere*" passage as a reference to the tension between God (the superego) and the devil (the suspended superego) in a "satanic pact" in which permission is granted to "violate the precepts of the superego" making it possible for the "suppressed material to rise to consciousness" (Bakan 1958: 210–211). Thanks are due to Don Capps for reminding me of this passage in Bakan's book.

   In the same 1896 letter in which he first staked claim on Virgil's words, Freud also stated, reporting on a recent period of depression "my bad time has run its course . . . [I] am not in the least interested in life after death" (Masson 1985: 204–205). In a previous letter, he had described his period of depression: "what I am lacking completely are high spirits and pleasure in living; instead, I am busy noting the occasions when I have to occupy myself with the state of affairs after my death" (Masson 1985: 204). Masson responds to these remarks with a brief footnote: "meaning unclear" (204). But Rizzuto finds much to say about this material. She finds evidence of "religious thinking modulated by negation, displacement and sublimation" (254); she finds Freud defensive and disingenuous in denying an interest in life after death, and she argues that "he could not stop the return to consciousness of derivatives of unconscious God representations. His preoccupation with God and the underworld appeared in displaced, and sublimated form" in the reference to Virgil's words (Rizzuto 1998: 254). I read these remarks of Freud's somewhat differently. I see them as evidence that in 1896, shortly after the death of his father, even as he was formulating the Oedipus complex, he was also formulating an alternate view.
4. Freud provides hints about the gendered meaning of the landscape in "Introductory Lectures on Psychoanalysis," noting that pubic hair "is depicted in dreams as woods and bushes." He adds "the complicated topography of the female genital parts makes one understand how it is that they are often represented as landscapes, with rocks, woods, and water" (*SE* 15: 156). Hyman reiterates Freud's gender analysis: "All of

these dark woods, narrow defiles, high grounds, and deep penetrations are unconscious sexual imagery and we are exploring a woman's body—that of Freud's mother" (Hyman 1962: 333; cf. Shengold 1991: 50). Yet this is not simply an oedipal fantasy.

5. He was reading Dante at this time (Jones 1953: 380). See Shengold, who notes that both Freud's and Dante's masterpieces were composed by men in their early forties writing of their younger selves; both works describe a pilgrimage toward knowledge and both works recount journeys of the soul (1991: 47–48). I find parallels as well to Augustine's *Confessions.* Like Augustine's masterpiece, Freud's Dream Book is unquestionably an introspective confession of personal sins and desires, artfully arrayed with the intent of bringing the reader closer and closer to the "truth."
6. *Es ist Zeit, dass Ahasver irgendwo zur Ruhe kommt*" (E. Freud and L. Freud 1960: 459).
7. Might these subversions of the royal road be evident as well in hints and hesitations Freud provides about the geography of the journey itself? His hesitation is evident in this passage from the beginning of chapter 7 of *The Interpretation of Dreams:* "Before starting off along this new path, it will be well to pause and look around, to see whether, in the course of our journey we have overlooked anything of importance . . . the easy and agreeable portion of our journey lies behind us. Hitherto, unless I am greatly mistaken, all the paths along which we have traveled have let us to the light-toward elucidation and fuller understanding. But as soon as we endeavor to penetrate more deeply into the mental process involved in dreaming, every path will end in darkness . . . we must be careful (*SE* 5: 511). Freud's references to "uncertainties" and "incompleteness"; and his concern that "every path will end in darkness" may be reflections of anxieties about the counter thesis. See James DiCenso (1999), *The Other Freud,* for an analysis of other examples of Freud's complex and liberating strategies for deconstructing some of his own more rigid theses.
8. Derrida notes that it is difficult to decide whether "'one must' . . . records an unsurpassable limit . . . or whether it is a 'one must' of duty that institutes what one *must* do which is not to go beyond, or if you prefer, what one *must not* do, which is to go beyond because that has no meaning" (Derrida 1998: 14). The "unsurpassable limit" seems the most likely choice to me; Capps (personal communication 1999) opts for the "one must of duty."
9. Derrida hints at the same conclusion, linking scar, knot, navel, thread, and umbilical cord: "What forever exceeds the analysis of the dream is indeed a knot that cannot be untied, a thread that, even if it is cut, like an umbilical cord, nevertheless remains forever knotted, right on the body, at the place of the navel. This scar is a knot against which analysis can do nothing" (Derrida 1998: 11).
10. Kofman too sees a connection between *The Interpretation of Dreams* and "Medusa's head": "the intimate, shameful secrets that Freud fears to expose to the public, because of the horror they are very likely to arouse are thus inseparably linked with his Jewishness and with femininity, with castration anxiety. In this sense, *The Interpretation of Dreams* is another "Medusa's head" (1985: 32).
11. Some theorists addressing this turning aside at the "navel of the dream" find fault with Freud for this gesture. Sarah Kofman, for example, argues that while Oedipus solved the riddle of the feminine, Freud could not. "Only the man who has no fear of the incest transgression can go looking for it there. Oedipus alone was able to answer the riddle of the Sphinx, the enigma of femininity, by going to steal from the very womb of Mother Nature her most inviolable secrets" (1985: 94). In turning aside at this point, Kofman insists, Freud abandons the psychoanalytic project: He "gives way before the mother who alone holds the secret, the solution to the riddle" (94). Elements of Kofman's reading are correct: Freud *did* turn aside at the "navel of the dream," and the navel *is* a reference to the mother's body. Yet this turn-

ing aside is an important site for interpretation rather than a reason to reject Freud: The gesture is an indication that Freud saw the limitations of his dominant narrative paradigm.

References

Bakan, David. 1958. *Sigmund Freud and the Jewish Mystical Tradition.* Boston: Beacon.

Bloom, Harold. 1995. "Freud: Frontier Concepts, Jewishness, and Interpretation," in Cathy Caruth, ed., *Trauma: Explorations in Memory,* pp. 113–127. Baltimore: Johns Hopkins University Press.

Bonaparte, Marie, Anna Freud, and Ernst Kris, eds. 1954. *The Origins of Psycho-Analysis: Letters to Wilhelm Fliess, Drafts and Notes, 1887 - 1902,* trans. Eric Mosbacher and James Strachey. New York: Basic Books; *Aus den Anfängen der Psychoanalyse. Briefe an Wilhelm Fliess, Abhandlungen und Notizen aus den Jahren 1887 - 1902,* London: Imago, 1950.

Brooks, Peter. 1989. "Freud's Masterplot," in David Richter, ed., *The Critical Tradition: Classic Texts and Contemporary Trends,* pp. 710–20. New York: St. Martin's Press.

Capps, Donald. Personal communication, 1999.

Dante, Alighieri. 1961. *The Divine Comedy,* trans. and commentary, John Sinclair. New York: Oxford University Press.

Derrida, Jacques. 1998. *Resistances of Psychoanalysis,* trans. Peggy Kamuf, Pascale-Anne Brault, and Michael Naas. Stanford: Stanford University Press.

DiCenso, James. 1999. *The Other Freud.* New York: Routledge.

Freud, Ernst, and Lucie Freud, eds. 1960. *Sigmund Freud Briefe: 1873 - 1938.* Frankfurt am Main: S. Fischer Verlag.

Freud, Ernst, ed. 1992. *Letters of Sigmund Freud 1873 - 1939,* trans. Tania Stern and James Stern. New York: Dover.

Freud, Sigmund. 1942. *Traumdeutung. Gesammelte Werke* (GW). Zweiter und Dritter Band. Frankfurt am Main: S. Fischer Verlag.

———. 1953–1974. *The Standard Edition of the Complete Psychological Works of Sigmund Freud* (SE), volumes 1–24, trans. and ed. James Strachey. London: Hogarth Press.

———. 1955. "Extracts from the Fliess Papers," *SE* 1: 175–282.

———.1953. *The Interpretation of Dreams, SE* 4–5: 1–722.

———. 1963. *Introductory Lectures on Psychoanalysis, SE* 15: 1–239.

———. 1955. "Medusa's Head," *SE* 18: 273–274.

———. 1964. *New Introductory Lectures, SE* 22: 3–183.

———. 1958. "Theme of the Three Caskets," *SE* 12: 291–301.

Gay, Peter. 1999. "Psychoanalyst Sigmund Freud (Great Minds of the Century)," *Time* vol. 153, no. 12 (March 29, 1999): 64–69.

Geller, Jay. 1997. "Identifying 'Someone who is Himself One of Them': Recent Studies of Freud's Jewish Identity." *Religious Studies Review* 23: 323–331.

Hyman, Stanley Edgar. 1962. *The Tangled Bank.* New York: Atheneum.

Jones, Ernest. 1953. *Sigmund Freud, Life and Work,* vol. 1. London: Hogarth.

Jonte-Pace, Diane, 1996. "At Home in the Uncanny: Freudian Representations of Death, Mothers, and the Afterlife." *Journal of the American Academy of Religion* 64: 61–88.

———. 2001. *Speaking the Unspeakable: Religion, Misogyny, and the Uncanny Mother in Freud's Cultural Texts.* Berkeley: University of California Press.

Kofman, Sarah. 1985. *The Enigma of Woman: Woman in Freud's Writings,* trans. Catherine Porter. Ithaca: Cornell University Press.

Masson, Jeffrey, trans. and ed. 1985. *The Complete Letters of Sigmund Freud to Wilhelm Fliess 1887 - 1904.* Cambridge, MA: Harvard University Press.

Rizzuto, Ana Maria. 1998. *Why Did Freud Reject God? A Psychodynamic Interpretation.* New Haven: Yale University Press.

Shengold, Leonard. 1991. *"Father Don't You See I'm Burning?": Reflections on Sex, Narcissism, Symbolism, and Murder: From Everything to Nothing.* New Haven: Yale University Press.
Simon, Bennett and Rachel Blass. 1991. "The Development and Vicissitudes of Freud's Ideas on the Oedipus Complex." In Jerome Neu, ed., *The Cambridge Companion to Freud,* pp. 161–174. New York: Cambridge University Press.
Sprengnether, Madelon. 1990. *The Spectral Mother: Freud, Feminism, and Psychoanalysis.* Ithaca: Cornell University Press.
Weiner, Marc. 1995. *Richard Wagner and the Anti-Semitic Imagination.* Lincoln: University of Nebraska Press.
Wittgenstein, Ludwig. 1966. *Lectures and Conversations in Aesthetics, Psychology, and Religious Belief.* Berkeley: University of California Press.

20

Using Content Analysis to Study Dreams

Applications and Implications for the Humanities

G. William Domhoff

Content analysis—the use of carefully defined categories and quantitative techniques to find meaningful regularities in texts—is very different from the usual approaches to dreams. It does not make use of free associations, amplifications, autobiographical statements, or any other information from outside the dream reports themselves. It has led to numerous findings on the relationship of dream content to gender, age, mental health, culture, and individual differences. It can be used in conjunction with any theory or for descriptive empirical studies. It is most convincing when the content analyst knows nothing about the dreamer.

The application of content analysis to dream reports holds out considerable potential for questions of interest to scholars in the humanities and religious studies, in which this method has been used to study literary texts, Shakespeare's plays, fairy tales, folklore, and much else. For example, it often leads to the discovery of patterns in a series of dreams from one person that were not detected by other methods.

Content analysis is very simple in principle but difficult to carry out in practice. It consists of four basic steps: (1) creating relevant categories that can be understood and applied by any investigator; (2) tabulating frequencies for the categories; (3) using percentages, ratios, or other statistics to transform raw frequencies into meaningful data; and (4) making comparisons with normative samples or control groups. The usefulness of content analysis for the study of dreams has been increased exponentially by the constant improvements in personal computers. They make it possible to store and manipulate the large databases that are necessary to develop normative findings. They provide spreadsheets and other tools that make it easier and more accurate to analyze the codings from complex content analyses of hundreds of dream reports.

Although content analysis is simple in principle and has been used in many different disciplines, no general system is useful for texts ranging from literature to psychotherapy records to dream reports. Instead, specific systems have to emerge from a familiarity with the kind of text being analyzed. Furthermore, it is difficult to develop rules that always lead to similar codings by individual coders (reliability) and also relate to other cognitive states or behaviors (validity). Once a good system has been developed for a specific kind of text, it makes little or no sense for new investigators to try to develop their own systems, even if they think their questions are unique. It is far better to adapt established systems for their purposes.

This chapter focuses on the findings, implications, and future applications of two proven approaches to the content analysis of dreams, both of which are ready for immediate use and available via the Internet. The first method is a detailed coding system that provides over two dozen content indicators, along with normative findings for those indicators. It is modular and adaptable. The second is a computer-assisted system for making searches for phrases or strings of words within a database of over 10,000 dream reports, which adds up to a fast content analysis. When the two methodologies are used together, it may even be possible to build on the work of cognitive scientists to search for figurative meaning in dream reports.

These two new resources for the study of dream content may be especially appealing because of increasing doubts about other methods. Clinical studies of dreams are now compromised by studies showing that the social psychology of the psychotherapy relationship provides numerous opportunities for therapists to unwittingly shape the seemingly accurate interpretations of dreams that derive from free associations and amplifications (Loftus and Ketcham 1994; Ofshe and Watters 1994). Through the process of suggestion and persuasion, therapist and dreamer may be establishing a common belief system, rather than discovering the "meaning" of the dream. This possibility is supported by experimental studies showing that many participants can be convinced through dream interpretations that they had experiences from before age three that they do not remember (Mazzoni, Loftus, Seitz, and Lynn 1999; Tsai, Loftus, and Polage 2000). Similarly, the hypnotic investigation of dreams, as summarized by Moss, has been called into question by studies revealing the manipulative and capricious nature of the relationship between hypnotist and participant (Spanos 1996). As for symbolic dream interpretation, the continuing wide differences among Freudians, Jungians, and neo-Freudians show there has been no progress toward a common understanding of dream symbolism on the basis of systematic research. In fact, it can be argued that the rival schools of symbolic interpretation are particular applications of common metaphoric understandings to aspects of dreams. Even the methods used by phenomenological and existential theorists, such as Boss and Perls (Downing and Marmorstein 1973), who claim to reject symbolic interpretations, are actually metaphoric glosses of dreams, as can be seen by reading through their case examples.

The Hall/Van de Castle Coding System

The system of content analysis first outlined in the 1950s by psychologist Calvin S. Hall, and then finalized with the help of another psychologist, Robert Van de Castle, in the 1960s, is the most comprehensive and widely used coding system yet developed for the study of dreams (Hall 1951, 1953c, Hall and Van de Castle 1966). It consists of ten general categories that cover everything from characters to social interactions to such descriptive elements as intensity, size, and temperature. Most categories contain two or more subcategories. Characters, for example, consist of humans, animals, and mythical creatures, and the category for human characters is further subdivided by such features as gender, relation to the dreamer, and age. There are five subcategories for emotions, eight for activities, and twelve for objects. Not all categories need to be used in each study. The most frequently used categories are characters, social interactions, misfortune and good fortune, success and failure, and emotions.

The system rests on the nominal level of measurement, due to problems of reliability and psychological validity with rating scales. The raw frequencies are analyzed using percentages and ratios to correct for the varying length of dream reports from sample to sample and other problems that defeat many other systems for coding dream content. The system includes normative findings on men and women that have been replicated several times. Studies based on subsamples drawn from larger samples show that it takes 100 to125 dream reports to achieve results that can be repeated in future studies. The large number is due to the fact that most dream elements appear in less than half of all dream reports.

The entire coding system can be found on the Internet at www.dreamresearch.net, along with already-coded dreams to aid new researchers (Schneider and Domhoff). This Web site also includes a spreadsheet that computes the results for the content indicators once the codings are entered as well as significance levels, effect sizes, and confidence intervals. The results are displayed in tables and in graphs. In addition, dreamresearch.net contains information on how to do research projects and a library of past papers by Hall, Domhoff, and their students.

The type of findings produced by the system can be seen through a brief look at the male/female percentage, the animal percentage, and several different aggression indicators. The male/female percentage is derived by dividing the total number of male characters by the total number of male plus female characters. In virtually every sample from every culture that has been studied, the male/female percentage is about 67/33 for men and 48/52 for women, which means that women's scores are not the mirror image of men's. The same difference also appears in the dreams and stories of preschoolers and in dreams collected in the sleep laboratory (Domhoff 1996; Foulkes 1982). This unexpected regularity is not anticipated by any dream theory. It is also the largest gender difference in dreams.

The animal percentage (total animals divided by the total number of characters of any kind) provides another useful example because it has great variation by age and culture. The animal percentage is as high as 30 to 40 in young children, but only 6 for men and 4 for women in American society. It is as high as 30 in some hunting and gathering societies, and exceeds the American level in all of the dream samples collected by anthropologists in many different parts of the world.

Aggression, defined as a desire, intention, or action to annoy or harm some other character, is the most frequent type of social interaction in dreams, occurring at least once in 47 percent of men's dreams and in 44 percent of women's. It is the element that varies the most by age, gender, culture, and personality. Measures of aggression also show the largest difference between dreams written down at home and dreams collected in the sleep laboratory (Domhoff and Schneider 1999). The A/C ratio (total aggressions divided by total characters) yields a rate of aggression per character that is useful because it controls for both word length and the total number of characters in the sample. The physical aggression percentages (physical aggressions divided by physical plus nonphysical aggressions) reveal the second-largest gender difference and declines from the teenage years into adulthood, according to both cross-sectional and longitudinal studies. It is one of the few content indicators that changes after young adulthood is reached, which suggests there is a general consistency in dream content that is not expected by any dream theory.

One of the few differences between the dreams of mental patients and normal individuals is revealed by indicators concerning friendliness. First, patients have a lower friends percentage (total known characters divided by all human characters); their dreams are disproportionately populated by family members and strangers. Second, they have a lower F/C ratio (friendly interactions divided by total characters), which is not the same thing as the friends percentage because there may or may not be friendly interactions with friends, and there can be friendly interactions with family members and strangers (Domhoff 1996; Maharaj 1997).

Anthropologist Barbara Tedlock, in a paper reprinted as chapter 16 in this book, asserts that content analysis is not useful in anthropological studies because the dream reports cannot be taken at face value. Tedlock is right that there are many obstacles to collecting adequate samples in small traditional societies. However, the many good samples gathered by anthropologists do produce interesting results (unpublished studies by Hall reported by Domhoff). In addition to similarities in the male/female percentages, these samples are similar to the American norms in that there are more familiar than unfamiliar characters, more aggression than friendliness, more misfortune than good fortune, and more negative than positive emotions. At the same time, there are also content indicators that show differences from the American norms and variation from culture to culture. For example, there are wide variations in aggression percentages, especially in the physical aggression percentage, as shown in table 20.1. This table also shows that Dutch and Swiss samples have lower physical aggression percentages than the American norms. The findings in Thomas Gregor's detailed content analysis of Mehinaku dreams—which appears as chapter 7 in this book—also stand as a refutation to Tedlock's claims.

Tedlock's comments are puzzling because the article and the book that she cites as support for her claim present no cross-cultural findings. These two publications ap-

Table 20.1 Physical Aggression Percentages

Society	*Males*	*Females*
Yir Yiront	92	n/a
Baiga	86	n/a
Navaho	77	n/a
Skolt	70	68
Ifaluk	60	40
Tinquian	55	46
Alor	53	61
United States	50	34
Hopi	40	39
French Canadians	n/a	31
Dutch	32	14
Swiss	29	23

Table 20.2 The Consistency of the Dreams of "The Natural Scientist"

	Four Subsets (each n = 46)				*Three Subsets (each n = 62)*			*Two Subsets (each n = 93)*		*Total (n = 187)*
Characters										
Male/Female Percent	65%	76%	66%	74%	66%	74%	71%	70%	70%	70%
Familiar Characters	42%	34%	41%	34%	39%	38%	36%	38%	37%	38%
Animal Percent	15%	13%	08%	09%	14%	10%	10%	14%	09%	11%
Group Percent	21%	29%	14%	23%	26%	19%	21%	25%	19%	22%
Characters per dream	3.11	3.11	2.59	3.52	3.06	2.76	3.32	3.08	3.02	3.08
Aggression										
D-involved Aggression	57%	45%	67%	65%	55%	48%	67%	51%	66%	59%
Victimization Percent	58%	67%	60%	72%	53%	64%	71%	62%	68%	65%
Physical Aggression	33%	50%	38%	49%	34%	52%	45%	42%	45%	45%
A/C index	.15	.15	.18	.23	.15	.12	.25	.15	.21	.18
Aggressions per dream	.46	.48	.46	.80	.47	.34	.82	.46	.62	.55
Friendliness										
D-involved Friendliness	71%	65%	70%	73%	63%	64%	79%	68%	72%	70%
Befriender Percent	50%	40%	38%	68%	53%	29%	63%	44%	57%	52%
F/C index	.12	.16	.17	.19	.13	.16	.18	.14	.18	.16
Friendliness per dream	.37	.50	.43	.65	.39	.45	.61	.43	.54	.49
Settings										
Indoor Settings	53%	37%	40%	42%	52%	33%	44%	45%	41%	43%
Familiar Settings	75%	76%	68%	71%	73%	76%	71%	76%	70%	73%
Emotions										
Negative Emotions	89%	77%	70%	73%	86%	71%	76%	84%	72%	79%
D-involved Emotions	83%	46%	80%	60%	76%	64%	62%	68%	68%	68%
Emotions per dream	.39	.28	.22	.33	.34	.23	.34	.33	.27	.30

peared before Hall had done any cross-cultural content analyses. This suggests that Tedlock's strong emphasis on cultural variation makes it difficult for her to contemplate that a content analysis system devised to study dream reports provided by Americans could prove useful cross-culturally. She therefore presents an unnecessary choice between studying dream content or cultural beliefs relating to dreams. She also prejudges a hypothesis offered by Gregor on the basis of his empirical work with the Mehinaku: "with additional cross-cultural data it may be possible to show that the dream experience is less variant than other aspects of culture."

As surprising and interesting as many of these gender, age, and cross-cultural findings are, they are perhaps surpassed by the findings with lengthy dream journals from individuals. Although the early studies of dream journals pioneered by Wilhelm Stekel, Havelock Ellis, and Carl Jung produced many interesting findings, the great consistency in dream content over years and decades went undetected until journals were studied with the Hall/Van de Castle system. Since the results are similar in each case, despite the many different reasons why the dreamers kept personal journals, they are considered to be robust findings by those who advocate the study of archival records and other "unobtrusive" sources of data. Furthermore, most dream content is found to be continuous with waking thought in those cases where personal information can be obtained about the dreamer (Bell and Hall 1971; Domhoff 1996; Hall and Lind 1970; Hall and Nordby 1972).

Both of these points can be demonstrated with a natural scientist's dream journal from the summer of 1939. It was purchased from an antiquarian book dealer by psychiatrist J. Allan Hobson and used by him to illustrate the alleged bizarreness of the

Figure 20.1 *h*-profile for "The Natural Scientist."

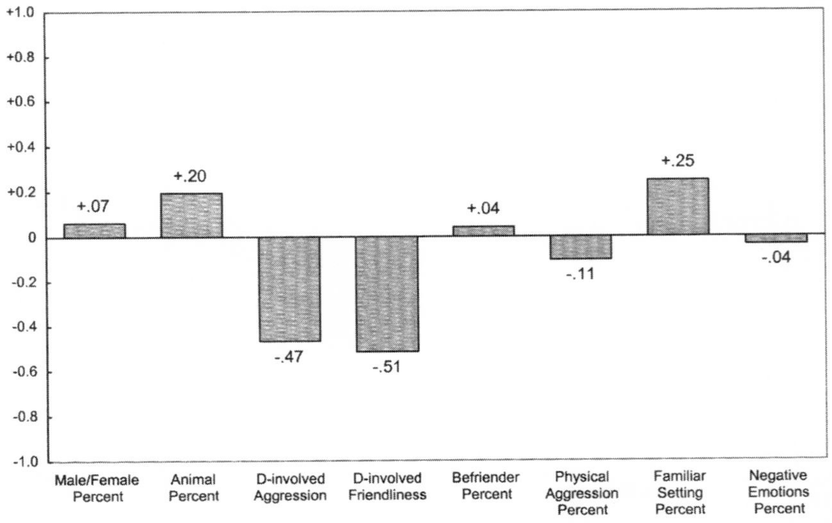

Note: *h* is a statistic that correct for the fact that the standard deviations cannont be calculated with percentage data. *h* is roughly twice as large as a percentage difference, An *h* of 0 to .20 is small, an h of .21 to .40 is moderate, and an *h* over .40 is large.

form and structure of dreams. Even with only 187 dreams that are over 50 words or more in length, the content is strikingly consistent over a three-month period, as shown in table 20.2. In addition, a graphic profile of how he compares to the male norms is provided in figure 20.1. This bar graph is based on the *h* statistic, which is roughly twice the size of a percentage difference. It shows that, in comparison to the Hall and Van de Castle male norms, the subject is nonaggressive, less likely to be involved in friendly interactions, more likely to be in familiar settings, and has a high animal percentage. These deviations from the norms fit with facts about his life found in an obituary in a scientific publication. These dreams can be found on www.dreambank.net under the pseudonym "Natural Scientist."

A comparison of the extant dreams of Freud and Jung led to interesting patterns, which went unnoticed despite the many commentaries upon them. Although there are only twenty-eight dream reports from Freud and thirty-one reports from Jung, far too few to be conclusive, earlier studies of dozens of dream journals by Hall and his students show that major themes can be discovered with as few as twenty to twenty-five dreams. The most striking differences concern the nature of their friendly and aggressive interactions. Freud's friendly interactions are far more frequent with males, whereas Jung has friendly interactions with both males and females. In every instance where Jung is involved in a friendly interaction he is the initiator, whereas Freud is the recipient of friendship in eight of eleven friendly interactions. In the case of aggressions, Jung is a typical male in that his aggressions are with males, not females, whereas Freud has an aggression with one in every four female characters and no aggressions with males. There is evidence that the waking preferences of the two men are compatible with these findings, and that the differences in the patterns of friendly and aggressive interactions might shed light on why they could not sustain their close working relationship (Domhoff 1996; Hall and Domhoff 1968).

While the results of studies with dream journals are encouraging, far more can be done with them. The ideal study would include a large number of dreams over a considerable span of years. Inferences from blind analyses would be tested by comparing them with information provided by both the dreamer and close friends of the dreamer. If inferences are denied by the dreamer, as sometimes has happened in past studies (Domhoff 1996, chapter 8), then the answers given by friends will provide a way to resolve the disagreement. If the friends agree with the content analyst, then it can be inferred that the dreamer has a "blind spot" on the issue. If the friends agree with the dreamer, then the content analyst is probably wrong, an outcome that can be very valuable in improving a theory.

A dream journal that is useful for studies of this kind is now available at www.dreambank.net. It contains over 3,300 dreams, culled over a period of 22 years, from a woman, Barbara Sanders, now in her fifties. She has also been interviewed over a two-day period about both her life and her dreams, and four of her female friends have been interviewed about those aspects of her life that appear in her dreams. The unpublished research on this series that has been completed to date demonstrates, once again, the astonishing consistency in dreams over long periods of time, which in this case is captured by a comparison of 125 dreams from the first half of the series with 125 from the second half.

Other unpublished work on the Barbara Sanders series shows that her dreams are continuous with her waking concerns, such as her interest in cats, of which she has several. Her dreams also portray her feelings about relatives and friends with striking accuracy. However, inferences based on a continuity principle have been disconfirmed on several topics, which opens up new avenues for adding depth and complexity to the understanding of dreams. For example, Barbara Sanders's cats are often underfed, lost, or deformed in her dreams, but not in waking life, where they are treated quite well. She rides horses fearlessly in her dreams but is not a good rider and fears them in waking life. Her dreams give the impression that she probably learned to shoot guns when she was growing up, and likes them, but neither inference is correct.

Most studies using the Hall/Van de Castle system have focused on everyday dream reports. However, the system can be adapted to study the occasional highly memorable or impactful dream that has carryover effects into waking life and is of great interest to clinicians and humanists. Then, too, the Hall/Van de Castle norms provide a basis for commenting on the rarity of such dreams, as do results from studies of lengthy dream journals. Many of the elements in highly memorable dreams can be classified as "good fortunes," which are defined as good things that happen to the dream character as a result of fate, as opposed to intentional striving by the character or beneficial actions by other dream characters. Sudden recovery from injuries or illness, the possession of extraordinary abilities, the unexpected discovery of valuable objects, and arriving in a very bountiful environment are all examples of good fortunes.

Highly memorable dreams also seem to be characterized by particular patterns of Hall/Van de Castle indicators. This can be seen by looking at the patterns in the three types of "impactful" dreams—transcendent, existential, and anxiety—identified in studies using one-month diaries from college students; these three types were then compared to everyday dreams (Busink and Kuiken 1996; Kuiken and Sikora 1993). Although the phenomenologists who developed this typology do not think a standardized coding system can be useful in studying such dreams, their examples show that these dreams fit the following coding patterns:

- Transcendent dreams are characterized by unusual or distorted settings, famous or mythical characters, friendly interactions, good fortunes, success, and positive emotions.
- Existential dreams are more likely to involve deceased characters, major misfortune, thinking instead of physical activity, and intense feelings of sadness or confusion.
- Anxiety dreams contain unfamiliar settings, unknown characters or animals, physical aggression directed at the dreamer, physical activities instead of thinking, and intense feelings of apprehension.
- Ordinary dreams are far more likely to have familiar settings, familiar characters, nonphysical aggressions, minor misfortunes, and no emotions.

Fast Content-Analysis via Dreambank.Net

Dreambank.net is a resource for dream researchers that contains over 10,000 dreams from individuals and groups. Most of the dreams are contained in a few lengthy dream journals contributed by older adult women, but there are also sets of dreams from children, teenagers, college students, and blind people (Schneider and Domhoff 1999). The search engine on the site makes it possible to do very fast content analyses of one or more of these sets of dreams and to create new subsets that contain a specific element, such as "bridges," or a specific activity, such as "weddings," that might be of interest for making metaphoric studies of dream content. This Web site also provides a private space where researchers can use the DreamBank search engine to analyze dream reports that are already in a digital format. A private space also can be reserved to make daily entries into a dream journal for those who want to use DreamBank to study their own dreams.

The phrases or strings of words that are entered into the DreamBank search engine obviously fulfill the first step in making a content analysis—the creation of clearly defined categories that lead to the same results each time. The program also carries out the second step of a content analysis, which is to provide a frequency count. The frequencies can be turned into percentages and ratios in ways that will be explained shortly. Finally, normative findings can be obtained, because the dream reports that were used to create the Hall/Van de Castle norms are part of the DreamBank, and they can be searched at the same time the sample of interest is being searched.

These points can be demonstrated through a simple study that asks whether people's concern with cats and dogs can be predicted on the basis of their dreams. The program is put in "OR" mode so that it will find any instance of a cat or a dog in a dream. Then two search expressions are entered: ^(cat|kitten|kitty|kittie)s?^ and ^(dog|doggy|doggie|puppy|puppie)s?^. Next the dreams of two cat lovers, Alta and Barbara Sanders, are selected for searching, along with those of a young girl, Melissa, who loves all animals, and one older woman, Arlie, who has little or no interest in animals. In addition, the 500 dreams from 100 college women that were used to create the female norms for the Hall/Van de Castle system are selected. The search produces the results that are presented in table 20.3.

As can be seen in the table, the results reveal the number and percentage of dreams that contain at least one dog (left-hand column), at least one cat (center column), and at least one dog or cat (right-hand column). The right-hand column provides an indication of a general interest in pet animals. As expected, Arlie is below the female normative sample, and the other three are above it. The determination of the degree to which a person is concerned with cats as compared to dogs

Table 20.3 Search Results for "Cat" and "Dog" in the DreamBank

<table>
<tr><th></th><th>^(cat | kitten | kitty | kitie)s?^</th><th>^(dog | doggy | doggie | puppy | puppie)s?^</th><th>Any Term</th></tr>
<tr><td>Alta: a detailed dreamer (n = 422)</td><td>55 (13.0%)</td><td>21 (5.0%)</td><td>67 (15.9%)</td></tr>
<tr><td>Arlie: a middle-aged woman (n = 212)</td><td>1 (0.5%)</td><td>3 (1.4%)</td><td>4 (1.9%)</td></tr>
<tr><td>Barb Sanders (n = 3116)</td><td>176 (5.6%)</td><td>105 (3.4%)</td><td>257 (8.2%)</td></tr>
<tr><td>Female Norms (n = 491)</td><td>9 (1.8%)</td><td>11 (2.2%)</td><td>19 (3.9%)</td></tr>
<tr><td>Melissa: a young girl (n = 67)</td><td>9 (13.4%)</td><td>11 (16.4%)</td><td>18 (26.9%)</td></tr>
<tr><td>Total (n = 4308)</td><td>250 (5.8%)</td><td>151 (3.5%)</td><td>365 (8.5%)</td></tr>
</table>

is accomplished by dividing the total number of dreams with at least one cat by the total number of dreams with at least one cat plus the total number with at least one dog. Alta and Barbara Sanders's high "cat percentages"—72 and 63—reveal that they much prefer cats to dogs, whereas young Melissa's cat percentage of 45 rightly suggests that she is interested in both cats and dogs. The cat percentage for the normative sample—45—shows that Alta and Barbara Sanders are well above the average woman in their cat percentages.

DreamSearch can be used in conjunction with Hall/Van de Castle codings in studying lengthy dream journals. The ideal starting point for such studies is the Barbara Sanders series, because 675 of the 3,300 dreams already have been coded, and there is ample information available on her life due to the interviews with her and her friends. By entering the name "Howard," for example, all the dreams of her ex-husband can be studied for possible themes or metaphors in the context of the Hall/Van de Castle codings for those dreams. The name "Derek" can be entered to study her dreams about a man in whom she had a romantic interest when she was in her late forties. The trajectory of her feelings can be compared with the codings for friendly, sexual, and aggressive interactions throughout the Derek subset.

Implications and Future Directions

The methods and findings presented in this chapter have two major implications for scholars in the humanities and related fields who want to contribute to the attempt to understand dreams or to use ideas and methods concerning dreams as part of other projects. First, the best-known dream theories cannot be used with confidence to understand dream content. There are too many findings from content analysis that are not consistent with their claims. For example, dreams are more patterned and consistent over time than Hobson (1988) and his colleagues (Hobson, Pace-Schott, and Stickgold 2000; Hobson, Stickgold, and Pace-Schott 1998) would expect and more similar across cultures than neo-Freudians (Fromm 1951) and most anthropologists might think. They are more consistent in late adulthood and more continuous with waking life than Jung would predict.

This skepticism about the best-known theories is reinforced by other types of systematic dream studies that are not discussed in this chapter. The developmental findings with children studied in sleep laboratories contradict Freud, Jung, and Hobson on key points (Foulkes 1982, 1999; Foulkes et al. 1990). So do many other laboratory and experimental studies. In the case of Freud, not a single hypothesis put forth by him on any topic related to dreams receives empirical support in the dream literature (Domhoff 2000b, 2000c; Fisher and Greenberg 1977, 1996). Freud and the other clinical theorists made an important contribution by suggesting that there is psychological meaning in dreams, and they put forth many ideas that stimulated future research, but continuing adherence to their theories is not likely to advance the understanding of dreams.

Second, the findings presented in this chapter should give us pause about the use of traditional methods of dream analysis. The findings from content analysis add to the numerous studies casting doubt on claims based on either psychotherapy sessions or hypnosis, because they are often very different from what those methods lead us to expect. Although symbolic interpretations might be useful someday if they are viewed as the product of figurative thought (Gibbs 1994, 1999; Grady, Oakley, and Coulson

1999), there is still much work to be done before it can be certain that waking figurative thinking is also present in dreaming.

What, then, are the future directions that theorizing about dreams might take? First, the developmental, content analysis, and laboratory findings are most consistent with an open-ended and loosely structured cognitive approach. Within that context, there is a wide range of opinion concerning the degree to which dream content is the product of coherent thought. Foulkes, who argues that dreaming is the form that consciousness takes during sleep, concludes that dreaming, like consciousness, is a cognitive achievement that only gradually becomes more or less coherent. In his view, much of dream content is the product of seat-of-the-pants, one-thing-after-another type of thinking, rather than deeply motivated metaphoric thought, and some of it is not completely sensible. On the other hand, Lakoff, one of the founders of cognitive linguistics, argues that dreams are often structured by conceptual metaphors.

Within a cognitive framework, future studies of dream content might start with the idea that dreams reflect concerns and interests and that they are generally consistent over time and continuous with waking thoughts. Such a theory can encompass wish-fulfillment dreams as well as the realistic post-traumatic stress disorder nightmares that often occur after deadly accidents, shocking assaults, or the witnessing of murders. Then the deviations and discrepancies from consistency and continuity could be used to nuance and modify the theory. Why, for example, would Barbara Sanders's dreams so accurately depict her feelings and concerns in regard to the key people in her life but so inaccurately portray the health of her cats, her feelings about horses, and her proficiency with guns? Why do some of those who are successful in ending their dependency on tobacco or alcohol nonetheless have upsetting dreams in which they find themselves back to their old habits and feeling terrible about it? More generally, why do some people dream of former lovers that they are no longer attracted to in waking life?

Finally, it seems critical to build on the insights of cognitive linguists to see if there is sense in those elements in dreams that are not captured by the content indicators or that do not seem to relate to the concerns, interests, and emotional preoccupations of the dreamer. Once again, it is the Barbara Sanders series that provides a good starting point in a search for conceptual metaphors and other forms of figurative thought in dreams. Through such detailed studies it will be possible to see if all aspects of dreams "make sense," as Freud, Jung, and Hall would maintain, while at the same time disagreeing among themselves about what that sense is. If such a search fails, then it may be that some aspects of dream content make no sense, as Foulkes and Hobson would argue, even while they disagree about the origins of dreams and the point where sense fades into nonsense.

References

Bell, A. and Hall, C. 1971. *The Personality of a Child Molester: An Analysis of Dreams.* Chicago: Aldine.

Boss, M. 1958. *The Analysis of Dreams.* New York: Philosophical Library.

———. 1977. *I Dreamt Last Night.* New York: Gardner Press.

Busink, R. and Kuiken, D. 1996. Identifying Types of Impactful Dreams: A Replication. *Dreaming* 6: 97–119.

Domhoff, G. W. 1996. *Finding Meaning in Dreams: A Quantitative Approach.* New York: Plenum.

———. 1999a. "Drawing Theoretical Implications from Descriptive Empirical Findings on Dream Content. *Dreaming* 9: 201–210.
———. 1999b. "New Directions in the Study of Dream Content Using the Hall and Van de Castle Coding System." *Dreaming* 9: 115–137.
———. 2000a. "Methods and Measures for the Study of Dream Content." In M. Kryger, T. Roth, and W. Dement, eds., *Principles and Practices of Sleep Medicine* (3rd ed., pp. 463–471). Philadelphia: W. B. Saunders.
———. 2000b. "The Misinterpretation of Dreams." *American Scientist* 88 (March-April): 175–178.
———. 2000c. "Moving Dream Theory Beyond Freud and Jung." Paper presented at the conference "Beyond Freud and Jung? The Interpretation of Dreams, Religion, and Culture." September 23, Graduate Theological Union, Berkeley, CA.
———. 2001. "A New Neurocognitive Theory of Dreams." *Dreaming* 11: 13–33.
Domhoff, G. W. and Schneider, A. 1999. "Much Ado about very Little: The Small Effect Sizes when Home and Laboratory Collected Dreams Are Compared." *Dreaming* 9: 139–151.
Downing, J. and Marmorstein, R. 1973. *Dreams and Nightmares: A Book of Gestalt Therapy Sessions.* New York: Harper & Row.
Fisher, S. and Greenberg, R. 1977. *The Scientific Credibility of Freud's Theories and Therapy.* New York: Basic Books.
———. 1996. *Freud Scientifically Appraised.* New York: John Wiley.
Foulkes, D. 1982. *Children's Dreams.* New York: John Wiley.
———. 1985. *Dreaming: A Cognitive-Psychological Analysis.* Hillsdale, NJ: Lawrence Erlbaum.
———. 1996. "Dream Research: 1953 - 1993." *Sleep* 19: 609–624.
———. 1999. *Children's Dreaming and the Development of Consciousness.* Cambridge, MA: Harvard University Press.
Foulkes, D., Hollifield, M., Sullivan, B., Bradley, L., and Terry, R. 1990. "REM Dreaming and Cognitive Skills at Ages 5–8: A Cross-Sectional Study." *International Journal of Behavioral Development* 13: 447–465.
Freud, S. 1900. *The Interpretation of Dreams,* trans. J. Crick. London: Oxford University Press.
Fromm, E. 1951. *The Forgotten Language.* New York: Grove Press.
Gibbs, R. 1994. *The Poetics of Mind: Figurative Thought, Language, and Understanding.* New York: Cambridge University Press.
———. 1999. "Speaking and Thinking with Metonymy." In K. Panther and G. Radden, eds., *Metonymy in Language and Thought* (pp. 61–75). Philadelphia: John Benjamins.
Grady, J., Oakley, T., and Coulson, S. 1999. "Blending and Metaphor." In R. Gibbs and G. Steen, eds., *Metaphor in Cognitive Linguistics* (pp. 101–124). Philadelphia: John Benjamins.
Gregor, T. 1981. "A Content Analysis of Mehinaku Dreams." *Ethos* 9: 353–390.
Hall, C. 1947. "Diagnosing Personality by the Analysis of Dreams." *Journal of Abnormal and Social Psychology* 42: 68–79.
———. "What People Dream about." *Scientific American* 184: 60–63.
———. 1953a. "A Cognitive Theory of Dream Symbols." *Journal of General Psychology* 48: 169–186.
———. 1953b. "A Cognitive Theory of Dreams." *Journal of General Psychology* 49: 273–282.
———. 1953c. *The Meaning of Dreams.* New York: McGraw-Hill.
———. 1969. "Content Analysis of Dreams: Categories, Units, and Norms." In G. Gerbner, ed., *The Analysis of Communication Content* (pp. 147–158). New York: John Wiley.
———. 1984. "A Ubiquitous Sex Difference in Dreams, Revisited." *Journal of Personality and Social Psychology* 46: 1109–1117.
Hall, C. and Domhoff, G. W. 1963. "A Ubiquitous Sex Difference in Dreams." *Journal of Abnormal and Social Psychology* 66: 278–280.
———. 1968. "The Dreams of Freud and Jung." *Psychology Today* 2: 42–45.

Hall, C. and Lind, R. 1970. *Dreams, Life and Literature: A Study of Franz Kafka*. Chapel Hill: University of North Carolina Press.

Hall, C. and Nordby, V. 1972. *The Individual and His Dreams.* New York: New American Library.

Hall, C. and Van de Castle, R. 1966. *The Content Analysis of Dreams.* New York: Appleton-Century-Crofts.

Hobson, J. Allan 1988. *The Dreaming Brain.* New York: Basic Books.

Hobson, J., Pace-Schott, E., and Stickgold, R. 2000. "Dreaming and the Brain: Towards a Cognitive Neuroscience of Conscious States." *Behavioral and Brain Sciences* 23(6).

Hobson, J., Stickgold, R., and Pace-Schott, E. 1998. "The Neuropsychology of REM Sleep Dreaming." *NeuroReport* 9: R1-R14.

Jung, C. 1974. *Dreams.* Princeton: Princeton University Press.

Kuiken, D. and Sikora, S. 1993. "The Impact of Dreams on Waking Thoughts and Feelings." In Alan Moffitt, Milton Kramer, and Robert Hoffmann, eds., *The Functions of Dreaming.* (pp. x, 610). Albany: State University of New York Press.

Lakoff, G. 1993. "How Metaphor Structures Dreams." *Dreaming* 3: 77–98.

———. 1997. "How Unconscious Metaphorical Thought Shapes Dreams." In D. Stein, ed., *Cognitive Science and the Unconscious* (pp. 89–120). Washington, D.C.: American Psychiatric Press.

Loftus, E. and Ketcham, K. 1994. *The Myth of Repressed Memory.* New York: St. Martin's Press.

Maharaj, N. 1997. "An Investigation into the Content and Structure of Schizophrenic Dreams." Ph.D. diss., Leiden University, Leiden, The Netherlands.

Mazzoni, G., Loftus, E., Seitz, A., and Lynn, S. 1999. "Changing Beliefs and Memories through Dream Interpretation." *Applied Cognitive Psychology* 13(2): 125–144.

Moss, C. S., ed. 1967. *The Hypnotic Investigation of Dreams.* New York: John Wiley.

Ofshe, R. and Watters, E. 1994. *Making Monsters: False Memories, Psychotherapy, and Sexual Hysteria.* New York: Charles Scribner's Sons.

Schneider, A. and Domhoff, G. W. 1995, updated 2000. "The Quantitative Study of Dreams" (website): www.dreamresearch.net/.

———. 1999, updated 2000. "DreamBank" (website): www.dreambank.net/.

Spanos, N. 1996. *Multiple Identities and False Memories: A Socio-Cognitive Approach.* Washington, D.C.: American Psychological Association.

Tedlock, B. 1991. "The New Anthropology of Dreaming." *Dreaming* 1: 161–178.

Tsai, A., Loftus, E., and Polage, D. 2000. "Current Directions in False-Memory Research." In E. David F. Bjorklund et al., eds., *False-Memory Creation in Children and Adults: Theory, Research, and Implications.* (pp. x, 254). Mahwah: Lawrence Erlbaum.

Van de Castle, R. 1969. "Problems in Applying Methodology of Content Analysis." In M. Kramer, ed., *Dream Psychology and the New Biology of Dreaming* (pp. 185–197). Springfield: Charles C. Thomas.

Webb, E., Campbell, D., Schwartz, R., Sechrest, L., and Grove, J. 1981. *Nonreactive Measures in the Social Sciences,* 2nd ed. Chicago: Rand-McNally.

21

The New Neuropsychology of Sleep

Implications for Psychoanalysis

J. Allan Hobson

In his 1895 *Project for a Scientific Psychology,* Sigmund Freud clearly stated his goal: to integrate the workings of the mind with the workings of the brain. But in his day, too little neurobiology was known to make his goal attainable, and he tried instead to understand such fascinating normal phenomena as dreaming in exclusively psychodynamic terms. A century later, Freud's brilliant but entirely speculative dream theory is in need of radical revision, if not complete overhaul, because dreams as well as other unusual states of consciousness can finally be approached from the solid foundation of modern neuroscience. In other words, the goals of Freud's *Project* are at last within our grasp. Ironically, an obstacle to progress is the tenacious adherence of orthodox psychoanalysis to a theory that, even by the standards of its originator, is now clearly outmoded.

In this chapter, recent positron emission tomography (PET) imaging and brain lesion studies in humans are integrated with new basic research findings at the cellular level in animals to explain how the formal cognitive features of dreaming may be the combined product of a shift in neuromodulatory balance of the brain and a related redistribution of regional blood flow. In rapid eye movement sleep (REM), the brain thus becomes activated but processes its internally generated data in a manner quite different from that of waking.

The New Neuropsychology and Psychoanalysis

The field of sleep and dream research has recently been invigorated by convergent new data from two complementary neuropsychological sources. (1–4) In brain imaging and brain lesion studies, the evidence for a strong pontine role in human REM sleep dream generation complements the cellular and molecular level data in animal studies and reveals an unexpectedly prominent role of the limbic system in the selection and elaboration of dream plots. The emerging picture of dreaming as the synthesis of emotional and sensorimotor data generated by the distinctive mechanisms of brain activation in REM sleep will be of interest to all who share Sigmund Freud's early vision of a psychology founded on the solid base of neuroscience (5) even as it forces revision of his highly speculative dream theory. (6)

Insofar as psychoanalysis remains committed to Freud's view of dreaming, or to any revisions of that view that retain the notion of disguise-censorship as the mechanism of dream bizarreness, the new results are without the faintest modicum of support. Also without support is the corollary assumption that dreaming affords privileged access to unconscious motives via the technique of free association to bizarre dream material.

If, instead, the modern psychoanalyst takes the more open view, afforded by the activation-synthesis hypothesis, that dreaming is a physiological projection test revealing—rather than concealing—emotionally salient concerns, the prospect is quite bright. The question is, can psychoanalysis afford to admit that Freud was wrong about the dream theory? Even if some would agree that it cannot any longer afford not to do so, the consequences of such an avowal are profound and far-reaching. Because the dream theory is so foundational, its renunciation forces a major reformulation on the whole field.

Brain-Based Differences Between Waking and Dreaming

The demonstration that the human brain activation pattern of REM sleep is distinctly different from that of waking has an important bearing on our conception of how conscious states are generated by the brain. It supports the hypothesis that quite different mechanisms underlie waking and dreaming consciousness and that those differentiated mechanisms are causally determinant of the differences in our subjective experiences of the two states. For some time, it has been the cognitive similarities between waking and dreaming that have been emphasized by dream psychologists. (7–11) These similarities have been ascribed to brain activation processes that were thought to be identical in the two states. This inference of identity was supported by evidence from neurophysiology of shared electrical and ionic mechanisms for cortical electroencephalogram (EEG) activation seen in both REM sleep and waking. (12) Besides being unable to account for the robust differences between wake and dream consciousness (13), this inference is now clearly in need of amendment on physiological grounds.

Brain-Mind States and the Study of Consciousness

One of the strongest supports for the scientifically hypothesized unity of brain and mind comes from the changes in conscious experience that we all experience when we doze off, fall deeply asleep, and—later—dream. The initial loss of contact with the outside world at sleep onset with its flurry of fleeting hypnagogic images, the deeply unconscious oblivion of sleep early in the night, and the gripping hallucinoid scenarios of late-night dreams all have such strong and meaningful underpinnings in brain physiology as to make all but certain the idea that our conscious experience is the brain-mind's awareness of its own physiological states. (See 15, 16.)

But whether they are accepted as firm proof of brain-mind identity or not, these simultaneous subjective and objective events encourage the concept of a unified system that we call the brain-mind. (13) And they further encourage a detailed accounting in the separable analytic domains of the neurophysiology and psychology of the events that change—or remain the same—as the brain changes state.

REM Sleep Dreaming Defined

Formal Features of REM Sleep Dreams

REM sleep dreams have several distinctive formal features that the underlying brain state must somehow determine. They include: sensorimotor hallucinations; bizarre imagery; the delusional belief that one is awake; diminished self-reflective awareness; orientational instability; narrative structure; intensification of emotion; instinctual behaviors; attenuated volition; and very poor memory. Table 21.1 summarizes these features. Our discussion is based on our psychophysiological theory of brain-mind isomorphism. We assume that any enhancement (or impairment) of any psychological function (e.g., dreaming) will be mirrored by enhancement (or impairment) of its physiological substrates function (e.g., REM sleep). We have emphasized these formal aspects of dreaming because they are noted in all REM sleep dreams regardless of their specific narrative content. We expect that REM sleep neurobiology will be able to explain more about such features than it now can about specific dream content.

Dream Motor Hallucinosis——Fictive Movement

The nature of the motor hallucinations of dreams deserves special comment, because it suggests that brain mechanisms subserving active motor behaviors are brought into play during REM. Thus, even office-bound intellectuals never dream of what they do every day: sitting at their desks reading, writing or analyzing data. (See 24.) Instead they ski, swim, fly, or play tennis in their dreams, whether they have recently done any of these things in their waking lives or not. In contrast to the deficits in memory functions discussed below, REM sleep dream consciousness routinely has *more* motor hallucinatory content than nonREM (NREM) consciousness, and perhaps even more than most waking fantasy. In this case we must look for what has been *added* to brain

Table 21.1 The Formal Features of REM Sleep Dreaming

Hallucinations—especially visual and motoric, but occasionally in any and all sensory modalities.
Bizarreness—Incongruity (imagery is strange, unusual, or impossible; discontinuity (imagery and plot can change, appear, or disappear rapidly); uncertainty (persons, places, and events often bizarrely uncertain by waking standards).
Delusion—we are consistently duped into believing that we are awake (unless we cultivate lucidity).
Self-reflection absent or greatly reduced relative to waking.
Lack of orientational stability—persons, times, and places are fused, plastic, incongruous, and discontinuous.
Narrative story lines explain and integrate all the dream elements in a confabulatory manner.
Emotions increased, intensified and predominated by fear-anxiety.
Instinctual programs (especially fight-flight) often incorporated.
Volition control greatly attenuated.
Memory deficits across dream-wake, wake-dream, and dream-dream transitions.

function in REM. We might expect to find an enhancement of those physiological processes that subserve internal visuomotor activation. We would then predict selective activation of the visual system, the basal ganglia, the motor cortex, or the subcortical motor pattern generators. The neurophysiological studies and PET data from humans confirm these predictions.

Dream Emotion

Emotion is a subjective experience that is intensified in dreams. To account for the documented prominence of anxiety-fear, elation, and anger in dreams (20–22) we would not be surprised to find selective activation of the limbic brain, and this is the prediction most strongly supported by the new neuropsychological evidence. (1–3) That dream emotion is usually consistent with the dream narrative (25) and bizarre incongruities between emotion and narrative are rarer than incongruities among other dream elements (21) can be explained by viewing dream emotion as a primary shaper of plots rather than as a reaction to them. (See 26.) Thus in a classic anxiety dream, the plot may shift from feeling lost, to not having proper credentials, adequate equipment, or suitable clothing, to missing a train. These plots all satisfy the driving emotion—anxiety—while being only very loosely associated with one other.

Dream Cognition

The distinctively discontinuous and incongruous nature of dream cognition can be measured as a construct termed bizarreness. (14, 17) Bizarreness in turn reflects the hyperassociative quality of REM sleep dream consciousness. The instability of time, place, and—most strikingly—person is a qualitatively unique feature of REM sleep dreams. A dream character may thus have the name of one of our friends but the wrong face, hairstyle, or clothing. Other dream characters are true chimeras, having some of the features of one individual and some of another. Even the sexual identity of dream characters is fluid, and this ambiguity can be anatomically explicit, not just psychological.

Dream Amnesia and Related Cognitive Deficits

The loss of memory in REM sleep makes dreaming consciousness much more difficult to recall than waking consciousness. This phenomenological deficit logically implies a physiological deficit: Some functional process, present and responsible for memory in waking is absent—or at least greatly diminished—in REM sleep.

In our attempt to explain dream amnesia, we look with interest at such functional deficits as the loss of noradrenergic and serotonergic modulation in REM sleep. This is because these very neuromodulators have been shown, in many human and animal studies, to be critical to learning and memory and to such memory-enhancing cognitive functions as perception and attention via their direct central nervous system (CNS) effects as well as their indirect peripheral mechanisms. (27–40) This REM-related aminergic demodulation is best viewed as a subtraction of noradrenenaline and serotonin from the varied neuromodulatory mixture facilitating waking cognition, a mixture that, of course, includes acetylcholine (e.g., 41), which remains abundant during REM.

The loss of orientational stability (which is at the cognitive root of dream bizarreness) and the loss of self-reflective awareness (which is the basis of the delusion that we are awake in our dreams) are two related deficits that could be caused by the aminergic demodulation of the brain in REM sleep. But we have wondered: Is there more to it than that? Could the frontal lobes be selectively inactivated during REM sleep? At least two of the new PET studies suggest that this is so. (1, 2)

REM Sleep Neurophysiology

In 1953 Eugene Aserinsky and Nathaniel Kleitman (42), working in Chicago, discovered that the brain-mind exhibited periodic self-activation during sleep. At regular 90- to 100-minute intervals they observed the spontaneous emergence of EEG desynchronization, accompanied by clusters of rapid saccadic eye movements (or REMs) together with acute accelerations of heart and respiration rates. When subjects were awakened and asked to report their antecedent mental activity, REM sleep was associated with longer, more vivid, more motorically animated, and more bizarre accounts than NREM. (7, 9, 13, 14, 18, 19, 43–53) Thus, while some dreaming can occur in other states of sleep (45, 46; for reviews see 9, 13, 19, 54), it is REM neurophysiology that most strongly supports dream psychology. (13) For this reason, we restrict our integrative efforts to the neuropsychology of REM sleep dreaming.

Human Neuropsychology

Until recently, the experimental study of human REM sleep dreaming has been limited on the physiological side by the poor resolving power of the EEG. Even expensive and cumbersome evoked potential and computer averaging approaches have not helped to analyze and compare REM sleep physiology with that of waking in an effective way. This limitation has probably reinforced the erroneous idea that the brain activation picture of REM sleep and waking are identical or, at least, very similar.

Fortunately, technological advances in the field of human brain imaging have now made it possible to describe a highly selective regional activation pattern of the brain in REM sleep. At the same time, experiments of nature—in the form of strokes—have allowed the locale of brain lesions to be correlated with deficits or accentuations of

Table 21.2 Imaging of Brain Activation in REM and the Effects of Brain Lesions on Dreaming

Region	*PET Studies of Activation in REM*	*Lesions Studies of Effects on Dreaming*
Pontine Tegmentum	Increase	No change
Limbic Structures	Increase	Decrease
Striate Cortex	Decrease	No change
Extrastriate Cortex	Increase	Decrease
Parietal Operculum	No change (right)	Decrease
Dorsolateral Prefrontal Cortex	Decrease	No change
Mediobasal Frontal Cortex	No change	Decrease

dream experience in patients. (4, 55) The remarkably complementary results of these two approaches are summarized in table 21.2.

PET Imaging Studies of REM Sleep Dreaming

Three very recent and entirely independent PET studies confirm the importance of the pontine brain stem in the REM sleep activation of the human brain. (1–3) This is an important advance because it validates, for the first time, the experimental animal data on the critical and specific role of the pontine brain stem in REM sleep generation. At the same time these new studies also provide important new data for our understanding of dream synthesis by the forebrain. Instead of the global, regionally nonspecific picture of forebrain activation that had been suggested by EEG studies, all of these new imaging studies indicate a preferential activation of limbic and paralimbic regions of the forebrain in REM sleep compared to waking or to NREM sleep. (1–3) One important implication of these discoveries is that dream emotion may be a primary shaper of dream plots rather than playing the secondary role in dream plot instigation that was previously hypothesized. (23)

Freud's Dream Theory Revised in the Light of Modern Sleep and Dream Research

There are five basic tenets to Freud's disguise-censorship dream theory that can now be contrasted with aspects of the activation-synthesis hypothesis.

1. The instigation of dreaming was, for Freud, caused by the upsurge of unconscious wishes following suspension of their wake-state repression. We would now say that dreaming is caused by brain activation during sleep. In NREM sleep, residual brain activation is at a low level, hence dreaming is less intense and less sustained, whereas in REM, brain activation is as vigorous as that in waking but that activation is both biochemically and regionally differentiated from waking.
2. The bizarre character of dreaming was, for Freud, determined by the disguise and censorship of the unconscious wishes. In order to protect consciousness from disruption (which would otherwise lead to awakening), such defensive processes as displacement, condensation, and symbolization were called into play. Even the visual hallucinosis of dreaming was viewed by Freud as a "regression to the sensory side" that served to neutralize the impact of the unconscious wishes on consciousness.

   We would now say that dreaming is bizarre because of the distinctive neurophysiology of REM sleep with its shift from top-down cortical control in waking to bottom-up phasic autoactivation epitomized by the ponto-geniculo-occipital (PGO) process. The distinctive regional activation pattern of the forebrain (with limbic, paralimbic, and parietal cortical regions taking precedence over the dorsolateral prefrontal cortex), and the global shift in the biochemical mode of information processing (caused by the noradrenergic and serotonergic demodulation) also contribute to dream bizarreness.
3. The visual nature of dreams is for activation-synthesis not defensive, as Freud asserted, but rather the direct result of both the bottom-up activation processes

(which convey information about brainstem eye movement commands). The degree to which primary versus secondary unimodal and multimodal cortices mediate dream vision and the relative influence of subcortical-cortical versus cortico-cortical activation processes remains to be clarified. But the answers to these fascinating questions have no direct bearing on the disguise-censorship postulate that is the heart of the Freudian dream theory.

While dreaming, we never sit and watch but are constantly moving through dream space. Thus dreams are not properly thought of as simply visual; more accurately, they are visuomotor. This feature was not recognized by Freud, even if he did correctly infer the necessity of inhibiting motor output to prevent the behavioral enactment of the fictive movement of dreams. This is a key point for activation-synthesis (and for any modern general theory of hallucinosis) because of the apparent link between brainstem motor pattern generators and cortical sensory processes. A strong implication is that far from being a feedback regression to the sensory side, dream hallucinosis results from a feed-forward conveyance of data about motor intentions to the sensory processors in the upper brain.

4. The emotional character of dreams was not easily dealt with by Freud's theory. He repeatedly sidestepped the obvious inconsistency between the presence of sleep-disruptive anxiety and his mechanistic postulate of disguise and censorship of the psychonoxious dream content. The presence of dream anxiety also inveighed against his "guardian of sleep" functional hypothesis. In other parts of Freudian theory, anxiety is viewed as a symptom of inadequate compromise between id and ego functions; Freud supposed it operated in a like manner in dreaming sleep.

Activation-synthesis has always regarded anxiety (which is the leading emotion in all dreams and all dreamers [20–22]) as the primary product of limbic lobe activation. This speculative hypothesis has now received powerful support from recent PET studies (showing amygdala, parahippocampal cortex, and anterior cingulate gyrus activation in human REM sleep) and clinical lesion studies (showing cessation of dreaming following destruction and disconnection of many of these same structures).

In this sense anxiety (and the two other prominent dream emotions, elation and anger) can be seen as major dream plot organizers and shapers of the emotional salience of dreams. For the reform-minded psychoanalyst, this should be heard as brain-music of divine inspiration, because it suggests that dreaming is a conscious state in which the impact of emotion on cognition is more clearly demonstrated than in waking. A major reason for this shift must be that, together with the limbic lobe activation, the seat of the executive control of cognition in the dorsolateral prefrontal cortex is deactivated in REM!

But let us make no mistake. This cortex versus limbic system construct in no way vindicates disguise-censorship, nor does it support any interpretive scheme that carries any trappings of that dogma. On the contrary, it favors the view that dreams are, in part, the transparent exposure of an individual's cognitive associations to—and means of coping with—anxiety (where anxiety is viewed as an inherent, existential emotion that is designed to interact with cognition in an adaptive if disruptive manner).

5. Amnesia for dreams was due to repression, according to Freud. Why repression was needed if the dreams had already been bowdlerized by disguise and censorship was

never made clear. Activation-synthesis says that both the dream forgetting following awakening and the defective episodic memory that occurs within dreams is a simple, state-dependent amnesia compounded by the global aminergic demodulation and the deactivation of working memory mechanisms in the dorsolateral prefrontal cortex. Activation-synthesis further asserts that the reason that dream recall is enhanced by spontaneous or stimulated awakenings from REM sleep is because the aminergic demodulation and prefrontal cortical deactivation of REM are suddenly reversed. As is well known, even these postarousal recollections are evanescent, probably because it takes several minutes to reinstate waking cognition.

The Function of Dreaming

If dream bizarreness indeed arises from the chaotic autoactivation process and the absence of top-down control from the frontal cortex in REM sleep, the apparent nonsense of dreams is most likely just that, and not the result of disguise and censorship as Freud's psychoanalytic dream theory proposed. (5) At the same time, the instigation of emotionally salient memories is probably also just that. Hence dreams may be both nonsensical (i.e., bizarre) and transparently meaningful (i.e., emotionally salient). (14) They are therefore potentially clinically and personally informative if one discounts the bizarreness and attends to the undisguised emotional content. This approach, which is straightforward and requires no interpretation, may be well undertaken without mediation, but it also may be facilitated by a sympathetic interlocutor.

Because dreams are so difficult to remember, it seems unlikely that attention to their content could afford much in the way of high priority survival-value. Indeed, it might instead be assumed that dreaming is an epiphenomenon of REM sleep whose cognitive content is so ambiguous as to invite misleading or even erroneous interpretation. From the neurobiological point of view it seems more likely that it is REM sleep itself, and not the subjective experience of dreaming, that has a functional significance for cognition that cannot easily be deduced from dream content. Among the many interesting theories that have been put forth, the restoration of cognitive capabilities such as attention and the enhancement of such learning processes as memory consolidation are of particular interest. (56–64) We regard the testing of this memory consolidation hypothesis as a most promising area of ongoing research on sleep and dreaming.

Periodically throughout sleep the brain self-activates. This self-activation is a complex, stereotyped process that is now well understood at the cellular and molecular levels. Like the circadian rhythm of sleep and waking, the ultradian 90 to 100 minute alternation of REM and NREM sleep is caused not by the ebb and flow of desire but by a biological clock composed of reciprocally interactive aminergic and cholinergic brain stem neurons. This oscillator causes the brain and mind to change its activation structure, and both the flow and mode of information processing is accordingly reversed. During REM sleep, dreaming assumes its most intense, sustained, and distinctive character because of the shift in the mechanism of activation from aminergic-cholinergic (in waking) to exclusively cholinergic (in REM sleep).

Any functions of dreaming must be clearly distinguished from the functions of REM sleep, many of which (like temperature control or immune function maintenance) could never be inferred from dream consciousness and have little or nothing to do with dream consciousness. In this sense it is already clear that dreaming is epiphenomenal with respect to the most fundamental biological adaptations of REM sleep.

What about more intermediate level functions, such as the regulation of neuromodulatory balance (via shifts in the balance of synthesis and degradation of crucial brain chemicals)? Such shifts could subserve optimal waking function (including protection from the breakthrough of REM-like psychotogenic processes). Here again, dream content might be quite irrelevant, telling us only what a subject's mental state might be like if he or she were to become delirious. In this sense, the interpretation of dreams in terms of unconscious motives would make about as much sense as interpreting the ravings of an alcoholic in the throes of delirium tremens or the demented ramblings of an Alzheimer's disease victim.

For the progressive psychoanalyst, this point might be reframed in a more general, heuristic manner: REM sleep dreaming is didactic! It shows the doctor and the patient what psychosis is like. It shows that the propensity to psychosis is natural and universal. It shows that all psychoses are both functional and organic. And it shows that all mental products have both a meaningful (read: emotionally salient) and nonsensical (read: chaotic) aspect.

But it is at the cognitive level that the most intriguing reframings must proceed. Abundant evidence is fast accumulating to indicate that both NREM and REM sleep benefit learning and memory. As these mental functions are the coin of the realm in any psychology, psychoanalysis, or psychotherapy, the door is open to an examination of dream content for direct evidence of the kind of social and psychological learning that all therapies, including psychoanalysis, want to promote.

Obstacles to Progress

Three fundamental problems must be overcome if psychoanalysis wants to counter its rapidly progressive marginalization:

1. The cult of Freud and the argument from authority. The reverence for Freud's self-styled heroism and for his texts has held the field back from revision in the light of modern cognitive neuroscience.
2. The rigid institutional structure and rigid adherence to methodological narrowness embodied by the suggestion that the only dreams that matter are those that are brought to the analyst and that the method of free association is the only legitimate means of understanding dreams and dreaming. This method is so clearly circular as to be practically worthless if scientific validity is a goal. When the data are out of register, the progressive analyst must be encouraged and supported rather than punished for dissidence. The ad hominem argument that anyone who is skeptical of psychoanalytic theory needs further analysis is one unfortunate offshoot of this methodological argument.
3. The socioeconomic parochialism of psychoanalysis, which makes it appear to some as a parlor game practiced by upper-middle-class doctors upon each other and their urban friends. To survive and to have any claim to universalism, psychoanalysis needs to democratize as well as to diversify. A corollary of this principle is that it is unconscionable to claim, as did Freud, that psychoanalysis is a research tool and then charge people for it as if it were medical treatment. And the joke of the century must be the claim that psychoanalysis can be effective only if its cost is kept high! That is certainly not true of the polio vaccine, or penicillin, or even lithium.

Conclusion

In my opinion, the new dream theory is so different from Freud's as to make the use of a word like "revision" a euphemism. Because there is essentially nothing left of the Freudian hypotheses, what is needed is not revision but complete overhaul. Instead what we see is a tenacious adherence to a faith in the interpretability of dreams using vague and unscientific terms like "metaphor" and "hermeneutics," or, what is worse, we see recourse to the relativistic claim of "narrative truth." This limits psychoanalysis to a literary exercise with no claim to the scientific legitimacy that Freud dreamed of in his 1895 *Project for a Scientific Psychology.*

References

1. Braun A. R., Balkin T. J., Wesensten N. J., Carson R. E., Varga M., Baldwin P., Selbie S., Belenky G., and Herscovitch P. *Brain* 120 1173–1197 (1997).
2. Maquet P., Peters J. M., Aerts J., Delfiore G., Degueldre C., Luxen A., and Franck G. *Nature* 383 163–166 (1996).
3. Nofzinger E. A., Mintun M. A., Wiseman M. B., Kupfer D. J., and Moore R. Y. *Brain Research* 770 192–201 (1997).
4. Solms M. *The Neuropsychology of Dreams: A Clinico-Anatomical Study.* Mahwah: Lawrence Erlbaum Associates, 1997.
5. Freud S. *Project for a Scientific Psychology.* In Strachey J., ed., *The Standard Edition of the Complete Psychological Works of Sigmund Freud,* vol. 1. London: Hogarth Press, 1895: 347–447.
6. Freud S. *The Interpretation of Dreams.* J. Strachey. New York: Basic Books, 1900.
7. Antrobus J. S. *Psychophysiology* 20 562–568 (1983).
8. Foulkes D. *European Journal of Cognitive Psychology* 2 39–55 (1990).
9. ———. *Journal of Sleep Research* 2 199–202 (1993).
10. ———. *Sleep Research Society Bulletin* 3 2–4 (1997).
11. Moffitt A. *Impuls* 3 18–31 (1995).
12. Llinas R. and Pare D. *Neuroscience* 44 521–535 (1991).
13. Kahn D., Pace-Schott E. F., and Hobson J. A. *Neuroscience* 78 13–38 (1997).
14. Hobson J. A. *The Dreaming Brain.* New York: Basic Books, 1988.
15. Hobson J. A. *The Chemistry of Conscious States.* Boston: Little Brown, 1994.
16. Hobson J. A. "Consciousness as a State-Dependent Phenomenon." In Cohen J. and Schooler J., eds. *Scientific Approaches to the Question of Consciousness.* Mahwah: Lawrence Erlbaum Associates, 1997: 379–396.
17. Hobson J. A., Hoffman E., Helfand R., and Kostner D. *Human Neurobiology* 6 157–164 (1987).
18. Porte H. S. and Hobson J. A. *Journal of Abnormal Psychology* 105 329–335 (1996).
19. Foulkes D. *Dreaming: A Cognitive-Psychological Analysis.* Mahwah: Lawrence Erlbaum Associates, 1985: 221.
20. Domhoff G. W. *Finding Meaning in Dreams: a Quantitative Approach.* New York: Plenum, 1996: 356.
21. Merritt J. M., Stickgold R., Pace-Schott E., Williams J., and Hobson J. A. *Conscious Cognition* 3 46–60 (1994).
22. Nielsen T. A., Deslauriers D., and Baylor G. W. *Dreaming* 1 287–300 (1991).
23. Hobson J. A. and McCarley R. W. *American Journal of Psychiatry* 134 1335–1348 (1977).
24. Hartmann E. *Sleep Research* 25 136 (1996).
25. Foulkes D., Sullivan B., Kerr N. H., and Brown L. "Dream Affect: Appropriateness to Dream Situations." In Koella W. P., Obal F., Scholz H., and Vizzer P., eds. *Sleep 86.* New York: Gustav Fisher Verlag, 1988: 131–134.

26. Seligman M. E. P. and Yellen A. *Behavioral Research and Therapy* 25 1–24 (1987).
27. Abel T., Alberini C., Ghirardi M., Huang Y., Nguyen P., and Kandel E. R. "Steps Toward a Molecular Definition of Memory Consolidation." In Schacter D. L., ed. *Memory Distortion.* Cambridge: Harvard University Press, 1995: 298–325.
28. Cahill L., Prins B., Weber M., and McGaugh J. L. *Nature* 371 702–704 (1994).
29. Clark C. R., Geffen G. M., and Geffen L. B. *Neuroscience and Biobehavioral Review* 11 353–364 (1987b).
30. Clark C. R., Geffen G. M., Geffen L. B. *Neuropsychologia* 27 131–139 (1989).
31. Coull J. T., Middleton H. C., Sahakian B. J., and Robbins T. W. J. *Psychopharmacology* 95 A24 (1992).
32. Frith C. D., Dowdy J., Ferrier N., and Crow T. J. *Psychopharmacology* 87 490–493 (1985).
33. Kandel E. R. *Journal of Neuropsychiatry* 1 103–125 (1989).
34. Kandel E. R. and Schwartz J. H. *Science* 218 433–443 (1982).
35. Mattay V. S., Berman K. F., Ostrem J. L., Esposito G., VanHorn J. D., Bigelow L. R., and Weinberger D. R. *Journal of Neuroscience* 16 4816–4822 (1996).
36. McGaugh J. L. *Psychological Science* 1 15–25 (1990).
37. McGaugh J. L. "Emotional Activation Neuromodulatory Systems and Memory." In Schacter, D. L., ed. *Memory Distortion.* Cambridge: Harvard University Press, 1995: 255–274.
38. Quatermain D. "The Role of Catecholamines in Memory Processing." In Deutsch J. A., ed. *The Physiological Basis of Memory.* New York: Academic Press, 1983: 387–423.
39. Robbins T. W. and Everitt B. J. "Arousal Systems and Attention." In Gazzaniga M., ed. *The Cognitive Neurosciences.* Cambridge: MIT Press, 1994: 703–720.
40. Witte E. A., Gordon-Lickey M. E., and Marrocco R. T. *Society of Neuroscience Abstracts* 18 537 (1992).
41. Hasselmo M. E. and Bower J.M. "Acetylcholine and Memory." *Trends in Neuroscience* 16 218–222 (1993).
42. Aserinsky E. and Kleitman N. *Science* 118 361–375 (1953).
43. Antrobus J. S., Kondo T., and Reinsel R. *Conscious and Cognition* 4 275–299 (1995).
44. Casagrande M., Violani C., Lucidi F., Buttinelli E., and Bertini M. *International Journal of Neuroscience* 85 19–30 (1996).
45. Cavallero C., Cicogna P., Natale V., Occhionero M., and Zito A. "Slow Wave Sleep Dreaming." *Sleep* 15 562–566.
46. Foulkes D. *Journal of Abnormal and Social Psychology* 65 14–25 (1962).
47. Foulkes D. and Schmidt M. *Sleep* 6 265–280 (1983).
48. Ogilvie R., Hunt H., Sawicki C., and Samahalski J. *Sleep* 11 11–27 (1982).
49. Porte H. S. and Hobson J. A. *Journal of Abnormal Psychology* 105 329–335 (1996).
50. Goodenough D. R., Lewis H. B., Shapiro A., Jaret L., and Sleser I. *Journal of Personal and Social Psychology* 2 170–179 (1965b).
51. Rechtschaffen A., Verdone P., and Wheaton J. *Canadian Psychiatry* 8 409–414 (1963).
52. Stickgold R., Pace-Schott E., and Hobson J. A. *Conscious Cognition* 3 16–29 (1994).
53. Waterman D., Elton M., and Kenemans J. L. *Journal of Sleep Research* 2 8–12 (1993).
54. Foulkes D. *Experimental Neurology* 19 28–38 (1967).
55. Doricchi F. and Violini C. "Dream Recall in Brain-Damaged Patients: A Contribution to the Neuropsychology of Dreaming through a Review of the Literature." In Antrobus J. S. and Bertini M., eds. *The Neuropsychology of Sleep and Dreaming.* Mahwah: Lawrence Erlbaum Associates, 1992: 99–143.
56. Askenasy J. J. M., Karni A., and Sagi D. "Visual Skill Consolidation in the Dreaming Brain." In Hayaishi O. and Inoue S., eds. *Sleep and Sleep Disorders: From Molecule to Behavior.* New York: Academic Press, 1997: 361–377.
57. Cai Z. J. *Behavioral and Brain Research* 69 187–194 (1995).
58. Crick F. and Mitchison G. "REM Sleep and Neural Nets," *Behavioral and Brain Research* 69 147–155 (1995).

59. Giuditta A., Ambrosini M.V., Montagnese P., Mandile P., Cotungo M., Zucconi G. G., and Vescia S. *Behavioral and Brain Research* 69 157–166 (1995).
60. Hennevin E., Hars B., Maho C., and Bloch V. *Behavioral and Brain Research* 69 125–135 (1995).
61. Hobson J. A. and Stickgold R. *Current Biology* 5 35–36 (1995).
62. Kavanaugh J. L. *Neuroscience* 79 7–44 (1997).
63. Smith C. *Behavioral and Brain Research* 69 137–145 (1995).
64.———. *Behavioral and Brain Research* 78 49–56 (1996).

22

Consciousness in Dreaming

A Metacognitive Approach

Tracey L. Kahan

Consciousness

Over a century ago, William James wrote: "The universal conscious fact is not 'feelings exist' and 'thoughts exist' but '*I* think' and '*I* feel'" (James 1890: 226). In other words, central to consciousness is the self-as-observer, what James called 'the knower.' As Baars explains, "the self is that which has access to consciousness" (1997: 153). (Also see Dennett, 1978.) The notion of self-as-observer implies dual levels of awareness: The contents of experience (participant perspective) are the object of awareness (observer perspective).

Consider the following narrative, for example:

> I am traveling with M. B. next to a river, moving slowly in the direction opposite the current. On the opposite bank, I see a huge, solitary pine tree growing very close to the edge of the bank. Its lower branches have been removed to avoid their dragging in the water. I find myself wondering who cut these branches off. The tree is beautifully shaped—tall, symmetrical, with enough space between the limbs to see the full silhouette against the sky. *I think to myself, "I really should say something to M. about how beautiful and striking this tree is," but I decide not to say anything.* We continue upriver. (Kahan 2001; emphasis added)

In this narrative, the individual is simultaneously experiencing the beauty of the tree (participant perspective) and noticing the thoughts she has about sharing this experience with her companion (observer perspective). This situation is similar to what Ernest Rossi termed "self- reflectiveness" (SR), which he defined as "the examination of one's thoughts, feelings, or behavior." (p. 139). Self-reflectiveness involves the dual levels of awareness alluded to by James, "an experiencing self immersed in its own pattern of awareness and . . . the secondary level of awareness examining the experiencing self" (Rossi 1972: 139).

Metacognition

Self-reflectiveness also is one dimension of what cognitive psychologists call "metacognition," or the awareness of one's cognitive processes. Metacognition also may include the deliberate direction of one's thought processes (Nelson and Narens 1990). Thus, in addition to self-reflectiveness, metacognition includes intentionality and self-regulation. Alan Rechtschaffen describes the relationship among these skills as follows: "Volitional control, at least phenomenologically, immediately implies reflectiveness, i.e., one part of the mind tells another part where to go [*intentionality*], observes its progress [*self-reflection (monitoring)*], and corrects its deviations [*regulation*]" (1978: 99; emphasis added).

In the earlier "tree" narrative, for example, there is evidence of intentionality and behavior regulation as well as the aforementioned self-reflection. The storyteller's remark that she "should say something" about the tree demonstrates intentionality, in this case the intention to express herself. Her decision "not to say anything" illustrates behavior regulation in that she chooses between two possible courses of action (saying something versus saying nothing). And we see self-reflection in her comment "I find myself wondering who cut these branches off."

The Metacognitive Model

The metacognitive model proposed by Nelson and Narens (1990, 1994) is one way to characterize the interplay between self-awareness, intentionality, and behavior regulation, considered by many theorists to be key components of consciousness (Baars 1997; Dennett 1978; Flavell 1979; Kihlstrom 1987; Nelson 1996; Varela, Thompson, and Rosch 1995).

In their metacognitive model, Nelson and Narens first distinguish between a person's ongoing phenomenal experience and his or her goals and intentions. According to the metacognitive model, phenomenal experience occurs at the "object-level" and goals or intentions at the "meta-level" (see figure 22.1). Information flows between the object and meta levels in both directions. "Metacognitive monitoring" occurs when information flows from the object level to the meta level, such as when we examine our ongoing experience in relation to our goals and intentions. For example, an actor notices where he is on the stage in relation to his goal of remaining visible to the audience. "Control" (or behavior regulation) occurs when information flows from the meta level to the object level, such as when we select a behavior that promises to fulfill our intentions. So the same actor *intentionally* turns to face the audience in order to be seen. Consider the following narrative, for example:

> "I am in Bishop and I go to the high school. I tell them I am a student and that I need to see a guidance counselor. The secretaries are doing nothing; they are sitting around in a dingy caramel-colored office, ratting their hair, chomping gum and chatting . . . I decide to go look for myself and find someone to help me. I have my resume with me, and I say that I need help with it. I think to myself how incompetent this person is that is helping me and they say that I need to put completely different jobs on there. I decide to leave . . ." (C. Doherty 2001, unpublished data).

At the object level, the narrator is describing her experience of visiting a high school. At the meta level, her intention is to find a guidance counselor to review her resume.

Metacognitive monitoring is exemplified by her observation that the secretaries are doing nothing and cannot help her achieve her goal. And, finally, control, or behavior regulation, is seen in the narrator's decision to go and find someone to assist her.

Accuracy per se is not a critical aspect of this model. As Nelson explains, "the individual participant can be treated as an *imperfect* measuring device of his or her own cognitions, in which the individual's metacognitive monitoring is assumed to sometimes contain errors or distortions . . ." (1996: 106). So a child who is monitoring how well he understands a difficult story may decide he needs to reread a particular passage only once in order to increase understanding when, in fact, he may have needed to reread that passage three times to achieve his comprehension goal.

Metacognition in Sleep

Until recently, metacognition, like consciousness more generally, was viewed as a potentiality of the *waking* mind alone. What are now called metacognitive skills (self- reflectiveness, intentionality, and self-regulation) were presumably *absent* during sleep. (See Rechtschaffen 1978; Hobson 1988.) In the next section, we consider the evidence for the claim that metacognitive skills are, indeed, suspended during sleep.

Metacognition Does Not Occur During Sleep

As noted above, the prevailing view has been that metacognition occurs *only* during our waking hours; that self-reflection, intentionality, and behavior regulation are absent or seriously deficient during dreaming. (See Kahan and LaBerge 1994; Levin 2000; Purcell, Moffitt, and Hoffmann 1993, for recent discussions of "deficiency theories.") No less than William James (1890), the founder of psychological science in the United States, held that self-reflection, or "self-consciousness," to use James's term, characterizes waking but does not occur during sleep. As Kunzendorf (1987–1988) explains:

Figure 22.1 The Metacognitive Model, adapted fro Nelson and Narens (1994).

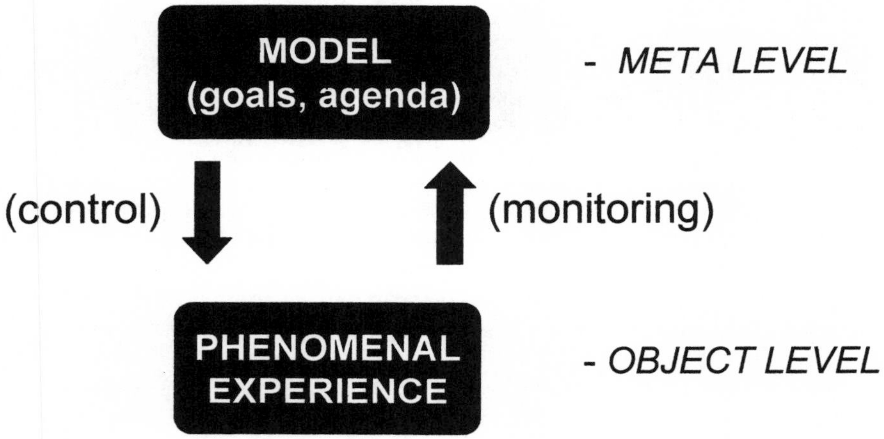

> James' recollective theory of self-consciousness implies that dream images and waking images are not only different, but literally "dissociated," from each other. Because dreams contain their own quality of familiarity *but not the waking quality of self-consciousness,* dream memories are dissociated from waking memories. Accordingly, these two dissociated sets of memories result in two dissociated experiences of self-consciousness: a waking self alternating with a sleeping self. (5, emphasis added)

Freud (1953) also saw dreaming and waking as inherently different. According to Freud, ego control was suspended during sleep, and the dreaming mind regressed to the more primitive cognitive style, or "primary process thinking," associated with the unconscious mind. (Also see Koukkou and Lehman 1983.) In contrast to the "secondary processes" of rationality, order, and clarity that characterize waking mentation, dreaming was seen as illogical, bizarre, and involving magical thinking (e.g., Domino 1976). In describing the dissociation between waking and dreaming, Freud and other theorists who followed him went so far as to assert that dreaming processes parallel those of psychosis. (See especially Hobson 1988: 9, 229–230; Hobson 1994; Shafton 1995: 235–238.)

James's and Freud's assertions regarding the absence of high-order cognitive skills during dreaming have profoundly shaped contemporary research in cognitive dream psychology. (See especially Foulkes and Cavallero 1993; Haskell 1986; Hunt 1986.) Underlying all of these claims is the assumption that dreaming is *dissociated* from waking and that dreaming cognition is "deficient." The assertion that dreaming does not, cannot involve self-reflectiveness or volition has served as an unstudied, a priori assumption underlying much of the theoretical and empirical work on the mind in sleep (Arkin, Antrobus, and Ellman 1978; Blagrove 1992; Crick and Mitchison 1983; Ellman and

Table 22.1 Theorists Who Claim that Metacognition Does Not Occur in Dreaming

Theorist	*Claim*
James (1890)	Dreams do not contain the waking quality of self-consciousness.
Freud (1953)	Ego control is suspended during sleep, and dreaming is characterized by primary process thinking.
Rechtschaffen (1978)	Dreaming is "inherently" non-reflective (pp. 98–101).
Kunzendorf (1987–1988)	Self-consciousness is a defining characteristic of waking experience, but not dreaming experience (p. 6).
Weinstein et al. (1988)	The loss of reflective awareness is a central aspect of the dream experience (p. 445).
Hobson (1988)	Both orientation in the world and self-critical perspective are lost [due to the] loss of aminergic modulation associated with REM dreaming (p. 210).
Foulkes (1990)	Dream experience seems to be the prototype of passive awareness (p. 47) . . . the experiential price of falling asleep seem to be the relinquishment of the ability to exercise voluntary control over the contents of consciousness (p. 49).
Koukkou & Lehmann (1993)	Dreaming cognition is regressive, to an earlier developmental stage.
Hobson & Stickgold (1994)	Assume that dream consciousness and cognition are both highly state dependent phenomena (p. 1).

Antrobus 1991; Empson 1989; Foulkes 1985, 1990; Globus 1987; Green and McCreery 1994; Hartman 1973; Hobson 1988; Hobson and Stickgold 1994; Kahn and Hobson 1993; Koukkou and Lehmann 1983; Kunzendorf 1987–88; Rechtschaffen 1978; Sartre 1940; Weinstein, Schwartz, and Ellman 1988; Winson 1990.) (See table 22.1 for examples of the specific claims made by some of these theorists.) It is noteworthy that many of these theorists assert that there are *absolute* differences in cognition and metacognition across the dreaming and waking. In other words, a quality of waking cognition (e.g., self-reflection, intentionality, or self-regulation) is presumed absent in dreaming. Underlying these claims is the assumption that dreaming is generated by a different neurocognitive system than that which generates waking cognition/experience; hence, the notion that dreaming is "dissociated" from waking (Freud 1953; Hobson, 1988; Hobson and Stickgold 1994; Hobson, Pace-Schott, and Stickgold 2000; Koukkou and Lehmann 1983; Rechtschaffen 1978; also see Kahan 2000 and Nielsen 2000 for recent discussions of "one-generator" versus "two-generator" models of dreaming).

What Is the Evidence that Metacognitive Skills Are Suspended in Sleep?

Only a few of the above-mentioned theorists have offered *empirical* support for their claims. Just how convincing *is* the evidence that metacognitive skills are rare or absent in dreaming; that dreaming is "just degraded cognition" (Shafton 1995: 95)? We now turn to what is, arguably, the most influential of this empirical work.

In an article that is frequently cited as evidence for the deficiencies in dream cognition, Alan Rechtschaffen declares that dreaming is *inherently* nonreflective and lacking volition (1978: 98–101). Echoing Freud, Rechtschaffen claims that there is a suspension of ego control during dreaming that "results in the inherent nonreflectiveness of dreaming consciousness, including the typical absence of lucidity (awareness of dreaming)" (cited by Kahan and LaBerge 1994: 248). Surprisingly, Rechtschaffen's primary evidence for the nonreflectiveness of dreams comes from his own dream experiences and his study of the dream reports of four undergraduate students. (See Rechtschaffen 1978: 98–100.) For example, Rechtschaffen writes: "I cannot remember a dream report which took the form, 'Well, I was dreaming of such and such, but as I was dreaming this I was imagining a different scene which was completely unrelated'" (1978: 102). Rechtschaffen's anecdotal observation that he has never experienced "imagining" while dreaming does not constitute evidence that imagining is impossible in dreams; nor do the experiences of four individuals constitute valid evidence that *all* dreaming is nonreflective. It is a testament to Rechtschaffen's credibility as a sleep scientist, and the popularity of the "deficiency" paradigm, that this article, now over 20 years old, is still routinely cited as evidence for dreaming's lack of reflective awareness and other metacognitive skills (Crick and Mitchison 1983; Empson 1989: 92; Globus 1987: 80–84; Green and McCreery 1994: 12; Hobson 1988).

Even the second edition of the comprehensive volume *The Mind in Sleep* (Ellman and Antrobus 1991) includes little mention of "self-awareness," "self-reflection," or intentionality during dreaming. In their chapter on the qualitative aspects of sleep mentation, Weinstein, Schwartz, and Arkin (1991) do describe, albeit briefly, the seminal studies of dream self-reflection conducted by Purcell, Mullington, Moffitt, Hoffmann, and Pigeau (1986). But the authors do not discuss the implications for "discontinuity theories" of Purcell et al.'s findings that the normative level of self-reflection in dreaming is higher than generally assumed and that dream self-reflection can be increased through attentional training. Weinstein et al. also discourage further consideration of the potential for metacognition during dreaming by arguing that dreaming, particularly dreaming during phasic REM (rapid eye movement), involves a *suspension* of reflective self-awareness.

Activation-Synthesis Model of Dreaming

A well known and controversial contemporary dream theory is the activation-synthesis (AS) model, originally developed by J. Allan Hobson and Robert McCarley (Hobson and McCarley 1977, and updated by Mamelak and Hobson in 1989). The AS model begins with two basic assumptions. First, certain phenomenological features "define" dreams: intense emotions, scene shifts, plot coherence, amnesia for the experience, loss of orientation in the world, bizarre transformations, and the suspension of a self-critical perspective (Hobson 1988). A second major assumption of the AS model is that the phenomenological or psychological qualities of dreams are the direct consequence of the particular neurophysiological changes that occur during REM sleep (formal isomorphism). According to the model, the psychological experience of dreaming represents the forebrain's "best effort" to organize, integrate, and impose meaning on the random cerebral activation initiated by the brain stem during REM sleep (Hobson 1988: 210; Hobson 1990; Hobson and Stickgold 1994; Mamelak and Hobson 1989). For example, the suspension of a self-critical perspective and the associated delusional acceptance of the dream experience as "real" are presumably the result of a switch from the (waking) mode of information processing dominated by the aminergic system to a mode of information processing dominated by the cholinergic system (Hobson and Stickgold 1994: 13).

Notwithstanding the continuing evolution of the activation-synthesis model (see Hobson et al. 2000), the assumption of a formal isomorphism between dreaming features and REM raises several issues. (Also see Foulkes 1993; Nielsen 2000; Solms 2000). One is whether the "formal characteristics of dreaming" mentioned earlier constitute the necessary psychological features of dreaming; the community of dream researchers has not, in fact, reached consensus on how to define dreaming or on what constitute the normative characteristics of dreams. (See especially Hunt 1989: 69–76 for detailed discussion of problems in the definition of dreaming; also see Foulkes 1990 and Snyder 1970 for empirical studies of the phenomenological features of normative dreaming).

A second basic issue with the activation-synthesis model is that identifying dreaming with REM sleep has been, and continues to be, highly controversial. Numerous theorists have questioned the equation of REM with dreaming, particularly in light of unequivocal evidence of non-REM (NREM) dreaming, including dreaming so vivid that it is indistinguishable from REM dreaming. (See Bulkeley 1997; Domhoff 1999; Foulkes 1999; Kahan 2000; Nielsen 2000; Purcell et al. 1993; Van de Castle 1994 for recent discussions of REM versus NREM dreaming.) And the recent neuropsychological evidence offered by Mark Solms indicates that REM is neither necessary nor sufficient for dreaming to occur (Solms 1997, 2000). Even the earliest, classic, experimental studies of dreams acknowledged NREM dreaming: "it was immediately clear to Dement that dreaming is not entirely confined to the REM phase. . . . And some of the reports from non-REM sleep were *indistinguishable by any criterion* from those obtained from post-REM awakenings" (cited by Hobson 1988: 143; emphasis added).

Evidence for the AS Model of Dreaming/Waking Neurocognition

In research recently conducted by Hobson and his colleagues, the stated goal is to offer evidence for their neurobiological model of dreaming-waking phenomenology (see especially Hobson et al. 2000; Hobson and Stickgold 1994; Kahn and Hobson 1993; Kahn, Pace-Schott, and Hobson 1997 for reviews of this work).

For example, in an ambitious and ongoing study of the phenomenal qualities of dreams, Hobson and his colleagues have evaluated the qualitative and organizational features of home dreams. Narrative reports were obtained from different sleep stages, where REM and NREM sleep were identified from sleep records obtained via the "Nightcap." The Nightcap is a device designed by Hobson that uses eye movement and head movement activity to distinguish REM and NREM sleep. (See especially Mamelak and Hobson 1989.) The Nightcap does not distinguish between NREM stages ¾ (slow-wave) sleep and NREM stage 2 sleep.

Stickgold, Pace-Schott, and Hobson (1994), used the Nightcap to collect sleep samples from eleven subjects over ten nights. Of the 149 sleep-stage-defined reports, 59 percent (88) were from spontaneous REM awakenings and 41 percent (61) were from spontaneous NREM awakenings. The authors found that reports from REM sleep awakenings were typically longer than reports from NREM: 24 percent of REM reports were longer than 500 words, while only one NREM report was this long. At the same time, it is notable that 10 percent of the NREM reports were more than 200 words). Further, 83 percent of the REM reports (N = 88) contained sleep mentation, compared with 54 percent of the NREM reports (N = 33) (p. 24).

Reporting on the qualitative aspects of the data collected by Stickgold et al. (1994), Hobson and Stickgold (1994) conclude that REM dreams are "more perceptually vivid, more motorically animated, and more emotionally charged than NREM reports and that NREM reports tended to be more thought-like and contained more representations of current concerns than did REM sleep reports" (2). The authors then say that "it seemed reasonable to conclude that the activation level of the brain was the *major* determinant of these observed differences" (3). However, the empirical work of an Italian group, Bosinelli, Cicogna, and Cavallero, indicates that the content and memory sources of REM and NREM dreams are much more similar than different. (See especially Cavallero and Cigogna 1993; Cicogna, Cavallero, and Bosinelli 1991.) Also, the level of brain activation needed to support dreaming is not exclusive to REM sleep, as John Antrobus's work has also demonstrated. (See especially Antrobus 1990, 1991; Cavallero and Cigogna 1993; Solms 1997, 2000.)

In related articles (Hobson and Stickgold 1994; Kahn et al. 1997), this argument is extended to include the presumed qualitative differences in *waking*, REM, and NREM. However, the evidence cited for the hypothesized cross-state differences does not include direct comparisons of metacognitive processes, such as self-reflection, volition, or self-regulation, *across* waking and sleep.[1]

David Foulkes's Cognitive Approach to Dreaming

David Foulkes, another prolific and influential dream researcher, approaches dreaming from a cognitive-developmental perspective (Foulkes 1985, 1990, 1993, 1999). Foulkes is essentially a "continuity" theorist, one who argues that the same cognitive system is responsible for waking and dreaming cognition. However, with respect to metacognitive skills such as self-reflection, Foulkes's position has been that we can only *represent* self-reflection in dreams in a reproductive fashion. That is, we might "remember" an instance of self-reflection from waking, but we do not engage in self-reflection in a spontaneous fashion *within* the dream (Foulkes 1990: 51). Foulkes argues that dreaming is a conscious construction of a *model* of the waking self-in-world. Referring to his own dreams, Foulkes acknowledges (1990: 51) that there is reflection *in* dreams about ongoing events but little self-reflection about how current dream events relate to one's sense of self (autobiographical history). Thus, Foulkes agrees with other theorists who have argued that dreaming lacks "self-consciousness" because, typically, we are not fully aware that the dream experiences we are having are a "construction" of the imagination, and we are not fully aware of our current waking conditions when we are dreaming (e.g., Kunzendorf 1987–88: 6; Rechtschaffen 1978; Weinstein et al. 1988: 440).[2]

In summary, the "deficiency" theorists emphasize the presumed differences between waking and dreaming cognition, and assert that dreaming lacks the waking cognitive skills of self-reflection, intentionality, and behavior regulation. But are these metacognitive skills absent in dreaming? None of the research just reviewed directly tested this hypothesis.

Metacognition Does Occur During Sleep

Metacognition in Lucid Dreaming

In a "lucid dream," one is *aware* of dreaming *while* dreaming (Godwin 1994; Green and McCreery 1994; LaBerge 1985; Van Eeden 1913). In addition to this self-reflection on "state," which is their defining feature, lucid dreams often include other compelling examples of metacognition in sleep. For example:

> I have my skates with me. . . . On the floor that I will be skating on are blankets and hoops, like nets. I think the set-up must be for some sort of skating game. I am disappointed but will stay anyway. I remember that I have not skated since grade nine. I walk about, then fix the heel of my skate onto my foot properly as I think of the latest past events. Then I realize that the latest events have all been dreams. *I know that I am dreaming.* I get full of energy and run. I find myself running in the woods. I am naked. It is sunny out. I think to myself "Joe told me I would have a lucid dream, and I did!" I pass through skinny trees that look like alders. I can't feel them going through me. I stick out my right hand and watch the tree images pass through my arm (or my arm pass through the trees). When I want to touch the trees I grab them and bend them. They do not feel very solid; they feel the way a rotting tree feels. Briefly, while still running, I think of changing the scene by closing my eyes. I open them again quickly to find I am still in the same scene. I keep on moving. . . . (Gillis, reported by Sacksteder 1993: 13)

In this narrative, we see *intentionality* ("I think of changing the scene by closing my eyes"), *behavior regulation* ("When I want to touch the trees I grab them and bend them"), *reasoning* ("I think the set-up must be for some sort of skating game"), and *self-reflection on thoughts* ("I think to myself 'Joe told me I would have a lucid dream"), as well as the aforementioned *self-reflection on state* ("I know that I am dreaming"). Without question, such lucid-control dreaming exemplifies metacognition during sleep.

In laboratory studies of lucid dreaming, intentionality is especially important because participants must be able to induce awareness of dreaming while dreaming (lucidity) and also to remember the activities they agreed to carry out in the lucid dream. For example, in research reported by LaBerge and Zimbardo (2000), the dreamers had to remember their presleep intention to trace a circle (*volition*) and then actually engage in that activity in the lucid dream (*behavior regulation*). (See Hearne 1978 and LaBerge, 1985, 1990, for discussion of other studies in which particular tasks are carried out in the lucid dream.) An obvious advantage of laboratory studies of lucid dreaming is that, because these studies include standard measurements of sleep physiology, investigators can determine the sleep stage and other physiological correlates of lucid dreaming (Brylowski, Levitan, and LaBerge 1989; LaBerge, Levitan, and Dement 1986). The physiological recordings also indicate when the participant "signaled" that she became lucid, as well as when she began and ended the pre-agreed-upon task. This permits researchers to correlate the psychophysiological measures with the onset of lucidity (self-reflection) and with the deliberate execution of the task (self-reflection and intentionality). (See Baars 1997 and Kahan and LaBerge 1994 for further discussions of lucid dreaming as metacognition.) Such research has established that lucid dreaming occurs in bona-fide sleep, typically REM sleep (LaBerge, Nagel, Dement, and Zarcone 1981), and that the onset of lucidity (awareness of dreaming) is accompanied by an increase in the density of eye movements within REM (see LaBerge 1990 for further discussion of the psychophysiology of lucid dreaming).

Curiously, in spite of the obvious metacognitive skills involved in lucid dreaming, many influential dream theorists have been disinclined to revise their view of dreaming cognition to include metacognitive capabilities. Harry Hunt, for example, remarks: "the experience of lucid dreaming is just as distinct from 90 percent of our waking experience (which all too often is precisely marked by its lack of vividness and subjective sense of significance) as it is from 90 percent of our dreaming experience" (1989: 120).

A similar observation is made by Rechtschaffen: "the fact of occasional lucidity in dreams is useful as a demonstration of what most dreams are not" (1978: 100). The implication of Hunt's and Rechtschaffen's remarks is that lucid dreaming is not only unusual, but stands in stark contrast to nonlucid dreaming, with its lack of self-reflection and volitional control. (Also see Foulkes 1990, 1991.) More recently, even noted "deficiency" theorist Allan Hobson has acknowledged that lucid dreaming may occur with some frequency for certain individuals, but he has also taken the position that lucid dreaming should be considered a unique dream state, with its own neurophysiological correlates. (See Hobson et al. 2000.) Again, lucid dreaming is set apart from "most" dreaming, which many theorists continue to believe is deficient in the high-order cognitive skills that characterize waking cognition. However, researchers like Stephen LaBerge and Jayne Gackenbach have established that lucid dreaming is far from infrequent and that most people who are motivated to develop lucid dreaming skills are able to do so. (See Gackenbach and LaBerge 1988).

Metacognition in Nonlucid Dreaming

What of metacognition in *non*lucid dreaming, where there is no explicit awareness of dreaming while dreaming? Interestingly, many theorists have asserted that high-order cognitive skills do occur in nonlucid dreaming (Cartwright 1981; Cicogna et al. 1991;

Fitch and Armitage 1989; Foulkes 1985; Kahan 1994; Levin 2000; Mason et al. 1997; Moffitt 1995; Purcell et al. 1986; Rossi 1985; Snyder 1970). (See table 22.2 for representative claims.) And a number of empirical studies have investigated the occurrence of metacognition in nonlucid dreaming (e.g., Bradley, Hollifield, and Foulkes 1992; Kahan 1994; Kahan and LaBerge 1996; Kahan, LaBerge, Levitan, and Zimbardo 1997; Purcell et al. 1993; Purcell et al. 1986; Snyder 1970).[3]

Snyder (1970) conducted a large-scale study comparing the phenomenology of waking and dreaming. This work is described in a chapter by Schwartz, Weinstein, and Arkin (1978) in the first volume of *The Mind in Sleep* (Arkin et al. 1978). Snyder collected 635 reports from REM sleep from 58 adult men and women over 250 subject nights and rated numerous aspects of their content. (See Schwartz et al. 1978: 147–151.) Snyder concluded that dreams are "not so dreamy after all" (150) and that cognition across waking and dreaming is essentially continuous. According to Schwartz et al., "[T]he broadest generalization possible about the nature of dream experience is its more or less faithful reflection of daily life" (148). Of particular interest is Snyder's observation of volition in dreams: "references to making decisions (either their mere contemplation or actual implementation) were present in 10–50 percent of subjects' dreams," and of "reflective contemplation: silent observation and detached musing about dream events external to the self appeared in about 17–75 percent of dreams. . . . In general, all of these four cognitive elements, volition, reasoning, memory processes, and reflection were least often observed in the group of short dreams and most often seen in the dreams of over 300 words" (149).

Table 22.2 Theorists Who Claim that Metacognition Does Occur in Dreaming

Theorist	*Claim*
Snyder (1970)	The ongoing "reflectiveness" in REM dreaming is similar to that of waking.
Cartwright (1981)	The qualitative aspects of dreaming and waking mentation are similarly rhythmic.
Foulkes (1985)	Dreaming includes the same range of cognitive abilities as waking.
Rossi (1986)	There is a continuity of dialectical conscious processes between waking and dreaming.
Purcell et al. (1986)	Self-reflection does characterize dreaming, especially REM dreaming.
Fitch & Armitage (1989)	Sleep mentation is on a continuum with, and directly affects, waking cognition (p. 873)
Cicogna et al. (1991)	Abstract self-reference does occur during dreaming and is not restricted to REM sleep.
Moffitt (1995)	[Dreaming shows] similar variation in the organization of consciousness as does waking awareness, from nonmindedness through singlemindedness to fully reflective awareness of self and state (p. 29).
Mason et al. (1997)	Reflective awareness occurs during REM and slow-wave sleep.

Curiously, Schwartz et al. discount Snyder's research on the basis of "many methodological flaws" (150), yet they acknowledge (151) that the same basic patterns were observed by Kramer, Winget, and Whitman (1971). The fact that Snyder's findings did not, at the time, inspire widespread research into the relationship between waking and dreaming cognition underlines the general acceptance of the historical view that dreaming and waking are dissociated. And although Snyder did investigate dream phenomenology (Snyder, Karacan, Thorp, and Scott 1968; Snyder 1970), he did not continue this line of inquiry. It is interesting to note that thirteen years later, in the second volume of *The Mind in Sleep,* Schwartz and colleagues again discuss the qualitative aspects of sleep mentation (Weinstein et al. 1991) and argue that self-reflection is altogether suspended in REM sleep.[4]

Sheila Purcell, Alan Moffitt, and their colleagues at Carleton University developed a scale for measuring dream self-reflectiveness based on Rossi's developmental theory of self-reflectiveness (Rossi 1972, 1985). Purcell et al. utilized their dream self-reflectiveness (DSR) scale in two studies (both reported in Purcell et al. 1986). The first experiment assessed the level of DSR in dreams sampled from different sleep stages; the second experiment determined whether DSR could be increased through attentional training. In the first study, twelve individuals who remembered more than five dreams per week (high-frequency dream recallers) and twelve individuals who recalled fewer than one dream per week (low-frequency dream recallers) spent four nights in the sleep lab. Each night dream reports were requested following scheduled awakenings from stages 4, 2, and REM sleep, and upon awakening. The narrative reports were later scored by two raters for the highest level of self-reflection exhibited in the dream. For each participant, a mean SR score was computed for all dreams recalled from a given sleep. The main finding was that mean SR was higher for the seventy-one reported REM dreams (M = 4.22) than for the fifty reported stage 2 dreams (M = 3.45) or for the nineteen reported stage 4 dreams (M = 3.74). Self- reflectiveness in stage 2 and stage 4 dreams did not differ. There were also individual differences in DSR: high-frequency dream recallers had higher DSR scores than did low-frequency dream recallers, and the DSR score was more highly correlated with word count for high-frequency dream recallers.[5]

The typical SR score was 3 ("dreamer completely involved in dream drama; no other perspective"), a finding that could be used to argue that dreams often do not involve self-reflection. However, dream metacognition is clearly seen in reports with DSR scores of 5 (internal commentary), 7 (self-reflection: dual perspectives of participant and observer), 8 (volition), or 9 (lucid dreaming). (The scale value of 6 is more appropriately considered a measure of dream bizarreness than of dream self-reflection.) Summing across these four scale values (5, 7, 8, or 9), then, metacognitive skills were observed in roughly 40 percent of REM dreams, 20 percent of stage 2 dreams, and 25 percent of stage 4 dreams. (See Purcell et al. 1986: 42). In Experiment 2, Purcell et al. demonstrated that the level of DSR could be increased experimentally, particularly for the Schema group, which combined reality testing ("Am I dreaming now") and prospective memory training (remembering to engage in schema rehearsal whenever a leather bracelet worn during the study was noticed). The research of Purcell et al. (1986) is compelling because it indicates that dreams sampled in the laboratory include a higher incidence of metacognition than was previously claimed, that dream SR is correlated with self-reported dream recall frequency, and that the level of dream SR can be increased through experimental manipulation of intention and attention. At the same time, several methodological limitations need to be acknowledged. First, and most important, is the questionable construct validity of the DSR scale. This scale confounds several different metacognitive skills (self-reflection, intentionality, control), and also includes scale values that have little to do with self-reflection (e.g., scale value 6, which measures transformations, an aspect of dream bizarreness). Thus, this scale is not measuring what it was designed to measure: the *continuum* of self-reflection (see Kahan 1994 for further discussion of issues in measuring dream self-reflection.) Second, all of the participants in Experiment 2 were from the same college class, and this class was instructed by one of the primary investigators. This selection procedure increases the likelihood that demand characteristics and experimenter bias impacted the results. These students, who were assigned to one of five different groups for the experiment, may well have discussed the experiment among themselves. Also, participants may have chosen to report only those dreams they felt were consistent with the implied goal of increasing dream self-reflection; indeed, groups with higher SR had fewer dreams. Nevertheless, the Purcell et al. (1986) studies are important because they represent the first experimental work to directly investigate self-reflection in dreaming. (Also see Darling, Hoffmann, Moffitt, and Purcell 1993 for research on the stability of DSR scores across temporal units of the same dreams collected by Purcell et al. 1986.)

In a subsequent, more carefully controlled study, Purcell et al. (1993) essentially replicated their earlier findings regarding the distribution of dream self-reflection scores, with the notable difference that the modal dream SR score was now 5 ("dreamer thinks over an idea or has definite communication with someone"), compared with the earlier modal dream SR score of 3 ("dreamer completely involved in dream drama") (Purcell et al. 1986). (See Kahan 1994 for a study that reveals a similar distribution of DSR scores.)

Purcell et al. (1993) also developed a nine-category scale to measure intentionality in dreaming (dream control), with higher numbers representing greater intentionality. For example, a category 8 rating indicates the dream involved intentional regulation of some aspect of the dream mechanics, and a category 9 rating is given when intentional control is evident *and* the dreamer is aware of dreaming (lucid-control dreaming).

Ninety-five participants kept dream journals for three weeks in the context of one of three instructional conditions similar to those used by Purcell et al. (1986). The Baseline group was asked only to keep the dream journal. The Attention Control group completed a report skills questionnaire in addition to recording any dreams. The Schema group recorded their dreams and completed the dream control questionnaire (week 2) and the self-reflectiveness scale (week 3). The Schema group, which engaged in schema rehearsal (e.g., "Am I dreaming now?") whenever they noticed the leather bracelet they were assigned to wear, was the only group taught dream control. Each group included roughly the same number of self-reported frequent and infrequent dream recallers. Overall, frequent dream recallers showed more dream control (M = 5.1) than did infrequent recallers (M = 4.8), and, for all subjects, the mean level of dream control increased across the three weeks. These results again demonstrated that metacognitive skills—volition, in this case—do occur in dreaming and that metacognition can be increased simply by increasing one's attention to the reporting of dreams and reinforcing the intention to notice the process or content characteristics of one's dreams. Purcell et al. further conclude that their results "are supportive of a feedback loop between [waking and dreaming] states, mediated by attention and intention, by which both states can co-evolve" (1986: 244–245). (Also see Moffitt et al. 1988.)

Kahan (1994) compared two approaches to the measurement of dream self-reflectiveness and volition: third-person ratings (using the Moffitt DSR scale) and participants' first-person ratings of the content and process dimensions of their dreams. Eighteen female and twelve male college students made journal entries five days a week for three weeks in order to raise their level of dream recall. During the next two weeks, participants recorded and evaluated eight dreams (four dreams per week), using the Dream Rating Scale (after Johnson 1988; Johnson, Foley, Suengas, and Raye 1988; Johnson, Kahan, and Raye 1984). Third-person ratings were made by first transcribing the participants' 239 reports and then scoring them for dream self-reflectiveness using the Moffitt DSR scale. The distribution of SR scores obtained by Kahan (1994) was remarkably similar to that reported by Purcell et al. (1993: 228). Consistent with Purcell et al., the judges in Kahan's (1994) study scored Category 8 ("control") for 1.3 percent of the dream narratives and Category 9 ("lucidity") for .8 percent of the dream narratives. These percentages contrast with the incidence of control (volitional dreaming), particularly self-control, when rated by participants: 72 percent of the dreams were rated as including "control over own thoughts" and 64 percent were rated as including "control over their own feelings." (See Kahan 1994, table 1.) Overall, participants reported the same metacognitive skills as were noted by judges in the narrative reports. However, the incidence of these metacognitive skills was higher when participants assessed their own dream experiences using the Dream Rating Scale, compared with the judges' ratings of participants' narrative reports. Kahan's findings suggest that the incidence of metacognition may be seriously underrepresented in the narrative reports and underscore the need to develop alternative measures of dream metacognition.

Kahan (1994) also observed that 23 percent of the dream reports were rated as including some awareness of control but no awareness of dreaming, and 15 percent of the reports were rated as including some awareness of dreaming but no awareness of control. (See table 22.3.) Thus, although the awareness of dreaming (lucidity) and volition in dreaming (dream control) are highly correlated, these two dimensions of metacognition are dissociable. (Also see LaBerge 1985; Purcell et al. 1993.) So, although increased self-focus has been found to increase self-regulation in dreaming (Purcell et al. 1993) and in waking (Carver and Scheier 1981), increased self-focus may not typically include an explicit awareness of *state.*

In summary, the research reviewed above offers evidence that dreaming does involve metacognition, including self-reflection, intentionality, and self-regulation. This work presents a clear challenge to the traditional view that metacognition is absent in dreaming. As such, these studies are important in their own right. At the same time, a number of methodological and theoretical issues have yet to be resolved. For example, what constitutes the most valid (and reliable) measure(s) of dream metacognition? First-person ratings of the process aspects of dreaming? Third-person ratings of the narrative report? Some combination of the two? (See, e.g., Wilson 1994.) And should dreams be sampled in the home setting, the laboratory setting, or both? From a theoretical standpoint, does the occurrence of self-reflection in dreaming mean that dreaming and waking are *continuous?* Continuity implies relatively greater similarity (than dissimilarity) across waking and dreaming, including nonlucid dreaming, and that the same range of cognitive (and metacognitive) skills occurs across waking/dreaming. The underlying assumption here is that the *same* cognitive system that operates during waking also operates during sleep/dreaming. (See Antrobus 1991; Cavallero and Foulkes 1993; Foulkes 1985, 1993, 1999; Hall and Norby 1972; Hunt 1989; Kerr 1993; Levin 2000; Moffitt 1995.)

The question of how dream metacognition and waking metacognition are related cannot be answered without assessing the variety and frequency of reflective and other metacognitive activities in dreaming relative to waking (Kahan and LaBerge 1994, 1996). This call was issued by Cavallero and Foulkes (1993: 137): "If we take the possibility of continuities in waking and dreaming mentation seriously, we not only must study both in a comprehensive study of the human mind, but also must study them comparably."

The next section discusses recent research in which the goal was to obtain comparable samples of metacognition in dreaming and in waking.

Metacognition Across Dreaming and Waking

Notwithstanding the methodological challenges associated with obtaining "equivalent" measures of waking and dreaming experience (see Kahan and LaBerge 1994 for a discussion of this issue), a clear understanding of cross-state cognition and metacognition requires that measures of the content and process characteristics of dreaming be compared with measures of waking experience that are as comparable as possible. If a person's metacognitive skills in dreaming are assessed retrospectively, for example, then the same person's metacognitive skills in waking should also be evaluated retrospectively.

In a series of studies (Kahan and LaBerge 1996; Kahan et al. 1997; Kahan and LaBerge 2000) involving, over time, increased rigor in the methods used to sample dreaming and waking experiences, the objective was to obtain comparable measures of metacognitive skills across waking and sleep. The next section first describes the method used in each study to obtain samples of waking and dreaming metacognition. Then, a comparison of the findings across the three studies is made in order to highlight consistent patterns in the incidence of different aspects of metacognition across waking and sleep.

Kahan et al. (1997) obtained samples of waking and dreaming metacognition from thirty-eight "practiced/lucid" dreamers and fifty "novice" dreamers. The practiced dreamers were members of an organization that provides educational and research opportunities related to lucid dreaming. The eighteen male and twenty female individuals reported average dream recall of eight dreams per week, with a range of zero to twenty eight, prior to the study, and 84 percent of the participants reported having had at least one lucid dream in the prior six months. Upon awakening from a dream that was clearly remembered, these "practiced" dreamers provided a narrative report of the dream and completed the Metacognitive, Affective, and Cognitive Experience (MACE) questionnaire, which assessed the incidence emotion and eight dimensions of metacognition: Choice, Internal Commentary, Unexpected Attention, Sustained Attention, Public Self-Consciousness, Event-Related Self-Reflection, Event-Unrelated Self-Reflection, and Unusual Experiences. (See Kahan et al. 1997: 137.) For the waking sample, participants again provided a narrative report of their experience, this time for the fifteen minutes prior to their reading of the instructions for the study, and then completed the MACE.

The "novice dreamers" were twenty-six male and twenty-four female college students; only 6 percent of these individuals reported having had at least one lucid dream in the past six months. For the dream sample, all subjects chose a weekend morning to report a well-remembered dream and also complete the MACE. For the waking sample, half of the participants were called by an experimenter at a random time during the day; the remaining participants stopped their activities at 2 P.M. on a prearranged day and reported and rated their waking experiences. Novice dreamers assessed the presence of emotion and seven dimensions of metacognition: Choice, Internal Commentary, Unexpected Attention, Sustained Attention, Public Self-Consciousness, Event-related Self-Reflection, and Thwarted Intention.

In the Kahan and LaBerge (1996) study, the narrative reports of dreaming and waking from forty of the original fifty "novice" dreamers in the Kahan et al. (1997) study were assessed by two independent raters. The raters used the MACE to evaluate the incidence of metacognition in the narrative reports, permitting a comparison of first- and third-person ratings of metacognition across the samples of dreaming and waking experience.

The third study (Kahan and LaBerge 2001) involved twenty-six individuals, with an age range of eighteen to fifty-two, whose average dream recall was between five to eight dreams per week. Participants again used the MACE to judge the presence or absence of emotion and various metacognitive activities in sleep and waking. However, Kahan and LaBerge increased the rigor of the methods used to sample waking and dreaming experiences. A variation of the event sampling procedure employed by Kerr, Foulkes, and Schmidt (1982) was used to obtain six event samples from each participant, four from sleep and two from waking. Also, the timing of the samples was controlled with the use of specially designed equipment.

Two samples were obtained from REM sleep and two from NREM sleep using the DreamLight®, a computerized device developed by Stephen LaBerge to induce lucid dreams. The DreamLight is intended for home use and is similar to Hobson's Nightcap. (See Mamelak and Hobson 1989; Stickgold et al. 1994.) Sensors in the DreamLight mask relay information about vertical eye movements and head movements to the computer, which uses this information to predict REM or NREM sleep. Studies in the sleep lab that compared standard polysomnographic measures with sleep staging from the DreamLight have established that the DreamLight is generally reliable in discriminating REM sleep, NREM sleep, and waking (LaBerge and Levitan 1995).

Waking samples were obtained with the aid of a preprogrammed beeper (the Programmable Electronic State Tester or PEST®), also developed by Stephen LaBerge. The participant wore the beeper on a chosen day and also kept an envelope containing the reporting materials handy. When the beeper vibrated, the participant stopped his or her activities and provided a one-page description of the events of the roughly fifteen-minute period just prior to the sounding of the beeper. The participant also completed the MACE questionnaire.

In each of these studies, samples of waking and dreaming experiences were obtained and the participants evaluated various dimensions of metacognition using the MACE questionnaire. Table 22.3 presents the percentage of "yes" responses to each question for experiences sampled from NREM, REM, and waking. Several interesting patterns emerge in these data. First, metacognition occurs with considerable frequency in dreaming, including NREM dreaming. Second, four types of metacognition occurred with comparable frequency across waking and both REM and NREM dreaming (Sudden Attention, Unusual Difficulty, and Self-Reflection on External Events), and three types of metacognition occurred with comparable frequency across waking and REM sleep (Internal Commentary, Sustained Attention, and Public Self-Consciousness). Only three of the measured dimensions occurred with higher frequency in waking than in REM sleep (Choice, Self-Reflection on own thoughts and feelings, and Self-Reflection on own behavior). Thus, these data indicate that metacognition in dreaming, especially dreaming sampled from REM sleep, is more similar to waking cognition than it is different

Questions concerning the incidence of emotion and six dimensions of metacognition were common to all three studies, thereby permitting an informal cross-study comparison of these dimensions: Choice, Internal Commentary, Unexpected Attention, Sustained Attention, Public Self-Consciousness, and Self-Reflectiveness. In the first two studies (Kahan and LaBerge 1996; Kahan et al. 1997), the question about self-reflection asked whether any instance of self-reflection occurred: "Did you think about your own thoughts, feelings, attitudes, motivations, or behavior?" In the third study, which sampled both REM and NREM dreams (and waking experiences), three different questions were asked about the incidence of self-reflection: "Did you think about your own thoughts or feelings?" "Did you think about what you were doing?" "Did you think about what was happening around you?" (See table 22.3.)

Metacognition More Often Attributed to Waking Than to Dreaming Experiences

Across all three studies, as well as across third-person and first-person ratings (Kahan and LaBerge 1996), "choice" was less often associated with dreaming experiences than with waking experiences (See table 22.4.) Novice dreamers (Kahan and LaBerge

Table 22.3 Percentage of "Yes" Responses to MACE Questions about Different Aspects of Metacognitive Experiences[a] Sampled from NREM Sleep, REM Sleep, and Waking (N = 26)

	When Samples Were Obtained				
Dimension	*NREM (NR)*	*REM (R)*	*Waking (W)*	*R:W Ratio*	*NR:W Ratio*
Choice[b]	19%	52%	69%	.75	.28
Internal commentary[d]	38%	60%	58%	1.03	.66
Sudden attention[e]	25%	33%	38%	.87	.66
Focused attention[d]	37%	63%	75%	.84	.50
Public self-consciousness[d]	19%	38%	27%	1.41	.83
Emotion[e]	62%	75%	75%	1.00	.83
Self-reflection (on):					
Own thoughts/feelings[c]	19%	27%	44%	.61	.43
Own behavior[c]	29%	44%	65%	.68	.45
External events[e]	38%	52%	42%	1.24	.90

[a]These dimensions represent those that were evaluated in two other two studies (Kahan & LaBerge 1996; Kahan et al. 1997), as well as in this study (Kahan & LaBerge 2001).
[b]Waking > REM > NREM, $p < .05$.
[c]Waking > REM = NREM, $p < .05$.
[d]Waking = REM > NREM, $p < .05$.
[e]Waking = REM = NREM, $p < .05$.

1996; Kahan et al. 1997; Kahan and LaBerge 2000) attributed "choice" to about 46 percent of their dreams, and practiced/lucid dreamers (Kahan et al. 1997) to about 53 percent of their dreams. The same percentages for waking reports were 79 percent (novice dreamers) and 69 percent (practiced dreamers), respectively. Overall, participants rated about 50 percent of their dreaming versus 74 percent of their waking experiences as including "choice." Independent raters observed "choice" in 10 percent of participants' dream reports and in 30 percent of participants' waking reports (Kahan and LaBerge 1996). Choice may have been overrepresented in the first two studies because the sampling method required participants to select the time they provided their waking sample. As such, their experiences during the prior fifteen minutes necessarily involved making a choice.

The incidence of Self-Reflection was, in general, also lower in dreaming than in waking. Novice dreamers (Kahan and LaBerge 1996; Kahan et al. 1997; Kahan and LaBerge 2000) attributed "Self-Reflection"(SR) to about 45 percent of their dreams, and practiced/lucid dreamers (Kahan et al. 1997) to about 40 percent of their dreams. For waking reports, these percentages were 54 percent and 55 percent, respectively. The third study (Kahan and LaBerge 2000) asked about three different objects of self-reflection. A higher percentage of waking experiences were rated as including SR "on own thoughts or feelings" (44 percent) or "on own behavior" (65 percent), as compared with the same ratings of dreaming experiences (19 percent and 29 percent, respectively). On the other hand, SR on external events was more often attributed to REM dreaming (52 percent) than to waking (38 percent) or NREM (38 percent) experiences. Thus, it may well be that the incidence of self-reflection varies with the "object" of the reflection and/or the sleep stage from which experiences are sampled.

Table 22.4 Aspects of Metacognition Tending to Have a Higher Frequency in Waking than in Dreaming

Dimension	*Sample*[a]	*(N)*	*Dreaming Episode(s)*	*Waking Episode(s)*	*D:W Ratio*
Choice	Pract (P)	(38)	.53	.79	.67[b]
	Novice #1 (N1)	(50)	.46	.84	.55[b]
	P + N1	(88)	.50	.82	.55[b]
	Novice #2	(40)	.40	.83	.48[b]
	Judges	(2)	.10	.30	.33[b]
Self-reflection	Pract	(38)	.40	.55	.71
	Novice #1	(50)	.48	.62	.77
	P + N1	(88)	.44	.59	.75[b]
	Novice #2	(40)	.53	.63	.84
	Judges	(2)	.33	.50	.66

[a]Samples were the Practiced Dreamers (N = 38) (Pract) and the Novice Dreamers (N = 50) (Novice #1) described in Kahan et al. 1997, and the Novice Dreamers (N = 40) (Novice #2) and Independent Judges (N = 2) (Judges) described in Kahan & LeBerge 1996. The Novice #2 sample is a subset of the Novice #1 sample; the Judges' ratings were made of the dream reports provided by the Novice #2 sample.
[b]Comparison between dreaming and waking is significant at $p < .05$.

In short, of the six dimensions that were measured in all three studies, only Choice and certain types of Self-Reflection were consistently attributed to waking experience more often than to dreaming experience.

Metacognition More Often Attributed to Dreaming Than to Waking Experiences

In all three studies conducted by Kahan and her colleagues, Public Self-Consciousness (PSC) was consistently attributed to dreaming experiences (40 percent of all dreams) more often than to waking experiences (26 percent of all waking experiences). (See table 22.5.) However, the comparison of PSC in dreaming versus waking reached significance only for the Practiced/Lucid dreamers and for the analysis that combined the Novice and Practiced Dreamers. (See Kahan et al. 1997). PSC in waking may well have been underestimated given that the procedure for sampling waking experience, especially in the first two studies, inclined participants to make their waking reports and ratings when they were alone. Even in the third study, in which the waking samples were taken following a beeper signal, participants could elect to wait until the next signal if the timing was inconvenient, for example, if the individual was driving and could not pull over easily. Perhaps participants were also inclined to defer to the next signal when they were with other people.

A similar pattern was observed for Emotion, which, although it is not a metacognitive skill, is often considered to be a "defining" feature of dreaming (Hartmann 1998; Hobson 1988; 1993; Kramer 1993). Emotion was more often attributed to dreaming experiences (89 percent of all dreams) than to waking experiences (76 percent) when participants reported and rated a dream they remembered well upon awakening in the morning (spon-

Table 22.5 Aspects of Metacognition and Emotion Tending to Have Higher Frequencies in Dreaming than in Waking

Dimension	*Sample*[a]	*(N)*	*Dreaming Episode(s)*	*Waking Episode(s)*	*D:W Ratio*
Public self-consciousness	Pract (P)	(38)	.53	.32	1.66
	Novice #1 (N1)	(50)	.34	.22	1.55
	P + N1	(88)	.44	.27	1.63[b]
	Novice #2	(40)	.35	.23	1.52
	Judges	(2)	.20	.20	1.00
	Pract	(38)	.87	.71	1.22
Emotion	Novice #1	(50)	.92	.80	1.15
	P + N1	(88)	.89	.76	1.17[b]
	Novice #2	(40)	.93	.83	1.12
	Judges	(2)	.38	.35	1.09

[a]Samples were the Practiced Dreamers (N = 38) (Pract) and the Novice Dreamers (N = 50) (Novice #1) described in Kahan et al. 1997, and the Novice Dreamers (N = 40) (Novice #2) and Independent Judges (N = 2) (Judges) described in Kahan & LeBerge 1996. The Novice #2 sample is a subset of the Novice #1 sample; the Judges' ratings were made of the dream reports provided by the Novice #2 sample.
[b]Comparison between dreaming and waking is significant at $p < .05$.

taneous dream recall) (Kahan and LaBerge 1996; Kahan et al. 1997). However, in the DreamLight study, for dreams sampled from late-night REM and NREM sleep, emotion was attributed to dream reports and waking reports equally often (62 percent, 75 percent, and 75 percent for NREM, REM, and waking experiences, respectively).

Metacognition Attributed to Dreaming and Waking Experiences with Comparable Frequencies

In all three studies, the incidence of "Internal Commentary" was comparably high for dreaming and waking experiences. (See table 22.6.) Overall, 75 percent of all dreaming and 71 percent of all waking experiences were rated by participants as including "Internal Commentary."

No consistent trend was observed for either Sustained Attention or Sudden Attention. In general, 69 percent of the dreaming and 69 percent of the waking experiences were rated as including "Focused Attention." However, two out of the three samples (Practiced Dreamers in Kahan et al. 1997, and participants in Kahan and LaBerge 2000) attributed focused attention to waking experiences more often than to dreaming experiences. The opposite relationship was observed in the sample of novice dreamers (Kahan et al. 1997). In general, 60 percent of the dreaming and 47 percent of the waking experiences were rated as including "Sudden Attention." However, this time, two of the samples (Practiced Dreamers and Novice Dreamers in Kahan et al. 1997) attributed sudden attention more often to *dreaming* than to waking experiences. In the third study, sudden attention was attributed to dreaming and to waking with

Table 22.6 Aspects of Metacognition and Emotion Tending to Have Comparable Frequencies in Dreaming and Waking

Dimension	*Sample*[a]	*(N)*	*Dreaming Episode(s)*	*Waking Episode(s)*	*D:W Ratio*
Internal commentary	Pract (P)	(38)	.92	.87	1.06
	Novice #1 (N1)	(50)	.88	.80	1.1
	P + N1	(88)	.90	.84	1.07
	Novice #2	(40)	.90	.83	1.08
	Judges	(2)	.63	.68	.93
Focused attention	Pract	(38)	.76	.84	.91
	Novice #1	(25)	.68	.48	1.42[c]
	Novice #2	(40)	.55	.58	.95
	Judges	(2)	.48	.58	.83

[a]Samples were the Practiced Dreamers (N = 38) (Pract) and the Novice Dreamers (N = 50) (Novice #1) described in Kahan et al. 1997, and the Novice Dreamers (N = 40) (Novice #2) and Independent Judges (N = 2) (Judges) described in Kahan & LeBerge 1996. The Novice #2 sample is a subset of the Novice #1 sample; the Judges' ratings were made of the dream reports provided by the Novice #2 sample.
[b]Comparison between dreaming and waking is significant at $p < .05$.
[c]Comparison involved only the 25 Novice Dreamers who selected the time for recording the waking episode, because the "will-call" instructions for the other 25 participants artificially elevated the incidence of focused attention in the waking condition (Kahan & LaBerge 1996).

comparably low frequencies (25 percent, 33 percent, and 38 percent for NREM, REM, and Waking experiences, respectively). (See table 22.3.)

In summary, this series of studies clearly demonstrates that metacognition does occur in dreaming, including NREM dreaming. Across the three studies, a consistent cross-state relationship was observed for a number of metacognitive skills (e.g., Choice; Self-Reflection; Public Self-Consciousness; Internal Commentary) as well as for emotion. The patterns for Sustained Attention and Focused Attention were less reliable. The findings of Kahan and her colleagues indicate that dream metacognition occurs with considerable frequency, that the differences in metacognitive skills across waking and dreaming are more likely quantitative than qualitative, and that metacognition in dreaming, especially dreaming sampled from REM sleep, is more similar to waking cognition than it is different. Kahan's research also suggests we need a more nuance understanding of the relationship between waking and dreaming cognition. There are *both* similarities and differences in cognition and metacognition across waking and sleep, and additional research is needed to map these cross-state variations. (Also see Kahan and LaBerge, 2001.)

Dreaming Cognition, Waking Cognition: Some Considerations for Future Research

When designing future research on cross-state variations in consciousness and cognition, both methodological and theoretical issues warrant consideration.

Methodological Issues.

First, it is important to consider the ways in which theoretical biases might impact one's measurement approach. For example, if we make the a priori assumption that reflective awareness or intentionality does not characterize dreaming experience, then we are less likely to work to develop reliable methods for measuring such events. Similarly, if we assume that reflectiveness or intentionality do characterize dreaming, participants may be inclined to overstate the presence of these events in order to "please" the investigators. Or if we believe that waking is uniformly "conscious" and rational and that we can simply assume the characteristics of waking as the backdrop against which we compare dreaming, then we are not likely to make an effort to systematically compare the cognitive, metacognitive, or affective characteristics of dreaming and waking.

Second, what constitute the most valid (and reliable) measures of metacognition across sleep and waking? For example, what is the most appropriate waking situation to compare with dreaming? Some investigators have compared dreaming with waking imagery (Levin 2000; Strauch and Meier 1996), whereas others have compared dreaming with waking *experience* (Kahan and LaBerge 1996, 2001; Kahan et al. 1997). What are the most appropriate research techniques for sampling dreaming and waking consciousness? (See Pekala 1991.) Are questionnaire-based measures that utilize affirmative probes, such as those employed by Kahan and her colleagues and Hobson and his colleagues (Hobson and Stickgold 1994) more valid and reliable than third-person ratings of narrative reports? (See Kahan 1994.) How many participants and how many samples are needed to obtain "stable" measures? Should measures taken in the home setting or the lab setting? How critical is the need for converging measures of phenomenology, cognition, and psychophysiology? As Howard Gardner (1994: 44–45) has suggested: "If cognitive scientists want to give a complete account of the most central features of cognition [and consciousness], they (or other scientists) will have to discover or construct the bridges connecting their discipline to neighboring areas of study—specifically, to neuroscience at the lower bound, so to speak, and to cultural studies at the upper."

Converging measures of phenomenology, cognition, and neurophysiology would be helpful, not for purposes of reducing one level of analysis to another, but in order to understand the correspondences between these different levels and whether there are neurophysiological or state constraints on consciousness. (Also see Antrobus 1991; Kahan and LaBerge 1994; Nelson 1996; Varela et al. 1995.)

Theoretical Issues

Future research also should consider individual difference factors beyond dream recall frequency. It may well be that some of the findings from the "discontinuity" and "continuity" camps could be accounted for by individual differences. David Foulkes's longitudinal studies of children's dreaming, for example, clearly demonstrate that the cognitive sophistication of dreaming is related to waking cognitive development (Foulkes 1995, 1999). There is also a development course for the acquisition of metacognitive skills, although not all individuals develop all aspects of metacognition. (See Byrnes 2001; Foulkes et al. 1991; Kuhn 2000.) Furthermore, cognitive and other characteristics of dreams have been shown to be related to individual differences in, for example, experiencing level (Hendricks and Cartwright 1978), waking affective insight (Nielsen, Kuiken, and McGregor 1989), creativity (Domino 1982; Levin and Lamontoro 1997–98), attitude toward dreams (Tonay 1993), need for cognition (Blagrove and Hartnell 2000), daydreaming style (Starker 1984–85), mental boundaries (Hartmann, Rosen, and Rand 1998), absorption in imaginings (Schredl, Jochum, and Souguenet 1997), and current concerns (Saredi, Baylor, Meier, and Strauch 1997).

The characteristics of an individual's dreams are also influenced by his or her presleep intentions or motivation, as demonstrated in LaBerge's research on lucid dreaming and the work of Purcell, Moffitt and their colleagues on nonlucid dreams. Interest and practice in "cultivating" dreaming skills (lucid control dreaming, problem-solving dreams, or "teaching" dreams) will, therefore, have an impact on the level of dream recall as well as the specific characteristics of those dreams (Cartwright and Lamberg 1992; Hunt 1989; LaBerge 1985; Tedlock 1992; Young 1999). As Purcell et al. (1986: 436) write: "attention paid to dreaming sets in motion the process by which waking and dreaming self-reflectiveness may become codetermining."

One's religious practices and cultural values also shape the incidence and forms of dreaming, including dream consciousness. "Attention" and "intention" are more likely to be applied to dreams and dreaming when one's religious or cultural communities encourage dreaming and dream sharing (Bulkeley, 1994; Bulkeley 2000; Hunt 1989; Jung 1965; Kuiken and Sikora 1993; Moffitt et al. 1988; Young 1999).

Buddhist scholar Serinity Young (1999: 119), for example, points to the power of dreams to transform one's waking experience: "Dreams can reveal to an individual insights so powerful that the concerns or realities of waking life are lost in the blinding light of this new awareness. Such a dream shapes their reality, shapes their understanding of the waking world."

On a related note, anthropologist Barbara Tedlock (1992) has argued that we need to put the discussion of dreaming/waking cognition and experience in the context of our Western cultural perspective on dreaming as "unreal" and waking experience as "real." Cognitive scientists, in particular, would do well to consider their bias toward waking cognition as the "pinnacle" of cognitive achievement. It is possible that dreaming cognition and consciousness surpass that of waking precisely because there are unlimited possible worlds and possible selves that can be represented in dreaming.

Conclusion

This chapter explored whether dreaming cognition and consciousness are discontinuous or continuous with waking. With a focus on the metacognitive skills of self-reflection, intentionality, and behavior regulation, we reviewed evidence for the divergent claims that metacognition is either absent or present in dreaming. Recent work on both lucid and nonlucid dreaming clearly indicates that metacognition does occur in dreaming, and with considerable frequency. This research shows that the same range of metacognitive skills occurs in dreaming as in waking, although certain metacognitive skills (e.g., choice and self-reflection on one's own thoughts, feelings, or behaviors) occur less often in dreaming than in waking.

Future research on cross-state cognition and consciousness must replicate these findings and also push both the methodological and theoretical boundaries of previous research. We need to investigate how individual differences as well as cultural and religious factors shape consciousness both within and across waking and sleep. (Also see Hunt 1995.) By considering these "boundaries" in future investigations of consciousness in dreaming and waking, and continuing to hone our methodologies, ultimately we may design a more accurate map of the entire territory of human consciousness. As Havelock Ellis remarked, "dreams are real while they last; can we say more of life?"

Notes

The preparation of this chapter was partially supported by a Santa Clara University Thomas Terry Research Grant. I am grateful to Stephen LaBerge for our years of collaboration and to all of the students who have assisted in various phases of my research. I also warmly thank Kelly Bulkeley, Harry Hunt, Ross Levin, Mark Blagrove, Don Kuiken, and Roseanne Armitage for their continued interest in my work. Appreciation goes to Dorothea French and Diane Dreher for encouraging me in my writing, to Robert Numan for providing helpful comments on an earlier draft of this chapter, and to my husband, Steve Leinau, for his support and good-humored tolerance of my many hours at the computer. This chapter is respectfully dedicated to the memory of Alan Moffitt.

1. Recently Hobson and his colleagues have focused on dream bizarreness as the most distinctive feature of dreaming and have attempted to account for dream bizarreness in terms of REM neurophysiology. (See Hobson 1988; Hobson and Stickgold 1994; Kahn and Hobson 1993; Kahn, Pace-Schott, and Hobson 1997). However, their own empirical work provides only equivocal support for this claim, and other research on dream bizarreness indicates that bizarreness is overrepresented in spontaneously recalled home dreams as compared with dreams sampled in the sleep laboratory (e.g., Bonato, Moffitt, Hoffmann, Cuddy, and Wimmer 1991; Cipolli, Bolzani, Cornoldi, De Beni, and Fatioli 1993; Robinson-Riegler and McDaniel 1994). This research raises questions about the claim that bizarreness is, in fact, the central defining feature of dreaming, as claimed by Hobson and his team (e.g., Hobson and Stickgold 1994:10).

2. Foulkes's claims regarding metacognition in dreaming are unfortunate for cognitive dream psychology. In spite of his "call" to include dreaming in the domain of cognitive psychology and the necessity for quality empirical work on dream cognition (e.g., Foulkes 1993), a ready extension of his theoretical position is that there is little value in investigating dream cognition, since it merely "reflects" waking cognition. Thus, anything that cognitive psychologists might wish to know about cognition is essentially revealed by studying waking cognition, thereby avoiding the expense of a sleep laboratory and the methodological challenges inherent in dream research. However, this seemingly sensible conclusion flies in the face of earnest arguments, including those made by Foulkes himself, of why cognitive psychologists *should* study dreaming. (See Foulkes 1985, 1991b, 1999; Foulkes and Cavallero 1993; Haskell 1986; Hunt 1986).
3. For whatever individual cases are worth, the "tree" narrative discussed earlier was a report from a nonlucid dream.
4. Weinstein, Schwartz, and Ellman (1988) define "reflective self-awareness" as "an awareness that one was having an internal, mental experience with no external referents" (p. 211). This is the traditional definition of *lucid* dreaming (Van Eeden 1913) and should not be confused with Purcell and associates' concept of "self-reflection" as an "examination of one's thoughts, feelings, and behaviors" (Purcell et al. 1986: 424). Weinstein and coworkers' claim that heightened REM activation is associated with a suspension of the awareness of state is especially curious in light of evidence that the onset of lucid dreaming is associated with phasic REM. (See LaBerge and Dement 1986; LaBerge 1988, 1990).
5. The comparisons across high- and low-frequency dream recallers included an N of forty eight, because data from Experiment 1 were combined with data from the baseline condition of Experiment 2.

References

Antrobus, J. R. 1990. "The Neurocognition of Sleep Mentation: Rapid Eye Movements, Visual Imagery, and Dreaming. In R. R. Bootzin and J. F. Kihlstrom, eds., *Sleep and Cognition* (pp. 3–24). Washington, D.C.: APA.

———. 1991. "Dreaming: Cognitive Processes during Cortical Activation and High Perceptual Thresholds." *Psychological Review* 98: 96–121.

Arkin, A. M., Antrobus, J. S., and Ellman, S. J., eds. 1978. *The Mind in Sleep: Psychology and Psychophysiology.* Hillsdale, NJ: Lawrence Erlbaum Associates.

Baars, B. 1997. *In the Theater of Consciousness: The Workspace of the Mind.* New York: Oxford University Press.

Blagrove, M. 1992. "Dreaming and Thinking." Paper presented at the 9th International Conference of the Association for the Study of Dreams, Santa Cruz, CA.

Blagrove, M., and Hartnell. 2000. "Lucid Dreaming: Associations with Internal Locus of Control, Need for Cognition and Creativity." *Personality and Individual Differences* 28: 41–47.

Bonato, R. A., Moffitt, A. R., Hoffmann, R. F., Cuddy, M. A., and Wimmer, F. L. 1991. "Bizarreness in Dreams and Nightmares." *Dreaming* 1(1): 53–61.

Bradley, L., Hollifield, M., and Foulkes, D. 1992. "Reflection during REM Dreaming." *Dreaming* 2(3): 161–166.

Brylowski, A., Levitan, L., and LaBerge, S. 1989. "H-Reflex Suppression and Autonomic Activation during Lucid REM Sleep: A Case Study." *Sleep* 12: 374–378.

Bulkeley, K. 1994. *The Wilderness of Dreams: Exploring the Religious Meanings of Dreams in Modern Western Culture.* Albany: State University of New York Press.

———. 1997. *An Introduction to the Psychology of Dreaming.* Westport, CT: Praeger.

———. 2000. *Transforming Dreams: Learning Spiritual Lessons from the Dreams You Never Forget.* New York: John Wiley and Sons.

Byrnes, J. P. 2001. *Cognitive Development and Learning in Instructional Contexts.* Boston: Allyn and Bacon.

Cartwright, R. 1981. "The Contribution of Research on Memory and Dreaming to a 24-Hour Model of Cognitive Behavior." In W. Fishbein, ed., *Sleep, Dreams and Memory* (pp. 239–247). New York: Scientific Books.

Cartwright, R., and Lamberg, L. 1992. *Crisis Dreaming: Using Your Dreams to Solve Your Problems.* New York: HarperCollins.

Carver, C., and Scheier, M. 1981. *Attention and Self-Regulation: A Control-Theory Approach to Human Behavior.* New York: Springer-Verlag.

Cavallero, C., and Cicogna, P. 1993. "Memory and Dreaming." In C. Cavallero and D. Foulkes, *Dreaming as Cognition* (pp. 38–57). New York: Harvester-Wheatsheaf.

Cavallero, C., and Foulkes, D., eds. 1993. *Dreaming as Cognition.* New York: Harvester-Wheatsheaf.

Cicogna, P., Cavallero, C., and Bosinelli, M. 1991. "Cognitive Aspects of Mental Activity during Sleep." *American Journal of Psychology* 104(3): 413–425.

Cipolli, C., Bolzani, R., Cornoldi, C., De Beni, R., and Fagioli, I. 1993. "Bizarreness Effect in Dream Recall." *Sleep* 16(2): 163–170.

Crick, F., and Mitchison, G. 1983. "The Function of Dream Sleep." *Nature* 304: 111–114.

Darling, M., Hoffmann, R., Moffitt, A., and Purcell, S. 1993. "The Pattern of Self-Reflectiveness in Dream Reports." *Dreaming* 3(1): 9–19.

Dennett, D. 1978. "Toward a Cognitive Theory of Consciousness." In D. C. Dennett, ed., *Brainstorms.* Cambridge, MA: Bradford Books/MIT Press.

Doherty, C. 2001. Unpublished data (by permission of the author).

Domhoff, W. 1999. "Drawing Theoretical Implications from Descriptive Empirical Findings on Dream Content." *Dreaming* 3(2/3): 201–210.

Domino, G. 1976. "Primary Process Thinking in Dream Reports as Related to Creative Achievement." *Journal of Consulting and Clinical Psychology* 44: 929–932.

———. 1982. "Attitudes towards Dreams, Sex Differences, and Creativity." *Journal of Creative Behavior* 16: 112–123.

Ellman, S. J., and Antrobus, J. R., eds. 1991. *The Mind in Sleep: Psychology and Psychophysiology,* second ed. New York: Wiley.

Empson, J. 1989. *Sleep and Dreaming.* London: Faber and Faber.

Fitch, T., and Armitage, R. 1989. "Variations in Cognitive Style among High and Low Frequency Dream Recallers." *Personality and Individual Differences* 10(8): 869–875.

Flavell, J. H. 1979. "Metacognition and Cognitive Monitoring." *American Psychologist* 34: 906–911.

Foulkes, D. 1985. *Dreaming: A Cognitive-Psychological Analysis.* Hillsdale, NJ: Erlbaum.

———. 1990. "Dreaming and Consciousness." *European Journal of Cognitive Psychology* 2(1): 39–55.

———. 1991a. "Dreaming: Lucid and Non." *Lucidity* 10(1 and 2): 272–274.

———. 1991b. "Why Study Dreaming: One Researcher's Perspective." *Dreaming* 1(3): 245–248.

———. 1993. "Dreaming and REM Sleep." *Journal of Sleep Research* 2: 199–202.

———. 1995. "Dreaming as Cognition." *Impuls* 3: 8–9.

———. 1999. *Children's Dreaming and the Development of Consciousness.* Cambridge: Harvard University Press.

Foulkes, D. and Cavarello, C., eds. 1993. *Dreaming as Cognition.* New York: Harvester/Wheatsheaf.

Foulkes, D., Hollifield, M., Bradley, L., Terry, R., and Sullivan, B. 1991. "Waking Self-Understanding, REM-Dream Self-Representation, and Cognitive Ability Variables at Ages 5–8." *Dreaming* 1(1): 41–51.

Freud, S. 1953 (1900). "The Interpretation of Dreams." In J. Strachey, ed. and trans., *The Standard Edition of the Complete Psychological Works of Sigmund Freud,* vols. 4 and 5. London: Hogarth Press.

Gackenbach, J. and LaBerge, S., eds. 1988. *Conscious Mind, Sleeping Brain: Perspectives on Lucid Dreaming.* New York: Plenum.

Gardner, H. 1994. *The Mind's New Science.* New York: Basic Books.

Globus, G. 1987. *Dream Life, Wake Life: The Human Condition through Dreams.* Albany: State University of New York Press.

Godwin, M. 1994. *The Lucid Dreamer: A Waking Guide for the Traveler between Worlds.* New York: Simon and Schuster.

Green, C. and McCreery. 1994. *Lucid Dreaming: The Paradox of Consciousness during Sleep.* London: Routledge.

Hall, C. and Norby, V. 1972. *The Individual and His Dreams.* New York: Signet.

Hartmann, E. 1973. *The Functions of Sleep.* New Haven: Yale University Press.

———. 1998. *Dreams and Nightmares: The New Theory on the Origin and Meaning of Dreams.* New York: Plenum Press.

Hartmann, E., Rosen, E., and Rand, W. 1998. "Personality and Dreaming: Boundary Structure and Dream Content." *Dreaming* 8(1): 31–39.

Haskell, R. E. 1986. "Cognitive Psychology and Dream Research: Historical, Conceptual, and Epistemological Consideration." *Journal of Mind and Behavior* 7(2, 3): 131–160.

Hearne, K. M. 1978. "Lucid Dreams: An Electrophysiological and Psychological Study." Ph.D. diss., Liverpool University, England.

Hendricks, M., and Cartwright, R. D. 1978. "Experiencing Level in Dreams: An Individual Difference Variable." *Psychotherapy: Theory, Research and Practice* 15: 292–298.

Hobson, J. A. 1988. *The Dreaming Brain.* New York: Basic Books.

Hobson, J. A. 1994. *The Chemistry of Conscious States: How the Brain Changes its Mind.* Boston: Little, Brown and Co.

Hobson, J. A., and McCarley, R. W. 1977. "The Brain as a Dream State Generator: An Activation-Synthesis Hypothesis of the Dream Process." *American Journal of Psychiatry* 134: 1335–1348.

Hobson, J. A., Pace-Schott, E., and Strickgold, R. 2000. "Dreaming and the Brain: Towards a Cognitive Neuroscience of Conscious States." *Behavioral and Brain Sciences: Special Edition on Sleep and Dreaming* 23 (6): 793–842.

Hobson, J. A., and Stickgold, R. 1994. "Dreaming: A Neurocognitive Approach." *Consciousness and Cognition* 3:1–15.

Hunt, H. 1986. "Some Relations between the Cognitive Psychology of Dreams and Dream Phenomenology." *Journal of Mind and Behavior* 7(2 and 3) : 213–228.

———. 1989. *The Multiplicity of Dreams: Memory, Imagination, and Consciousness.* New Haven: Yale University Press.

———. 1995. *On the Nature of Consciousness: Cognitive, Phenomenological, and Transpersonal Perspectives.* New Haven: Yale University Press.

James, W. 1890. *The Principles of Psychology,* vol. 1. New York: Dover.

Johnson, M. K. 1988. "Reality Monitoring: An Experimental Phenomenological Approach." *Journal of Experimental Psychology: General* 117: 390–394.

Johnson, M. K., Foley, M. A., Suengas, A. G., and Raye, C. L. 1988. "Phenomenal Characteristics of Memories for Perceived and Imagined Autobiographical Events." *Journal of Experimental Psychology: General* 117: 371–376.

Johnson, M. K., Kahan, T. L., and Raye, C. L. 1984. Dreams and Reality Monitoring." *Journal of Experimental Psychology: General* 113(3): 329–344.

Jung, C. G. 1965. *Memories, Dreams, Reflections.* Translated by R. F. C. Hull. Princeton: Princeton University Press.

Kahan, T. L. 1994. "Measuring Dream Self-Reflectiveness: A Comparison of Two Approaches." *Dreaming* 4(3): 177–193.

———. 2000. "The 'Problem' of Dreaming in NREM Sleep Continues to Challenge Reductionist (2-Gen) Models of Dream Generation (Commentary)." *Behavioral and Brain Sciences: Special Edition on Sleep and Dreaming* 23 6): 956–958.

———. 2001. Unpublished data.

Kahan, T. L., and LaBerge, S. 1994. "Lucid Dreaming as Metacognition: Implications for Cognitive Science." *Consciousness and Cognition* 3: 246–264.

———. 1996. "Cognition and Metacognition in Dreaming and Waking: Comparisons of First and Third-Person Ratings." *Dreaming* 6(4): 235–249.

———. 2000. "Metacognition in Dreaming and Waking." Paper presented at the 4th biannual conference, "Toward a Science of Consciousness," Tucson, AZ.

———. 2001. "Metacognition in Experiences Recalled from non-REM Sleep, REM Sleep, and Waking. Manuscript in preparation.

Kahan, T., L., LaBerge, S., Levitan, L., and Zimbardo, P. 1997. "Similarities and Differences between Dreaming and Waking Cognition: An Exploratory Study." *Consciousness and Cognition* 6: 132–147.

Kahn, D., and Hobson, J. A. 1993. "Self-Organization Theory of Dreaming." *Dreaming* 3(3): 151–178.

Kahn, D., Pace-Schott, E. F., and Hobson, J. A. 1997. "Consciousness in Waking and Dreaming: The Roles of Neuronal Oscillation and Neuromodulation in Determining Similarities and Differences." *Neuroscience* 78(1): 13–37.

Kerr, N. 1993. "Mental Imagery, Dreams, and Perception." In C. Cavallero and D. Foulkes, eds., *Dreaming as Cognition* (pp. 18–37). New York: Harvester-Wheatsheaf.

Kerr, N. H., Foulkes, D., and Schmidt, M. 1982. "The Structure of Laboratory Dream Reports in Blind and Sighted Subjects." *Journal of Nervous and Mental Disease* 170: 286–294.

Kihlstrom, J. 1987. "The Cognitive Unconscious." *Science* 237: 1445–1452.

Koukkou, M., and Lehmann, D. 1983. "Dreaming: The Functional State-Shift Hypothesis, a Neuropsychophysiological Model." *British Journal of Psychiatry* 142: 221–231.

Kramer, M. 1993. "The Selective Mood Regulatory Function of Dreaming: An Update and Revision." In A. Moffitt, M. Kramer, and R. Hoffmann eds., *The Functions of Dreaming* (pp. 139-195). Albany: State University of New York Press.

Kramer, M., Winget, C., and Whitman, R. 1971. "A City Dreams: A Survey Approach to Normative Dream Content." *American Journal of Psychiatry* 127: 1350–1356.

Kuhn, D. 2000. "Metacognitive Development." *Current Directions in Psychological Science* 9(5): 178–181.

Kuiken, D., and Sikora, S. 1993. "The Impact of Dreams on Waking Thoughts and Feelings." In A. Moffitt, M. Kramer, R. Hoffmann, eds., *The Functions of Dreaming* (pp. 419–476). Albany: State University of New York Press.

Kunzendorf, R. 1987–88. "Self-Consciousness as the Monitoring of Cognitive States: A Theoretical Perspective." *Imagination, Cognition, and Personality* 7: 3–22.

LaBerge, S. 1985. *Lucid Dreaming.* Los Angeles: J. P. Tarcher.

———. 1988. "The Psychophysiology of Lucid Dreaming." In J. Gackenbach and S. Laberge, eds., *Conscious Mind, Sleeping Brain: Perspectives on Lucid Dreaming* (pp. 135–153). New York: Plenum Press.

———. 1990. "Lucid Dreaming: Psychophysiological Studies of Consciousness during REM Sleep." In R. Bootzin, J. Kihlstrom, and D. Schacter, eds., *Sleep And Cognition* (pp. 109–126). Washington, D.C.: American Psychological Association.

Laberge, S., And Levitan, L. 1995. "Validity Established of Dreamlight Cues for Eliciting Lucid Dreaming." *Dreaming* 5(3): 159–168.

Laberge, S., Levitan, L., And Dement, W. 1986. "Lucid Dreaming: Physiological Correlates of Consciousness during REM Sleep." *Journal of Mind and Behavior* 7(2, 3): 251–258.

Laberge, S., Nagel, L., Dement, W., And Zarcone, V., Jr. 1981. "Lucid Dreaming Verified by Volitional Communication during REM Sleep." *Perceptual And Motor Skills* 52: 727–732.

Laberge, S. And Zimbardo, P. 2000. "Smooth Tracking Eye Movements Discriminate both Dreaming and Perception from Imagination." Paper Presented at the 4th Biannual Conference, "Towards a Science of Consciousness," Tucson, AZ.

Levin, R. 2000. *The Relation Of Waking To Nocturnal Fantasy.* Paper Presented at the 4th Biannual Conference, "Toward a Science of Consciousness," Tucson, AZ.

Levin, R., And Lamontoro, L. 1997–1998. "Visual-Spatial Aspects of Primary Process in Dreaming and Waking." *Imagination, Cognition, And Personality* 17: 15–30.

Mamelak, A. N., And Hobson, J. A. 1989. "Dream Bizarreness As the Cognitive Correlate of Altered Neuronal Behavior in REM Sleep." *Journal Of Cognitive Neuroscience* 1: 201–222.

Mason, L., Alexander, C., Travis, F., Marsh, G., Orme-Johnson, D., Gackenbach, J., Mason, D., Rainforth, M., And Walton, K. 1997. "Electrophysiological Correlates of Higher States of Consciousness during Sleep in Long-Term Practitioners of the Transcendental Meditation Program." *Sleep* 20(2): 102–110.

Moffitt, A. 1995. "Dreaming: Functions and Meaning." *Impuls* 3: 18–31.

Moffitt, A., Hoffmann, R., Mullington, J., Purcell, S., Pigeau, R., and Wells, R. 1988. "Dream Psychology: Operating in the Dark. In J. Gackenbach and S. Laberge, eds., *Conscious Mind, Sleeping Brain: Perspectives On Lucid Dreaming* (pp. 429–439). New York: Plenum.

Nelson, T. O. 1996. "Consciousness and Metacognition." *American Psychologist* 51(2): 102–116.

Nelson, T. O., and Narens, L. 1990. "Metamemory: Theoretical Framework and New Findings." In G. H. Bower, ed., *The Psychology Of Learning And Motivation* (vol. 26, pp.125–141). New York: Academic Press.

Nelson, T. O., And Narens, L. 1994. "Why Investigate Metacognition?" In. J. Metcalfe and A. P. Shimamura, eds., *Metacognition: Knowing About Knowing* (pp. 1–11). Cambridge, MA: Bradford Books.

Nielsen, T. A. 2000. "Cognition in REM and NREM Sleep: A Review and Possible Reconciliation of Two Models of Sleep Mentation." *Behavioral And Brain Sciences: Special Edition On Sleep And Dreaming* 23 (6): 851–866.

Nielsen, T., Kuiken, D., and Mcgregor, D. 1989. "Effects of Dream Reflection on Waking Affect: Awareness of Feelings, Rorschach Movement, and Facial EMG." *Sleep* (3): 277–286.

Pekala, R. J. 1991. *Quantifying Consciousness: An Empirical Approach*. New York: Plenum.

Purcell, S., Moffitt, A., and Hoffmann, R. 1993. "Waking, Dreaming, and Self-Regulation." In A. Moffitt, M. Kramer, R. Hoffmann, eds., *The Functions of Dreaming* (pp. 197–260). Albany: State University of New York Press.

Purcell, S., Mullington, J., Moffitt, A., Hoffmann, R., and Pigeau, R. 1986. "Dream Self-Reflectiveness as a Learned Cognitive Skill." *Sleep* 9: 423–437.

Rechtschaffen, A. 1978. "The Single-Mindedness and Isolation of Dreams." *Sleep* 1: 97–109.

Robinson-Riegler, B., and McDaniel, M. A. 1994. "Further Constraints on the Bizarreness Effect: Elaboration at Encoding." *Memory And Cognition* 2(6): 702–712.

Rossi, E. 1972. *Dreams and the Growth of Personality.* New York: Pergamon Press.

Rossi, E. 1985. *Dreams And The Growth Of Personality,* second ed. New York: Brunner/Mazel.

Sacksteder, R., ed. 1993. *The Lucid Dream Exchange.* (Available from Ruth Sacksteder, P. O. Box 12593, Berkeley, CA 94701.)

Saredi, R., Baylor, G., Meier, B., and Strauch, I. 1997. "Current Concerns and REM Dreams: A Laboratory Study of Dream Incubation." *Dreaming* 7(3): 195–208.

Sartre, J. P. 1980. *The Psychology Of Imagination.* Secaucus, NJ: Citadel Press.

Schredl, M., Jochum, S., And Souguenet, S. 1997. Dream Recall, Visual Memory, and Absorption in Imaginings." *Personality And Individual Differences* 22: 291–292.

Schwartz, D. G., Weinstein, L. N., and Arkin, A. M. 1978. "Qualitative Aspects of Sleep Mentation." In A. Arkin, J. Antrobus, and S. Ellman, eds., *The Mind In Sleep: Psychology and Psychophysiology.* Hillsdale: Lawrence Erlbaum Associates.

Shafton, A. 1995. *The Dream Reader.* Albany: State University of New York Press.

Snyder, F. 1970. "The Phenomenology of Dreaming." In Madow and L. Snow, eds., *The Psychodynamic Implications of the Physiological Studies on Dreams* (pp. 124–151). Springfield: Thomas.

Snyder, F., Karacan, I., Thorp, U. R., and Scott, J. 1968. "Phenomenology of REM Dreaming." *Psychophysiology* 4: 375 (Abstract).

Solms, M. 2000. "Dreaming and REM Sleep Are Controlled by Different Brain Mechanisms." *Behavioral And Brain Sciences: Special Edition On Sleep And Dreaming* 23 (6): 843–850.

———. 1997. *The Neuropsychology of Dreams: A Clinico-Anatomical Study.* Mahwah: Erlbaum.

Starker, S. 1984–85. "Daydreams, Nightmares, And Insomnia: The Relation Of Waking Fantasy To Sleep Disturbances." *Imagination, Cognition, And Personality* 4: 237–248.

Stickgold, R., Pace-Schott, And Hobson, J. A. 1994. "A New Paradigm for Dream Research: Mentation Reports Following Spontaneous Arousal from REM and NREM Sleep Recorded in a Home Setting." *Consciousness And Cognition* 3: 16–29.

Strauch, I., And Meier, B. 1996. *In Search of Dreams: Results of Experimental Dream Research.* Albany: State University of New York Press.

Tedlock, B. Ed. 1992. *Dreaming: Anthropological and Psychological Interpretations.* Santa Fe, NM: School Of American Research Press.

Tonay, V. 1993. "Personality Correlates of Dream Recall: Who Remembers?" *Dreaming* 3: 1–8.

Van De Castle, R. L. 1994. *Our Dreaming Mind.* New York: Random House.

Van Eeden, F. 1913. A Study of Dreams. *Proceedings of the Society for Psychical Research* 26: 431–461.

Varela, F. J., Thompson, E., and Rosch, E. 1995. *The Embodied Mind: Cognitive Science and Human Experience.* Cambridge, MA: MIT Press.

Weinstein, L., Schwartz, D., and Arkin, A. M. 1991. "Qualitative Aspects of Sleep Mentation." In S. J. Ellman and J. S. Antrobus, eds., *The Mind In Sleep: Psychology And Psychophysiology,* second ed. (pp.172–213). New York: Wiley.

Weinstein, L., Schwartz, D., and Ellman, S. J. 1988. "The Development of Scales To Measure The Experience of Self-Participation in Sleep." *Sleep* 11(5): 437–447.

Wilson, T. D. 1994. "The Proper Protocol: Validity and Completeness of Verbal Reports." *Psychological Science* 5(5): 249–252.

Winson, J. 1990. The Meaning Of Dreams. *Scientific American* 11: 86–96.

Young, S. 1999. *Dreaming In The Lotus: Buddhist Dream Narrative, Imagery, And Practice.* Boston: Wisdom Publications.

23

Dialogue with a Skeptic

Frederick Crews and Kelly Bulkeley

This exchange is a revised transcript of a conversation between Frederick Crews and myself at a public symposium titled "Beyond Freud and Jung? The Interpretation of Dreams, Religion, and Culture," sponsored by the Religion and Psychology Area (Area 5) of the Graduate Theological Union in Berkeley, California on September 23, 2000. Fred's comments and my response to them are a fitting conclusion to this book because they highlight the ongoing challenges that face anyone who seeks to explore and understand the realm of dreams.

Comments of Frederick Crews

Let me begin by asking what we are really after today, in this largely religious setting and company. Is it a cross-cultural study of dreams? If so, much can be accomplished. It's a wonderful field of intellectual endeavor, and books on the subject are pouring out. The latest, I believe, is *Dream Cultures: Explorations in the Comparative History of Dreaming,* edited by David Shulman and Guy G. Stroumsa (Oxford University Press, 1999). Books like that can tell us a great deal. However, they don't tell us about dreams and dreaming per se, much less about an alleged cross-cultural significance of dreams. Rather, they explore what different societies have made of dreams. There can be no methodological objection to such study. But if this present company is inclined to wax transcendental about dream meaning, drawing some kind of spiritual comfort from it, I will have to be counted in the opposition.

The problem is simple and fundamental. If we are inclined to make pronouncements about the meanings of dreams based on our own intuitions, our own presuppositions, we must face the awkward fact that every society has always found just what it wants to find in dreams. That being so, we ought to be wary of showing the same parochialism ourselves. Outside of the sleep laboratory, I don't believe we even get terribly reliable knowledge of the bare content of dreams. Unless you wake someone up immediately when you sense that he or she is dreaming, you are dealing with summarized dream reports, not with dreams, and those reports reach you with a significant time lag that provides the dreamer with time to interweave the sheer memory of images with all manner of cultural assumptions. Furthermore, dreaming itself can be influenced by expectations. It's a well-known fact, for example, that Freudian patients after a while dream Freudian dreams, Jungian patients dream Jungian dreams, and so forth. Nothing could be less surprising than this. But it's methodologically sobering, because it suggests how far away we are from an unbiased universal account of "the" purport of dreams.

Perhaps this is why I personally have never taken any interest in the young field of religion and psychology. What little I know of it comes straight from Kelly's book *Visions of the Night: Essays on Dreams, Religion, and Psychology* (SUNY, 1999), a copy of which he was kind enough to give me. I apologize, Kelly, if I exaggerate the typicality of what I find in those pages, but I have a feeling that yours is indeed mainstream work. The assumptions behind it, insofar as I can discern them, are challenging but also open to challenge in their own right.

Kelly talks in this book about what he calls "the numinous power" of human dreams. A provocative phrase! Numinous power, to me, means that dreams are connected to some higher order of invisible reality. And Kelly appears to feel the same way. Early on he discusses his own adolescent dreams and says that he awoke from them with a sense that the dreams were "trying to teach me another way of looking at the world." That's a phrase I want to return to. And Kelly says that when he began studying dreams, "they seemed to lead beyond the individual, beyond the ordinary boundaries of the dreamer's personal psyche."

I suppose this is mainstream language in the subfield of religion and psychology, though of course it's quite foreign to psychology as usually understood in university psychology departments. To me, it's ambiguous language, and not necessarily in a fruitful sense. Does Kelly mean that he was being led beyond the individual plane to mere anthropological diversity and relativism? Or, as I rather suspect, does he mean that he was being taken outside his individual self to a higher spiritual meaning, residing in a world soul of some kind? What power, what mystic personality, is doing the "teaching" and "leading" here? For me this is a basic stumbling block—because, frankly, I can't accept that the invoking of invisible powers and spirit guides, even if you privately believe in them, has a place in legitimate empirical inquiry. My hope, in our forum today, would be that this intention can be clarified and, if I have it right, cogently defended. When Kelly uses words like "numinous" and says that his dreams seemed to be trying to teach him another way, I do suspect that he means an intervention, through dreaming, from another plane of reality. Is this correct? If so, the empirical question that needs answering is "How do you know, how can you show us, that your mystical feelings are responding to an objective, external, culturally uninfluenced source of concern and care?" Of course, if everyone present shares the same fondness for a religious style of explanation, the problem vanishes. But I don't share it, so—show me!

Later in his book, Kelly takes a dream of Freud's famous patient Dora, whose notoriously failed treatment occurred in 1899, though Freud didn't publish his defense of it until 1905. The Dora case was meant to be a showcase for Freud's method and brilliant skill in dream interpretation. By today, however, the case history is usually regarded as a remarkable display of forced interpretation and bullying behavior on the therapist's part.

I think that Kelly shares in this general dissatisfaction, though on rather narrower grounds. He wants to revise Freud's understanding of Dora's dream in accordance with his own sense of dream-messages-from-above. Freud, he says, has missed an "existential" theme in Dora's report; the dream was really sending advice "that could enable Dora to live a more fulfilling life."

Uh-oh! All of my doubts and questions spring to life again here. It certainly sounds as if Dora was getting taught a lesson from outside, from some realm of divine presence. If this is Kelly's view of the matter, how does he know it's correct? What can he reply to the skeptic's impression that Dora is here being given the standard spiritualizing workup, without any consideration of alternative possibilities? Since every school of dream interpretation—and there are scads of them!—invariably finds that every dream perfectly fits its prior expectations, what evidence or argumentation can show us that Kelly's school is the correct one, in this case or in any other?

Well, I will leave Kelly to ponder these challenges while I try to sketch a context for the whole project of "going beyond Freud and Jung." Please refer now to my handout, "A Spectrum of Perspectives on Dreams and Dreaming" (figure 23.1). In a very simple way, it shows where the two famous theorists can be located on a continuum stretching from the most inductive and cautious to the most metaphysical and speculative approach to dream content.

At this latter pole, you will see, lies a theological attitude to dreams. I take the word "theological" seriously in its root meaning: knowledge of divinity. We're not talking about tentative hypotheses here but about confident pronouncements about the ultimate nature and purpose of reality. Humankind in its long and often delusional history has never been bashful about putting forward theological dogmas. As for dreams, a theological perspective supposedly tells us just what God or the gods intend by them.

Dreams, in a theological account, are indeed messages from the divine; they direct our conduct, prophesy the future, etc. God or the gods want you to win the next battle, turn away from other gods, avoid all that is sinful and taboo, make the right sacrifices, feel better about your troubles, and get into heaven where your ancestors, restored to top condition and equipped with harps, are already belting out celestial tunes. Of course theology gets a lot more sophisticated than this when it is practiced by powerful and subtle intellects. What it never does, however, is admit the embarrassing truth: People through the ages have had no rational basis whatsoever for their culture-bound

Figure 23.1 A Spectrum of Perspectives on Dreams and Dreaming

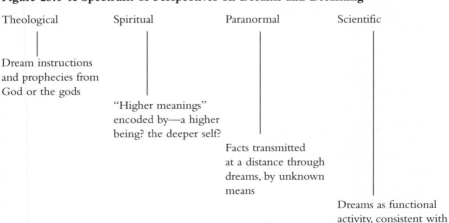

Theological
Dream instructions and prophecies from God or the gods

Spiritual
"Higher meanings" encoded by—a higher being? the deeper self?

Paranormal
Facts transmitted at a distance through dreams, by unknown means

Scientific
Dreams as functional activity, consistent with known laws of nature

notions of what God or the gods, if they exist at all, require of us. To be blunt about it, "theology" is a misnomer. It isn't knowledge at all, but just a body of shifting opinion that sounds right to members of a priestly class and to those who accept their word as authoritative.

At the opposite end of my spectrum lies science, where, obviously, I feel considerably more at home. A scientist would say that dreaming is a natural human function and that the content of dreams is also natural and available to study. Although dreams appear to be at least partly meaningful, that fact does not propel us into some kind of spiritual stratosphere. In waking life, after all, we use language, we think about the past and future, we express our hopes and fears. If all of these elements show up in dreams, the most we are entitled to assert is a degree of continuity between our waking life and our dream life.

Nearly all mammals apparently dream, so far as anybody can tell. Here once again is a fact that might make you want to think twice about dreams being divine messages. It's hard to see what kind of spiritual direction the marmots, say, are getting out of it. Our dreams are doubtless much more complex and interesting than those of other mammals. But that's just what we would expect from a routine functionalist perspective on the human brain, which is incomparably more intricate, with more neurons and more feedback loops, than any other brain we know about.

I think what is really interesting here is the middle terrain, which I have charted as spanning the spiritual and the paranormal. The paranormal refers to ideas of precognition, telepathy, and clairvoyance that go beyond the individual. But they don't go beyond the individual all the way to theological truths. Paranormal theory deals with rather mundane information that is transmitted in highly unusual ways. Thus a typical paranormal experience might be a sudden conviction that something bad has happened to a beloved person; one wakes up in the middle of the night overcome by dread and foreboding. Well, that bad accident, supposing that it actually did happen, wouldn't necessarily be connected with religious aspirations on anybody's part. But the paranormal theorist believes that this news can be transmitted through unknown means to a person who is dreaming, thanks to a psychic gift that is either common to humankind or available to "sensitives" alone.

The paranormal realm goes beyond science in a way that most scientists find unacceptable. Why? Because there is no physical medium of communication. Nothing that we know about the visible world allows us to grant that a dreamer can receive a message from, say, five thousand miles away—or even from the next room, for that matter.

Nevertheless, paranormal theory can be congenial to spiritual aspirations. If you want to believe that you're in contact with a higher realm, you'll need to posit a means of contact other than what has been available to science thus far. And so, quite frequently, we find people of a religious inclination leaning strongly toward paranormal sympathies. Of course they don't stop with the mundane information that paranormal experts usually dwell on, but go on to higher matters. Interestingly enough, the most widely used synonym for paranormal activity, from the early nineteenth century until now, has been "spiritualism." The connection is right there in the language. And Kelly: I note with interest that the bibliographical essay at the end of *Visions of the Night* appears distinctly hospitable toward paranormal possibilities.

Finally, we get to the spiritual range in my spectrum. Spirituality, as you may have gathered, is not my strong suit. What does the term mean? I defer to others, but my guess is that the spiritual has something to do with guidance toward a higher or more integrated state of being, a guidance that, traditionally, is supposed to come from outside the individual. But it's not absolutely necessary that it do so—and especially not here in California! Yet even if we reduce the spiritual to a form of talking to ourselves, it's still a matter of allowing our "better" self to instruct our "weaker" one. Perhaps the most scientifically respectable hypothesis about spiritual dreaming would be that, with our inhibitions temporarily disabled, our deeper selves tell our more troubled, less clear-minded selves what we should be doing, how we should be feeling, and what interpretation we should place on our lives. I don't actually buy this, but it's the least objectionable formulation that lets an element of guidance through the door.

Along the spectrum I have sketched, my own predilection is for the scientific point of view—the one that applies rational skepticism to the question of lawfulness in the world that we know, the empirical world. Why this preference? Simply because I'm interested in knowledge. Knowledge deserves the name only if it has been tested. To this end, it has to be presented in such a manner that an independent party, someone without a prior commitment, can examine the evidence and arrive at the same conclusion as the person who is propounding the idea. Science is all about testing for error. If you read a lot of philosophy of science, you will soon perceive that very little of it is concerned with how we get our ideas. Who cares whether or not an apple hit Newton on the head? The whole question is whether a given idea has been presented in a way that is accessible to neutral and very unsparing skeptical evaluation, and whether that idea has proved capable of surviving the most astute objections that can be leveled against it.

A scientific perspective won't allow us to make a shallow and self-serving distinction between dreaming, a mere physiological activity, and dreams, a realm of spiritual wonder. One sometimes reads, for example, that it's all very well for a theorist such as J. Allan Hobson to put forward ideas about dreaming as produced by electrical activity in the brain stem; meanwhile, it is said, the meaning of dreams falls outside the purview of science. Here, supposedly, we are in the more congenial realm of hermeneutics, where individual judgment matters more. But dream content is exactly as susceptible in principle to rational, skeptical, empirical investigation as the nature of dreaming itself is. It may be more difficult to ascertain the results that we're looking for. Indeed, I'm sure it is more difficult to talk accurately about dream content than it is to talk about the neurophysiology of dreaming. But exactly the same standards of rational skepticism must apply to both of these subject matters. This is not to say that dreams have no meaning, as Hobson has sometimes implied. It is to say that dream content demands the same kind of inductive study as dreaming itself, without preconceptions about messages emanating from beyond the dreamer.

What science cannot ever do is make room for miracles. A miracle is an intervention that overturns the laws of nature, and you can't allow miracles anywhere in science. It's not a question of our looking around at the world and deciding whether or not there's something miraculous about it. Science as an enterprise rules out miracles from the very beginning on methodological grounds. Some of you, less jaded than I about theology, may take some comfort from this observation. As my colleague Phillip Johnson [professor of law at the University of California, Berkeley] never tires of saying, if science starts from a naturalistic perspective and then gets only naturalistic results, it may be overlooking supernatural causes that would explain how and why we all got here. Be that as it may, the moment you invoke divine intervention, you have changed the rules of the science game in an impermissible way. And this means that you can't have a scientific view of dreams and dreaming that allows for any nonphysical means of transmitting thoughts and messages. Paranormal and spiritual accounts of dreaming are ruled equally out of bounds by this principle.

A scientific outlook today, for virtually everyone who takes it seriously, also entails a broad commitment to the Darwinian perspective on human affairs. That perspective tells us that we must regard ourselves as an evolved species whose cross-cultural, universal traits, such as they are, arose a long time ago under harsh tests of survival that we can scarcely imagine today. This is not to say that Darwinism obliges us to regard dreams as having a crucial survival value for our species. A good number of human traits, even universal ones, may have come into existence by taking a free ride on other features that were selected for our survival. Dreams themselves may be one such free ride—a by-product of the facts that humans think, both in waking and sleeping life.

Dreams, then, may not have a powerful adaptive function for the survival of the human individual; we don't really know. Nevertheless, an evolutionary perspective is important here, precisely because it was Darwin who eliminated teleology from science. From a Darwinian point of view, it is unimaginable that dream meaning can be imposed on us from above or outside the organism or its culture, as if the future were speaking to the present. The whole point of natural selection, after all, is that chance variations are continually tested against environmental conditions that change in unanticipated ways. Admonitory messages from friendly spirit guides would utterly sabotage this outlook.

Rational skepticism also entails a certain wariness of "discoveries" that fit too neatly with the predilections of the discoverer. It is perfectly all right to have such predilections and to go out and make assertions, but the closer they are to what one previously believed, the more imperative it is for others to insist that objective grounds for agreement be presented. Is the observer kidding himself? In science, he is presumed guilty until he can prove otherwise.

Here is why my own skepticism was aroused when I read that Kelly's dreams seemed to be leading him beyond his individual self. Was he, in his adolescence, being dragged reluctantly toward the spiritual by his dreams? Or was he the kind of fellow who, like most members of this assembly, harbors spiritual leanings anyway, and who therefore is more inclined to have (or think that he's having) dreams of this kind? In order to say that dreams have spiritual meaning, we need more evidence than a recollection of spiritual awakening in adolescence. Adolescence, as you know, produces awakenings of several kinds, and they can lead in radically opposite directions. We all remember being stirred up wildly in those years. We were the last to perceive—*n'est-ce pas?*—what was obvious to the rest of our family: that hormones might have had something to do with it. And Kelly, I must say, still seems reluctant to weigh that factor against a more ethereal interpretation of his teenage intensity.

Let me get around at last to Freud, who was professedly a Darwinian functionalist. He admired Darwin tremendously and thought of himself as carrying on Darwin's work. At first glance, then, you would want to put Freud all the way to the right of my spectrum here, as the Science Guy. He didn't believe dreams were prophetic, he didn't think they gave us any instructions for right conduct, and he thought they expressed the internal conflicts of the human subject. Dreams for Freud conveyed repressed desires and the defenses against those desires—defenses that the individual throws up because he is ashamed of his filthy wishes and fearful of the retaliation that would descend on him if he acted them out. The Freudian dream is a compromise formation, a vector between the unconscious urges of the individual and his largely unconscious defenses against those urges. And the ultimate function of dreams for Freud was to protect sleep by allowing for this symbolic discharge. It's a totally functionalist perspective, and even though it happens to be erroneous from beginning to end, there is nothing spiritual about it.

As for Jung, he took the Freudian unconscious and unabashedly endowed it with a soul. First he largely desexualized it, and then he linked up individual minds in what he called a "collective unconscious," which sends its ancestral wisdom across the ether to us. Through Jungian dreams, it says here, we can now be in contact with our wise elders from thousands of years ago. It's a form of channeling, precisely as ridiculous as the claims of Elizabeth Clare Prophet to be tuning into bulletins from a 30,000-year-old man. But since Jung nominally starts from secular observation of disturbed patients, he seems to go nearly all the way across my whole spectrum, from the scientific through the paranormal to the spiritual.

We tend to forget, however, that Freud himself was an enthusiast of the paranormal. He wrote four papers about the paranormal meaning of dreams—papers that caused great anxiety within his circle of disciples. Ernest Jones tried to get him to suppress this work, but Freud wouldn't do it. Admittedly, these papers of his are rather equivocal in what a Freudian might call their manifest content. But it is quite clear to anyone who studies Freud closely that he did believe in the paranormal and that he was casting about for ways of affirming and validating it. He would not leave the subject alone. Indeed, he actually performed paranormal experiments with his daughter Anna and with Sandor Ferenczi, who was himself a great believer in the paranormal—virtually a magician, if only in his own mind. So Freud goes from the scientific end of my spectrum as far as the paranormal, while Jung goes a little farther to the spiritual. Neither one of them, I would say, is truly theological, but Jung's leanings in that direction have been often noted.

What, then, should we make of the Jungian effort to revise Freud? A number of questions come to mind. First, if the Jungian unconscious is universal, how come it proves to be so very Germanic? Why should one cultural tradition be privileged above all the others? For example, why is it that the wise ancestors seem to transmit so many dumb sexist clichés about the eternal feminine? Again, what mechanism, other than a now-discredited Lamarckianism, has allowed the collective unconscious to become progressively wiser through the millennia? How can a source of telepathic information be located everywhere and nowhere? And if it's so smart, couldn't it have told its favorite Teutons, including Jung himself, to be a bit less enthusiastic about the Nazis? Jung never makes any attempt, so far as I know, to answer these questions. And this means, candidly, that his speculations are of no rational interest whatsoever. The beginning of wisdom is to stop reading Jung.

But this is not to let Freud off lightly. Rather than ask yourselves—as some of you, I gather, are doing—whether you prefer Jung's revised version of the Freudian unconscious, you would do well to consider what good evidence we have for that unconscious in the first place. As Bill Domhoff's excellent work shows [chapter 20 in this volume], there is not a single Freudian proposition about dreams that has received significant empirical support. I would add there is not a single Freudian proposition, period, that has received significant empirical support. And for evidence to back this controversial claim, I refer you either to my recent anthology, *Unauthorized Freud: Doubters Confront a Legend* (Penguin, 1999) or to a much more formidable study, Malcolm Macmillan's *Freud Evaluated: The Completed Arc* (MIT, 1997).

It is easy to see why people of a spiritual orientation gravitate to Jung. The harder-nosed, skeptical, atheistic types gravitate to Freud, who seems to them very stoical and tragic and scientifically disciplined. I thought this way myself thirty-five years ago. In fact, however, Freud was not scientifically inclined at all. What he gave us was the idiom of science, the tone of science. But if science is about the prudent, evidence-based correction of errors, there is no science in Freud. His whole method of ascertaining whether or not a proposition was valid was circular. For Freud, any given fact about a human being would always be evidence in favor of his theory. If it seemed to manifestly support his theory, then that was conclusive; but if it seemed to contradict his theory, he would import one of his defense mechanisms to explain how the observed fact was a point in his favor after all. Heads I win, tails you lose. Science cannot be conducted in such a manner.

Of course all this deprecation on my part appears to overlook what many people take to be Freud's rigorous determinism. Humanists who study psychology as a kind of hobby—and that was a good description of me a long time ago—tend to be impressed by Freud's insistence that everything in psychic life is caused by factors that, in principle at least, can be historically traced. That's what enabled Freud to explain adult neuroses in terms of very specific events that had happened in the early childhood of the patient, whether they were sexual molestations or repressions of shameful oedipal thoughts. But in the end, Freud's determinism proves to be utterly gratuitous. It simply expresses overconfidence in his own deductive abilities: "Nothing can escape me!" And indeed, nothing did. When Freud tells you that, in principle, every last detail of a dream can be explained in terms of unconscious conflict, you would do well to regard the claim as a warning flag. As is so often said, a theory that explains everything explains nothing.

Insofar as people with spiritual aspirations are drawn to Freud, who denied that he held any such aspirations himself, I suspect that it has to do chiefly with this overweening interpretative ambition of his. Why not have a go at it yourself? If Freud says that dreams are totally meaningful, and yet you don't care for the sexual and aggressive emphasis he places on them, then you may be tempted to make the following dubious move. Freud took us a certain way toward a true understanding of dreams, you may say, but unfortunately he didn't get the content quite right; here is the more appropriate spiritual content. Remember, that's exactly what Jung did, to grateful applause from people who understand nothing about the constraints of well-conducted science. It's an easy game to play: tennis with the net down. But Jung had the chutzpah to call it psychology. I fervently hope—but I can't be sure—that this isn't the spirit in which Freud and Jung are studied in religion-and-psychology programs. Say it ain't so, Kelly and the rest of you! Show me that, in your studies, a given psychological system isn't being favored simply because it flatters your spiritual yearnings. If you are headed "beyond Freud and Jung" in the same erroneous, anti-empirical direction as their own, you are that much farther away from a truly disciplinary point of view. Freud and Jung are quite irresponsible enough without needing "improvement" in such a manner. So: Is religion and psychology an authentic empirical discipline, or is it only—pardon the expression—a field of dreams?

Kelly Bulkeley's Reply

I take Fred's comments as a well-justified challenge to the scientific quality of present and future research in the study of dreams. One of the great virtues of science is its commitment to the free and open exchange of ideas. Scientific methodologies provide common principles, terms, and standards of measurement that enable people from widely varying backgrounds to share their findings and test the validity of each other's claims. To the extent that dream researchers share this goal of promoting better communication with people both inside and outside their field, the effort to enhance the scientific quality of dream research should be a vigorous one.

At the beginning of his discussion, Fred questions the possibility of gathering reliable data on dream content. This goes to the heart of whether dream research can be a scientific endeavor, because good, solid empirical data are the essential raw materials for any form of scientific investigation. I agree with Fred that this is a central question, and I would add that the methodological difficulties he cites are worse than he supposes. When he says, "Outside of the sleep laboratory, I don't believe we even get terribly reliable knowledge of the bare content of dreams," he gives more credit than is due to the scientific adequacy of sleep laboratory research on dreaming. It is now clear that the sleep laboratory has a strongly homogenizing influence on dream content. For example, people sleeping in a lab report fewer aggressive dreams and fewer sexual dreams than people sleeping outside a lab.[1] People who are frequent nightmare sufferers report having fewer nightmares when sleeping in a lab as compared to when they sleep at home.[2] Researchers have dubbed this general phenomenon "the lab effect."[3] The likely explanation is that when people enter the laboratory setting they remain aware as they go to sleep that professional researchers will be observing them all night long, and this awareness inhibits the reporting and/or experiencing of socially inappropriate dream content (such as engaging in aggressive or sexual activities). With nightmare sufferers, it seems the knowledge that trained researchers will be watching over them all night long provides a sense of security and safety, and this has the effect of diminishing the frequency of their bad dreams.

In light of this, dream researchers are faced with the vexing problem that even the sleep laboratory does not provide a perfect means of access to dream content. Indeed, Allan Hobson has frankly admitted in an interview that the most interesting dreams occur outside the lab.[4] A truly scientific portrait of human dream experience must therefore include data gathered from settings other than the sleep laboratory, even if this means that the dream reporting conditions cannot be as carefully controlled and minutely observed as is possible in a lab setting.

This formidable methodological challenge is compounded by the inescapable influence of linguistic, cultural, and psychological factors at work in both the formation and reporting of dream content. Although Fred assumes the possibility of distinguishing "the sheer memory of images" from secondary cultural accretions, as a practical matter such a distinction cannot be made. No technology exists that could give researchers access to the pure, culturally unsullied content of a person's dreams (although several science fiction writers and filmmakers have imagined what such technology could be used for[5]). The sleep laboratory, for all its success in creating a strictly controlled experimental environment, does not materially change this situation. A subject in the lab who is awakened from the midst of REM sleep and immediately asked for a dream report is still a person whose imagination has been deeply influenced by some particular culture, who is using a particular language to describe his or her dream, and who is participating in a particular mode of social interaction (namely, serving as a subject in a sleep lab experiment). There is no way around it: For better or for worse, all dream researchers, whether they work in or out of a sleep laboratory, are condemned to the use of personal, subjective, culturally saturated verbal reports as their primary source of empirical data on dream content.

Does this make it impossible to conduct dream research in a scientifically responsible fashion? Not at all. It remains quite possible to propose hypotheses about the nature and function of dreaming, to test those hypotheses by means of carefully designed empirical investigations, and then to analyze the results with a sharp and unsparing critical eye. The sources of data we currently have at our disposal, even if they are mediated by varying degrees of cultural influence, are perfectly sufficient for continuing the scientific process of developing a fuller understanding of dreams and dreaming.

The methodological challenge here is one that many other scientifically inclined researchers have faced, and their success in overcoming these challenges is worth noting. One such researcher is neuroscientist Antonio Damasio, author of *Descartes' Error* (Quill, 1994) and *The Feeling of What Happens* (Harvest, 1999). I believe the following quote regarding his work in the study of consciousness is directly relevant to our discussion of dream research methodology:

> Although the investigation of consciousness is condemned to some indirectness, this limitation is not restricted to consciousness. It applies to all other cognitive phenomena. Behavioral acts—kicks, punches, and words—are nice expressions of the private process of mind, but they are not the same thing. Likewise, electroencephalograms and functional MRI scans capture correlates of the mind but those correlates are not the mind. Inevitable indirectness, however, is not equivalent to eternal ignorance about mental structures or about the underlying neural mechanisms. The fact that mental images are accessible only to their owner organism does not deny their reliance on organic substance, and does not prevent our gradual closing in on the specifications of that substance. This may cause some worry to purists raised on the idea that what another person cannot see is not to be trusted scientifically, but it really should not worry anyone. This state of affairs should not prevent us from treating subjective phenomena scientifically. Whether one likes it or not, *all* the contents in our minds are subjective and the power of science comes from its ability to verify objectively the consistency of many individual subjectivities.[6]

I believe that this is the spirit by which future dream research should be guided. If we can make progress toward verifying "the consistency of many individual subjectivities," if we can do more to identify the broad patterns and deep structures that emerge in and through individual dream experiences, we will have done much indeed.

One of my current research projects is focused on the testing of a particular hypothesis about the function of dreaming, a hypothesis that draws together findings from religious studies, anthropology, neuroscience, and psychology. I would like to present this hypothesis in a somewhat roundabout fashion, by responding to several points that Fred makes in his comments. Each of these points highlights an important methodological principle that is relevant not only to my research but to the research of nearly everyone in this field.

To begin with, I want to respond to Fred's passing mention of the fact that *Visions of the Night* contains a bibliographical essay that in his view "appears distinctly hospitable toward paranormal possibilities." Why do I get the feeling that that's not a good thing? I am continually surprised by people who proudly pledge themselves to the scientific method and yet who claim that this or that class of phenomena cannot exist because it contradicts the present state of knowledge. Such an attitude must be rejected as a threat to future scientific progress. Science is nothing if it is not hospitable to the possibility that the present state of knowledge is partial, incomplete, or even mistaken; science is nothing if it is not open to the emergence of unexpected phenomena and new ways of understanding the world. Being open-minded toward the possible is the very essence of scientific inquiry.

What I imagine concerns Fred is the frequency with which "open-mindedness" becomes a code word for gullibility, fuzzy thinking, and self-serving fantasy. With the subject of paranormal phenomena, his concern is well justified, as I myself can testify. I remember an interview I did some years ago with a network television producer who, as the interview proceeded, became increasingly determined to induce me to say on camera that dreams can predict the future. I wouldn't oblige him, and the interview ended in mutual frustration.

It would be pleasing to think that humans have prophetic powers; it would relieve some of our worst fears and satisfy some of our most cherished fantasies; it might even make for good television ratings. But none of that makes it true, and as Fred rightly points out we should use extra caution when investigating phenomena that are so heavily laden with age-old wishes and desires.

As I have written elsewhere, I follow Aristotle's categorization of prophetic dreams into three groups: causes, tokens, and coincidences.[7] Dreams may be the cause of future actions, in that it sometimes happens that "the movements set up first in sleep should also prove to be starting-points of actions to be performed in the daytime."[8] Dreams may also be tokens (we might say symbols) of events to come in the future. Aristotle refers to dreams that reveal the imminent onset of an illness, before the person has become consciously aware of being sick. Aristotle says that in the quiet of sleep we become aware of slight "movements" and "beginnings" that are lost to us in the bustle of daily life: "it is manifest that these beginnings must be more evident in sleeping than in waking moments."[9] Having granted these two possibilities, Aristotle still believes that most allegedly prophetic dreams are mere coincidences, especially those that are "extravagant" or involve matters with no direct connection to the dreamer. It happens all the time, he argues, that people mistakenly connect two events that are in fact unrelated; this is not prophecy, just faulty reasoning. Aristotle's general attitude is thus quite skeptical toward the majority of prophetic dream reports. But at the same time, he is careful not to deny the possible legitimacy of at least some of these reports:

> [A]s to the divination which takes place in sleep, and is said to be based on dreams, we cannot lightly either dismiss it with contempt or give it implicit confidence. The fact that all persons, or many, suppose dreams to possess a special significance, tends to inspire us with belief in it, as founded on the testimony of experience; and indeed that divination in dreams should, as regards some subjects, be genuine, is not incredible, for it has a show of reason; from which one might form a like opinion also respecting all other dreams. Yet the fact of our seeing no probable cause to account for such divination tends to inspire us with distrust.[10]

I believe that this is the most appropriate and scientifically legitimate approach to take toward the subject of paranormal dreams. Perhaps someday researchers will be able to explain how, as so many people report, it is possible to dream of a faraway loved one who has suddenly taken ill or died. At the moment we cannot explain the seemingly prophetic power of such dreams except by dismissing them as mere coincidences or outright fabrications. My concern is that we not close the door to the possibility that an authentic scientific explanation for such dreams will be developed in the future.

Another point of Fred's I would like to discuss regards the probative value of the adolescent dreams I briefly describe at the beginning of chapter 1 of *Visions of the*

Night. Fred says, "in order to say that dreams have spiritual meaning, we need more evidence than a recollection of spiritual awakening in adolescence." Naturally, I agree. I did not present the dreams as decisive evidence in support of my general argument. Rather, I mentioned them as a way of describing how I came to be interested in the subject of dreams and how the questions I pursue in my research are intertwined with my own personal experiences. It seemed a simple matter of intellectual honesty to say as much.

Fred goes on to question whether my "ethereal" approach to the dreams did not overlook the "hormonal" factors that must have been involved in their formation. I don't believe so. On the contrary, it's clear to me that these dreams were deeply rooted in the sexual, aggressive, and ego-oriented desires surging through me during adolescence. What I discovered in the dreams, and what made them so significant for me, was a different way of *knowing* these desires—rather than struggling to fight and control them, I learned to understand their power and respect their intelligence, and I began to seek ways of better integrating them with my conscious sense of self. My "wild stirrings," as Fred puts it, were certainly stimulated by the same basic physiological changes that afflict everyone in adolescence, so in that sense there was nothing unique about my experience. Indeed, my dreams themselves were not especially unusual in their imagery or their impact on my waking life. As I soon found, when I began a serious study of dreams, people in many different cultures and periods of history, including people in contemporary Western society, have reported similar types of dreams, often occurring during times of major life change. Since that initial discovery I have tried in various ways to understand better the imaginative capacity that enables humans to experience such dreams, and I am quite convinced that natural physiological processes, not only in the brain but throughout the whole body, are a major factor in their formation.

A brief but important point of Fred's concerns my interpretation of a dream of Freud's famous patient Dora. How, Fred asks, do I know my view of her dream is correct? This is a crucial question, and one that leads into complex philosophical discussions of truth, meaning, and interpretive practice. Before going on, however, I would argue that practical methods of dream interpretation should be conceptually distinguished from theoretical models of dream function. The latter provide explanations, while the former discern meanings; the latter ask "How does dreaming in general work?" while the former ask "What does this particular dream mean?" Because the two pursuits have fundamentally different (though potentially compatible) aims, different standards must be used in evaluating whether they are successful in achieving what they set out to do.

I have written in detail about these matters in *The Wilderness of Dreams,* where I develop a hermeneutic approach to dreams based on the philosophical work of Hans-Georg Gadamer and Paul Ricoeur.[11] The basic premise of this approach is that there is no single correct meaning to any dream; there are many possible interpretations, some of which are more valid than others. The validity of an interpretation is determined by a process of critical testing and questioning, a process guided equally by rational skepticism and creative imagination. In chapter 13 of this volume, I describe four principles by which better and worse interpretations may be distinguished from each other:

1. The dreamer knows best what his or her dream means.
2. A good interpretation will account for as many of the dream's details as possible.

3. A good interpretation will make as many connections as possible between the dream's content and the dreamer's waking life.
4. A good interpretation will be open to new and surprising discoveries and will look beyond the obvious (what is already known) to find the novel and the unexpected (what is *not* already known).

Returning to the subject of Dora's dream, Freud's interpretation of it as measured by my four principles was a partial success on points two and three and a spectacular failure on points one and four. Although my alternative interpretation of Dora's dream cannot be tested by the first principle (this is the inherent limitation of historical dream research), I believe it satisfies points two, three, and especially four. Now, does this mean I claim to have discovered the one true and correct meaning of Dora's dream? No. It simply means I have offered an interpretation that is plausible, reasonable, consistent with the available data, and significant in terms of opening up new ways of understanding the dreamer's life.

For people who expect every question to have one simple answer, this approach is bound to be a disappointment. Likewise, for people (such as Freud) who believe they have a system to identify the true meaning of any and every dream, my approach is also bound to be frustrating. So be it. Dream interpretation is not equivalent to solving a mathematical equation, in which a single, unambiguous result is produced at the end of the process. Dream interpretation is much more comparable to art or literary criticism, in which close, detailed analysis is combined with empathetic intuition to produce a fruitful reading of a given text, a reading that asserts its reasoned integrity even as it remains open to critical correction and alternative possibilities. I would think this relatively modest and resolutely non-Freudian approach to dream interpretation would appeal to an English professor's humanistic sensibilities—but I could be wrong!

Now I come to Fred's most urgent question: Who or what is doing the "teaching" and "leading" in the dreams I am discussing? He highlights my use of the term "numinous power" to describe such dreams, and he asks whether this necessarily implies an occult connection to "invisible powers," "spirit guides," and/or "another plane of reality." Perhaps to his distress, my answer constitutes a version of what he disparagingly terms the least objectionable and most Californian (!) type of response, a response that refers to the transformative influence on waking consciousness of nonconscious mental powers. This brings me back to a research project I mentioned earlier. The hypothesis orienting this project is that certain extraordinary types of dreaming are generated by numinous powers that connect the dreamer to dimensions of energy, intelligence, and purpose far outside the normal boundaries of individual awareness.[12] I further propose that these extraordinary dreams function to promote greater cognitive flexibility, creative imagination, and adaptive well-being—in short, *they provoke greater consciousness.*

Can such a hypothesis be tested in a scientifically rigorous fashion? I believe it can be. For instance, current sleep laboratory research is providing important new insights into the amazingly intricate neural circuitry involved in all dream experience. The works of Allan Hobson, Mark Solms, Tore Nielsen, and the late Alan Moffitt[13] are especially helpful in formulating a sound neuropsychological understanding of dreaming in general, and such an understanding stands as the conceptual foundation for an investigation of the unusual types of dreams that are my chief concern. However, neuropsychology is not sufficient for the testing of my hypothesis—recall Hobson's admission that the most interesting dreams occur outside the sleep lab. Other sources of data are required, the most important of which are detailed historical and cross-cultural studies of dreaming (exemplified by several chapters in the present volume). A large professional literature has developed in this area to provide a wealth of information about "nonlaboratory" dream experiences, dreams that have occurred in relatively natural life settings. A careful comparative analysis of these dreams enables the development of a phenomenology of typical, cross-cultural themes and patterns in human dreaming. (Knowing Fred's aversion to Jung as well as Freud, I hasten to note that my approach aims to go much farther than Jung's does in establishing a broad empirical base for its phenomenological proposals.)

If such a phenomenology depended solely on historical and cross-cultural dream reports, it would be subject to the criticism that the reports did not provide a sufficiently representative sample of human dream experience to be accepted as evidence for a general theory of dreaming. This is where recourse to the content analysis methods first developed by Calvin Hall and Robert Van de Castle and recently reformulated by Bill Domhoff can be so useful.[14] In terms of methodology, content analysis stands somewhere between sleep laboratory research and historical/cross-cultural research. It provides a systematically gathered sample of thousands of dream reports and a well-tested method of quantitatively analyzing those reports in order to generate statistical portraits of what people dream about. This method is one of the best tools available for dream researchers to use in what the earlier quote from Antonio Damasio called the effort "to verify objectively the consistency of many individual subjectivities." If the content analysis method can be employed in conjunction with historical and cross-cultural studies on one hand and neuropsychological sleep laboratory research on the other, the stage will be set for a fair scientific testing of my hypothesis, as indeed it will be for any hypothesis about the nature and functioning of dreams.

An objection could still be raised about the theological implications of my hypothesis. If I understand Fred's comments on this point, he assumes that terms like "numinous" and phrases like "dimensions of power, intelligence, and purpose outside the normal boundaries of awareness" necessarily imply the existence of supernatural, nonmaterial divinities who wield ultimate control over human life. I believe this assumption is wrong. Even if we set aside all theological speculations about the existence of God as well as all psychoanalytic theories about the unconscious (as I know Fred would urge us to do!), the growing literature in neuropsychology and cognitive science clearly indicates that the human brain/mind system is built up of a remarkably complex and sophisticated array of neural patterns and processes, very few of which ever become an object of ordinary conscious awareness. There is nothing supernatural about that fact. Nor is there anything supernatural about people having dreams by means of which some of these ordinarily nonconscious neural patterns and processes enter into consciousness. Finally, there is nothing supernatural about the uncanny feeling regularly reported by people who have experienced such dreams, a remarkably sharp and vivid feeling that the dream seemed to come from powers outside themselves. If the "self" is understood here as referring to and individual's customary waking personality, then the feeling in certain dreams of a connection with numinous forces originating "beyond the self" has a clear empirical basis in the distinctive neuropsychological operations of the dreaming brain.[15]

Any claim about the adaptive value of dreaming must specify the evolutionary basis upon which such a function could have developed. As Fred points out, it could simply be that dreaming has no adaptive function whatsoever and is nothing more than an evolutionary "free rider" that sprouted up as a consequence of genuinely adaptive developments in other areas of brain functioning. Allan Hobson offers a similar suggestion in chapter 21 of this volume, saying it could be that "dreaming is an epiphenomenon of REM sleep whose cognitive content is so ambiguous as to invite misleading or even erroneous interpretation" (p. 328). This is a legitimate possibility, but much more research needs to be conducted before a decisive answer can be given one way or another. In fact, a great deal of evidence supports the contrasting position that dreaming does indeed have genuine adaptive value for the human species, and I believe the following areas of research will provide still more data in favor of this view:

1. Sexual dreams. Given the automatic physiological arousal of the genitals in REM sleep, could sexually arousing dreams serve an adaptive function in the development and stimulation of reproductive activity?
2. Nightmares. Given the frequency and intensity of terrifying dreams, particularly in childhood, could nightmares serve an adaptive function in the development of greater vigilance toward potential threats to self-preservation?
3. Dreams of the dead. Given the historically and culturally widespread phenomenon of vivid dreams in which a recently deceased loved one returns to visit the dreamer, could dreams of the dead serve an adaptive function in relieving the existential despair that comes with the evolution of a mind that knows it is fated to die?
4. Dreams of reassurance. Given the regular appearance during times of major life crisis (e.g., illness, accident, natural disaster) of striking dreams from which the dreamer awakens with a revitalized sense of confidence and optimism, could dreams of reassurance serve an adaptive function in activating people's emotional resources at just those moments when they are most vulnerable?[16]

Note that if the answer to any of these questions is yes, no specific teleological consequences are implied. The Darwinian imperative against teleology (which Fred emphasizes in his comments) will be satisfied if it can be shown that extraordinarily vivid "numinous" dreams make a significant contribution to the adaptive fitness and reproductive success of *Homo sapiens sapiens.* This should not, of course, be taken as foreclosing further theological speculation about the possibility that, in addition to their adaptive value, numinous dreams may have a genuinely teleological dimension. But that is a different discussion, and for the present I will simply conclude by saying that the investigation of extraordinary types of dreams can proceed in a way that is authentically scientific and compatible with a broadly Darwinian evolutionary perspective.

In other conversations I have had with people of a skeptical bent, their final comment often goes something like this: "All this research on extraordinary, 'numinous' dreams is fine and well, but *I* don't have any such dreams, and I know plenty of people who take no interest whatsoever in their dreams and live perfectly adapted, evolved, contented lives." I'm not sure Fred would say this, but I believe it is a common sentiment among his intellectual kindred, so I will close my comments by agreeing with the basic point that not everyone has these kinds of extremely vivid, hauntingly memorable, deeply affecting dreams. Although researchers still have much to learn about why some people are powerfully moved by their dreams and other people are not, we do know that the variability of dream experience is directly influenced by cultural factors. Some communities actively seek to enhance powerful dreams (for example, the Plains Indians described by Lee Irwin in chapter 5), while other communities develop practices that inadvertently suppress dream recall (as in the widespread use of alarm clocks by contemporary Westerners). My ultimate claim is that there *is something* to enhance or suppress: The numinous power of dreaming is observable, lawful, physical, and consistent in its nature with scientifically valid knowledge gleaned from other areas of study; it is grounded in the natural evolution of the mammalian brain and subsequently shaped and mediated by language, culture, and individual personality.

A field of dreams indeed!

Notes

1. See Domhoff, chapter 20 this volume, and Robert Van de Castle, *Our Dreaming Mind* (New York: Ballantine, 1994), pp. 235–237.
2. Ernest Hartmann, *The Nightmare: The Psychology and Biology of Terrifying Dreams* (New York: Basic Books, 1984).
3. For more on the lab effect see Kelly Bulkeley, *An Introduction to the Psychology of Dreaming* (Westport: Praeger, 1997), pp. 63–65.
4. Cited in "The Power of Dreams," documentary produced and shown by the Discovery Channel, 1994.
5. For example, Ursula K. LeGuin, *The Lathe of Heaven* (New York: Avon, 1971), and the film *Until the End of the World,* directed by Wim Wenders, 1995.
6. Antonio Damasio, *The Feeling of What Happens,* pp. 82–83.
7. Kelly Bulkeley, *Spiritual Dreaming: A Cross-Cultural and Historical Journey* (Mahwah: Paulist Press, 1995), p. 117.
8. "On Prophesying by Dreams," by Aristotle, in Richard McKeon (ed.), *The Collected Works of Aristotle* (New York: Random House, 1941), p. 626.
9. Ibid., p. 627.
10. Ibid., p. 626.
11. *The Wilderness of Dreams: Exploring the Religious Meanings of Dreams in Modern Western Culture* (Albany: SUNY, 1994), Sections III and IV.
12. My use of the term "numinous" relies in part on Rudolph Otto's elaboration in *The Idea of the Holy* (London: Oxford University Press, 1958) of encounters with the *mysterium tremendum.*
13. Hobson, chapter 21 this volume; Mark Solms, *The Neuropsychology of Dreams* (Mahwah: Lawrence Erlbaum, 1996); Tore Nielsen, "Mentation in REM and NREM Sleep: A Review and Possible Reconciliation of Two Models," *Brain and Behavioral Sciences,* forthcoming; Alan Moffitt and Robert Hoffman, "On the Single-Mindedness and Isolation of Dream Psychophysiology," in *Sleep and Dreams: A Sourcebook,* edited by Jayne Gackenbach (New York: Garland, 1987).
14. Calvin Hall and Robert Van de Castle, *The Content Analysis of Dreams* (New York: Appleton-Century-Crofts); G. William Domhoff, *Finding Meaning in Dreams: A Quantitative Approach* (New York: Plenum, 1996).
15. Another quote from Antonio Damasio's *The Feeling of What Happens* is in order:

    The unconscious, in the narrow meaning in which the word has been etched in our culture, is only a part of the vast amount of processes and contents that remain nonconscious, not known in core or extended consciousness. In fact, the list of the "not-known" is astounding. Consider what it includes:

1. all the fully formed images to which we do not attend;
2. all the neural patterns that never become images;
3. all the dispositions that were acquired through experience, lie dormant, and may never become an explicit neural pattern;
4. all the quiet remodeling of such dispositions and all their quiet renetworking—that may never become explicitly known; and
5. all the hidden wisdom and know-how that nature embodied in innate, homeostatic dispositions.

Amazing, indeed, how little we ever know. (p. 228)

16. I discuss these four areas of research in more details in the first four chapters of a general-audience book, *Transforming Dreams: Learning Spiritual Lessons from the Dreams You Never Forget* (New York: John Wiley & Sons, 2000).

About the Contributors

KELLY BULKELEY teaches religion and psychology at San Francisco Theological Seminary and Santa Clara University and is author of several books on dreams, including *Transforming Dreams* (John Wiley & Sons, 2000), *Visions of the Night* (SUNY, 1999), *An Introduction to the Psychology of Dreaming* (Praeger, 1997), and *The Wilderness of Dreams* (SUNY, 1994).

BERTRAM COHLER is a Professor on the Committee on Human Development at the University of Chicago and is the editor of several books on psychoanalysis and culture, including *The Course of Gay and Lesbian Lives: Social and Psychoanalytic Perspectives,* coedited with Robert M. Galatzer-Levy (University of Chicago Press, 2000) and *The Invulnerable Child,* coedited with E. James Anthony (Guilford Press, 1987).

FREDERICK CREWS is emeritus Professor of English at the University of California, Berkeley. He is the editor of *The Unauthorized Freud: Doubters Confront a Legend* (Penguin, 1998), as well as author of critical studies of Henry James, E.M. Forster, and Nathaniel Hawthorne and the satire *The Pooh Perplex* (Dutton, 1965).

JAMES J. DICENSO is Professor of Religious Studies at the University of Toronto and is the author of *The Other Freud: Religion, Culture, and Psychoanalysis* (Routledge, 1998).

G. WILLIAM DOMHOFF is Professor of Psychology and Sociology at the University of California, Santa Cruz. He has written *Finding Meaning in Dreams: A Quantitative Approach* (Plenum, 1996) and *The Mystique of Dreams* (University of California Press, 1985), as well as several books on power, race, and equality in contemporary America.

WENDY DONIGER is Professor of the History of Religions at the University of Chicago Divinity School. Among her many books on myth and religion are *The Bedtrick: Telling the Difference* (University of Chicago Press, 2000), *Splitting the Difference: Gender and Myth in Ancient Greece and India* (University of Chicago Press, 1999), and *Dreams, Illusion, and Other Realities* (University of Chicago Press, 1984).

NANCY GRACE is a musician and dream educator with a focus on art, religion, and consciousness. She is a member of the Board of Directors of the Association for the Study of Dreams.

THOMAS GREGOR is Chair of the Department of Anthropology at Vanderbilt University author of *Mehinaku: The Drama of Daily Life in a Brazilian Indian Village* (University of Chicago Press, 1980) as well as coeditor (with Donald Tuzin) of *Gender in Amazonia and Melanesia: An Exploration of the Comparative Method* (University of California Press, 2001).

MARCIA HERMANSEN is Assistant Professor of Islam at Loyola University of Chicago and is the translator of *The Conclusive Argument for God: Shah Wali Allah of Dehli's Hujjat Allah al-Baligha (Islamic Philosophy, Theology, and Science, Volume 25)* (E.J. Brill, 1995).

J. ALLAN HOBSON is Director of the Laboratory of Neurophysiology at Harvard Medical School and the author of *Dreaming and Delirium: How the Brain Goes Out of Its Mind* (MIT Press, 1999) and *The Dreaming Brain* (Basic Books, 1988).

LEE IRWIN is Chair of the Department of Religious Studies at Charleston College and the author of *Native American Spirituality: A Critical Reader* (Bison Books, 2000) and *The Dream Seekers: Native American Visionary Traditions of the Great Plains* (University of Oklahoma Press, 1994).

DIANE JONTE-PACE is Associate Professor of Religious Studies at Santa Clara University and is the author of *Speaking the Unspeakable: Religion, Misogyny, and the Uncanny Mother in Freud's Cultural Texts* (University of California Press, 2001) and coeditor with William Parsons of *Religion and Psychology: Mapping the Terrain* (Routledge, 2001).

TRACEY L. KAHAN is Associate Professor of Psychology at Santa Clara University and has written several articles on lucid dreaming, metacognition, and consciousness.

WAUD H. KRACKE is Professor of Anthropology at the University of Illinois, Chicago, and has written *Force and Persuasion: Leadership in an Amazonian Society* (University of Chicago Press, 1978) and several articles on psychoanalytic interpretation in anthropology.

JEFFREY KRIPAL is a Associate Professor of Religion at Westminster College and is author of *Kali's Child: The Mystical and the Erotic in the Life and Teachings of Ramakrishna* (University of Chicago Press, 1995) and *Roads of Excess, Palaces of Wisdom: Eroticism and Reflexivity in the Modern Study of Mysticism* (University of Chicago Press, 2001).

GEORGE LAKOFF is Professor of Linguistics at the University of California, Berkeley and the author of several books on language and metaphor, including *Women, Fire, and Dangerous Things: What Categories Reveal about the Mind* (University of Chicago Press, 1990) and *Metaphors We Live By,* cowritten with Mark Johnson (University of Chicago Press, 1984).

ROGER IVAR LOHMANN is Visiting Professor of Anthropology at the College of Wooster and is editor of a volume in preparation on cultural and experiential qualities of dreaming-as-traveling in Western Pacific societies.

SCOTT NOEGEL is Assistant Professor of Ancient Near Eastern Languages and Civilizations at the University of Washington-Seattle and is author of a forthcoming book on ancient dream interpretation, titled *Nocturnal Ciphers: The Allusive Language of Dreams in the Hebrew Bible and Ancient Near Eastern Literature.*

KASIA SZPAKOWSKA is Associate Professor of Near Eastern Languages and Cultures at the University of Swansea, Wales, and is author of *The Perception of Dreams and Nightmares in Ancient Egypt: Old Kingdom to Third Intermediate Period* (UMI, 2000).

JEREMY TAYLOR is a Unitarian Universalist Minister, Professor of Theology at the Starr King School for the Ministry, and author of *Dream Work* (Paulist Press, 1983), *Where People Fly and Water Runs Uphill* (Warner Books, 1992), and *The Living Labyrinth* (Paulist Press, 1998).

BARBARA TEDLOCK is Professor of Anthropology at State University of New York, Buffalo and the author of *The Beautiful and the Dangerous: Encounters with the Zuni Indians* (University of New Mexico Press, 2001), editor of *Dreaming: Anthropological and Psychological Interpretations* (Cambridge University Press, 1988), and coeditor with Dennis Tedlock of *Teachings from the American Earth: Indian Religion and Philosophy* (Liveright, 1992).

JANE WHITE-LEWIS is a Jungian analyst in private practice and the author of several articles on teaching inner-city high school students about dreams, myth, and symbolism.

SERINITY YOUNG is a Fellow at the Center for Writers and Scholars of the New York Public Library and has done fieldwork in India, Tibet, Nepal, Bangladesh, and Russia. She is author of *Dreaming in the Lotus: Buddhist Dream Narrative, Imagery, and Practice* (Wisdom Publications, 1999) and the editor of *The Encyclopedia of Women and World Religion* (Macmillan, 1999) and *An Anthology of Sacred Texts By and About Women* (Crossroads, 1994).

Index